STUDENT WORKBOO

Pearson's Comprehensive Medical Assisting

FOURTH EDITION

KRISTIANA D. ROUTH, RMA (AMT)
Allied Health Consulting Services • Girard, PA

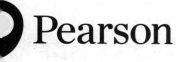

330 Hudson Street, NY, NY 10013

5 2020

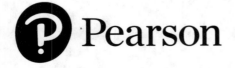

ISBN 10: 0-13-447299-3
ISBN 13: 978-0-13-447299-7

Contents

INTRODUCTION

This student workbook is designed as a study guide and practice tool to accompany the student text, *Pearson's Comprehensive Medical Assisting, Fourth Edition.* Use the study guide to reinforce what you have learned. Test your knowledge of medical terminology by completing the variety of activities in the Key Terminology Review section. Measure whether you have achieved the learning objectives in each chapter by completing the exercises in the Applied Practice and Learning Activities sections of the workbook. Apply your knowledge to real-life situations by answering the Critical Thinking Questions. Use outside and Internet resources to complete the research activity at the end of each chapter.

Each chapter of this student workbook includes the following:

Student Study Guide: This is material presented in the chapter. Fill in the blanks, or answer the questions by following PowerPoint presentations in class, or reading through your text.

Applied Practice: Use the knowledge you learned in the chapter to complete these activities.

Learning Activities: These questions/tasks allow you to measure whether or not you have achieved the learning objectives for the chapter.

Key Terminology Review: This section tests your knowledge of the medical terminology presented in the chapter.

Critical Thinking Questions: These challenging questions allow you to apply your knowledge to real-life situations.

Research Activity: Use outside sources to complete these activities and go beyond the classroom.

Procedure Skill Sheets: These boxed procedures, found in the back of the workbook, correspond to those in the student textbook and allow students to demonstrate the skills needed to become a medical assistant. A space is included for your instructor to document that you have successfully completed the skill. Each step is weighted to better indicate proficiency in the skill.

Note: Answer key located in Instructor's Manual.

Procedures

Procedure Number	Procedure Title	Date Mastered	Instructor's Signature
1-1	Locating a State's Scope of Practice for Medical Assisting		
3-1	Performing Compliance Reporting Based on Public Health Statutes		
3-2	Reporting Illegal Activity in the Health Care Setting		
3-3	Separating Personal and Professional Ethics		
5-1	Using Active Listening Skills		
5-2	Assisting an Angry or Anxious Patient		
5-3	Assisting the Hearing-Impaired Patient		
5-4	Communicating with a Patient When There Is a Language Barrier		
6-1	Managing a Fire in the Medical Office		
6-2	Ensuring Proper Use of an Eyewash Device		
6-3	Housekeeping Using OSHA Guidelines		
6-4	Completing an Incident Report		
7-1	Answering the Telephone and Placing Calls on Hold		
7-2	Taking a Telephone Message		
7-3	Taking a Prescription Refill Message		
7-4	Calling the Pharmacy for a Prescription Refill		
7-5	Placing a Conference Call		
8-1	Opening the Office		
8-2	Registering a New Patient		
8-3	Collecting Copayments		
8-4	Closing the Office		
9-1	Scheduling Established Patients		
9-2	Scheduling a New Patient Appointment		
9-3	Arranging a Referral Appointment		
9-4	Scheduling an Inpatient Surgical Procedure		

Procedure Number	Procedure Title	Date Mastered	Instructor's Signature
9-5	Scheduling an Outpatient Surgical Procedure		
10-1	Maintaining Equipment		
10-2	Performing Office Inventory		
10-3	Placing a Supply Order		
11-1	Composing a Business Letter		
11-2	Proofreading Written Documents		
11-3	Opening and Sorting the Daily Mail		
11-4	Creating and Sending a Business Letter Using E-mail		
12-1	Installing Computer Hardware		
12-2	Installing Computer Software		
12-3	Performing Data Backup		
12-4	Using the Internet to Access Health Information		
13-1	Completing a Request to Release Medical Records		
13-2	Correcting an Entry in the Electronic Health Record		
13-3	Creating a Patient's Medical Record		
13-4	Organizing a Patient's Medical Record		
13-5	Filing a Record Alphabetically		
13-6	Sending Automated Orders		
14-1	Calculating Patient Financial Responsibility		
14-2	Interpreting Information on an Insurance Card		
14-3	Verifying Eligibility		
14-4	Obtaining Insurance Company Authorizations		
14-5	Obtaining Managed Care Referrals		
14-6	Completing a CMS-1500 Claim Form		
14-7	Completing Electronic Insurance Claims		

Procedure Number	Procedure Title	Date Mastered	Instructor's Signature
15-1	Performing ICD-10-CM Diagnostic Coding		
16-1	Using Medical Necessity Guidelines		
16-2	Performing Procedural Coding		
17-1	Obtaining Accurate Patient Billing Information		
17-2	Using a Computerized Billing System		
17-3	Correcting Account Posting Errors		
17-4	Posting NSF Checks		
17-5	Posting Insurance Payments		
17-6	Responding to a Denied Insurance Claim		
17-7	Preparing Patient Statements		
17-8	Processing Credit Balances and Refunds		
17-9	Making Collection Calls		
17-10	Writing a Collection Letter		
17-11	Posting a Payment from a Collection Agency		
18-1	Preparing a Bank Deposit		
18-2	Paying Bills with Accounts Payable Software		
18-3	Preparing Manual Checks		
18-4	Reconciling a Bank Statement		
18-5	Working with an Outside Payroll Service		
19-1	Following Staff Meeting Procedures		
19-2	Developing a Patient Information Booklet		
33-1	Disposing of Biohazardous Material		
33-2	Performing Handwashing		
33-3	Applying and Removing Nonsterile Gloves		
33-4	Selecting and Using Personal Protective Equipment (PPE)		
33-5	Sanitizing Instruments		
33-6	Preparing Items for Autoclaving		

Procedure Number	Procedure Title	Date Mastered	Instructor's Signature
35-9	Positioning the Patient in the Sims Position		
35-10	Positioning the Patient in the Knee-Chest Position		
35-11	Assisting with a Complete Physical Examination		
36-1	Performing a Scratch Test		
36-2	Taking a Wound Culture		
36-3	Performing and Educating the Patient Regarding Blood Glucose Monitoring		
36-4	Testing for Occult Blood		
36-5	Assisting with a Sigmoidoscopy		
36-6	Instructing and Preparing a Patient for a Colonoscopy		
36-7	Performing a Pupil Check on a Patient		
36-8	Assisting with a Neurologic Examination		
37-1	Instructing a Patient on Breast Self-Examination		
37-2	Assisting with a Pelvic Examination and Pap Test		
37-3	Instructing a Patient on Testicular Self-Examination		
38-1	Assessing and Recording Distance Vision Acuity Using a Snellen Eye Chart		
38-2	Assessing and Recording Near Vision Acuity Using a Jaeger Card		
38-3	Assessing and Recording Color Vision Acuity Using the Ishihara Test		
38-4	Irrigating the Eye		
38-5	Instilling Eye Medication		
38-6	Irrigating the Ear		
38-7	Instilling Ear Medication		
38-8	Assisting with Audiometry		
38-9	Instilling Nasal Medications		
39-1	Measuring and Recording Pediatric Vital Signs		

Procedure Number	Procedure Title	Date Mastered	Instructor's Signature
39-2	Measuring and Recording the Weight and Length of an Infant		
39-3	Measuring and Recording Head Circumference		
39-4	Measuring and Recording Chest Circumference		
39-5	Documenting a Growth Chart		
39-6	Applying a Pediatric Urine Collection Device		
40-1	Communicating Effectively with the Older Adult Patient		
41-1	Performing Sterile Scrub/Surgical Hand Hygiene		
41-2	Donning and Removing Surgical Gloves		
41-3	Preparing a Sterile Field		
41-4	Performing within a Sterile Field		
41-5	Assisting with Minor Surgery		
41-6	Preparing the Patient's Skin for Surgical Procedures		
41-7	Performing Wound Care and Changing a Dressing		
41-8	Assisting with Suturing		
41-9	Removing Sutures and Staples		
41-10	Applying a Bandage over a Sterile Dressing		
42-1	Performing Adult Rescue Breathing and One- and Two-Rescuer CPR		
42-2	Performing Infant Rescue Breathing		
42-3	Demonstrating the Use of an Automated External Defibrillator		
42-4	Responding to an Adult with an Obstructed Airway		
42-5	Performing First Aid for a Person in Shock		
42-6	Performing First Aid for Diabetic Shock/Diabetic Coma		
42-7	Applying a Pressure Bandage to Control Bleeding		

Procedure Number	Procedure Title	Date Mastered	Instructor's Signature
42-8	Performing First Aid for a Patient Having a Seizure		
42-9	Responding to a Patient with Syncope		
42-10	Performing First Aid for a Patient with a Fracture		
42-11	Creating a Medical Emergency Plan		
42-12	Developing an Environmental Exposure Safety Plan		
43-1	Completing a Laboratory Requisition Form		
43-2	Maintaining Lab Test Results Using Flow Sheets		
43-3	Performing Quality Control Measures for a Glucometer		
43-4	Using and Cleaning a Microscope		
44-1	Performing a Throat Swab for Culture		
44-2	Obtaining a Sputum Specimen for Culture		
44-3	Preparing a Smear		
44-4	Preparing a Wet Mount Slide		
44-5	Performing a Gram Stain		
44-6	Performing Rapid Group A Strep Testing		
44-7	Performing CLIA-waived Microbiology Testing		
45-1	Instructing a Patient on Collecting a 24-Hour Urine Specimen		
45-2	Instructing a Patient on Collecting a Clean-Catch Midstream Urine Specimen		
45-3	Assisting with a Straight Catheterization and Collecting a Sterile Specimen		
45-4	Evaluating the Physical Characteristics of Urine		
45-5	Measuring the Specific Gravity of Urine with a Refractometer		
45-6	Testing the Chemical Characteristics of Urine with Reagent Strips		

Procedure Number	Procedure Title	Date Mastered	Instructor's Signature
51-4	Applying a Heating Pad		
51-5	Applying a Cold Compress		
51-6	Applying an Ice Bag		
51-7	Instructing a Patient to Use Crutches Correctly		
51-8	Instructing a Patient to Use a Cane Correctly		
51-9	Instructing a Patient to Use a Walker Correctly		
51-10	Performing a Patient Transfer from a Wheelchair		
52-1	Preparing Proper Medication Dosage: Applying Mathematic Computations to Solve Equations		
52-2	Preparing Proper Medication Dosage: Converting from One Measurement System to Another		
52-3	Preparing Proper Medication Dosage: Calculating Correct Dosage for an Injectable Medication		
52-4	Applying Mathematic Computations to Solve Equations: Calculating Correct Pediatric Dosage Using Body Surface Area		
52-5	Applying Mathematic Computations to Solve Equations: Calculating Correct Pediatric Dosage Using Body Weight		
54-1	Administering Medication Safely		
54-2	Administering Oral Medications		
54-3	Administering Sublingual or Buccal Medication		
54-4	Administering a Rectal or Vaginal Suppository		
54-5	Withdrawing Medication from Single-Dose or Multiple-Dose Vials		
54-6	Withdrawing Medication from an Ampule		
54-7	Reconstituting a Powdered Medication for Administration		

Procedure Number	Procedure Title	Date Mastered	Instructor's Signature
54-8	Administering a Z-Track Injection		
54-9	Reviewing Parenteral Medication Injection Sites		
54-10	Administering Parenteral Subcutaneous or Intramuscular Injections		
54-11	Administering an Intradermal Injection		
54-12	Preparing an Intravenous Tray		
55-1	Providing Patient Education on Disease Prevention: Smoking Cessation		
55-2	Coaching Patients with Consideration of Communication Barriers: A Hearing-Impaired Patient		
55-3	Creating a Community Resources Brochure		
55-4	Creating an Office Policies Brochure		
55-5	Working as a Patient Navigator: Facilitating a Referral for Community Resources		
56-1	Calculating Adult Body Mass Index		
56-2	Instructing a Patient According to Dietary Needs		
57-1	Assisting a Terminally Ill Patient		
59-1	Conducting a Job Search		
59-2	Preparing Your Résumé and References		
59-3	Preparing a Cover Letter		
59-4	Interviewing for a Job		
59-5	Preparing a Follow-Up Thank-You Letter		

CHAPTER 1
Medical Assisting: The Profession

STUDENT STUDY GUIDE

Use the following guide to assist in your learning of the concepts from the chapter.

I. The History and Training of Medical Assistants

  1. Steps in the History of Trained Medical Assistants

    A. Originally MAs received their training from _____ while on _____ _____.

    B. The increase in responsibility and _____ issues led to the need for medical assistants to be more formally trained.

    C. Before the formal training of medical assistants, _____ were in higher demand to assist physicians.

  2. The AAMA

    A. AAMA is the acronym for the _____ _____ _____ _____ _____.

    B. The AAMA was founded by _____ _____.

    C. The AAMA was organized in the year _____.

  3. Formal Training for the Medical Assistant and Accreditation of Medical Assisting Programs

    A. Certificate training varies in length from _____ _____ to 1 year. A certificate program may concentrate on either _____ or _____ skills.

    B. Diploma MA programs are often offered at _____ and community colleges.

    C. Medical assistant degree programs are approximately _____ month(s) to _____ year(s) in length.

    D. Accreditation is a(n) _____ process.

    E. Accreditation ensures that a school program meets or exceeds _____.

  4. The Medical Assisting Externship

    A. The externship is a(n) _____ component of an MA program.

    B. Externships take place in _____ _____, _____, or _____ settings.

II. Role and Responsibilities of the Medical Assistant

  1. Role of the Medical Assistant

    A. The role of the MA is to _____ the physician in providing

    _____ _____.

  2. Places of Employment for MAs (List four.)

    A. _____

    B. _____

    C. _____

    D. _____

  3. Responsibilities of the Medical Assistant

    A. Duties typically _____ from office to office.

    B. _____ and _____ of setting determine the types of duties the medical

    assistant will perform.

    C. Duties vary because of _____ and _____ regulations and guidelines.

  4. Administrative Duties (List five administrative duties of a medical assistant.)

    A. _____

    B. _____

    C. _____

    D. _____

    E. _____

  5. Clinical Duties (List five clinical duties of a medical assistant.)

    A. _____

    B. _____

    C. _____

    D. _____

    E. _____

  6. Delegation of Duties

    A. Because medical assistants are _____, their physician-employer is

    responsible for the work they _____.

    B. Delegating duties refers to _____ work-related

    _____ that the medical assistant is both responsible and

    _____ to complete.

    C. A physician may never _____ duties in such a way that a medical

    assistant is construed as _____ _____.

    D. _____ _____ vary regarding who can delegate

    duties to a medical assistant.

7. Professional Qualities of a Good Medical Assistant (List the nine professional qualities presented in this section of the textbook.)

A. _____

B. _____

C. _____

D. _____

E. _____

F. _____

G. _____

H. _____

I. _____

III. Professional Certifying Organizations

1. MA Certifying Organizations (List four.)

A. _____

B. _____

C. _____

D. _____

2. American Association of Medical Assistants (AAMA)

A. The AAMA is headquartered in _____.

B. The AAMA offers the _____ credential.

C. A candidate must be a graduate of either a(n) _____ or a(n) _____ accredited medical assisting program.

D. The AAMA requires _____ recertification points, to be obtained within a(n) _____-year period, in order to maintain certification.

3. American Medical Technologists (AMT)

A. _____ is the credential awarded to candidates who pass the AMT certification exam for medical assisting.

B. The RMA certification exam focuses on three areas. List them.

i. _____

ii. _____

iii. _____

4. National Center for Competency Testing (NCCT)

A. The NCCT issues the _____ credential.

B. A candidate must be a(n) _____ _____ graduate and must be eligible through one of the following routes.

i. Graduation within the past _____ year(s) from a medical assisting program at a(n) _____-authorized school

ii. Verification of at least _____ years of full-time work as a medical assistant within the past _____ year(s)

iii. Completion of _____ _____ service training as a medical assistant (or equivalent) within the past _____ year(s)

C. Continuation of certification requires _____ hour(s) per year of continuing education.

5. National Healthcareer Association (NHA)

A. The NHA was founded in the year _____.

B. The NHA grants two credentials: _____ and _____.

C. An applicant must be over _____ years of age; have a high school diploma or _____ equivalent; have completed a training program in the field of _____ _____ covered by the certification exam; or have at least _____ year(s) of verifiable, full-time, _____ work experience in the field.

IV. Career Opportunities

1. Expected Growth

A. Medical assistants rank among the _____-growing occupations over the decade _____ to _____.

B. In some states and settings, additional _____, _____, and certification may be required for medical assistants to fulfill certain _____.

2. Patient Navigators

A. Patient navigators help patients by _____ their health care needs, encouraging _____ to _____ plans, and encouraging and _____ patients regarding self-management skills.

B. The _____ of patient navigation is to streamline the _____ of health care services, improve _____, and ensure that patients are well educated regarding their _____ _____ _____.

KEY TERMINOLOGY REVIEW

Complete the following sentences using the correct key terms found at the beginning of the chapter.

1. The _____ was previously known as the Kansas Medical Assistants Society.

2. _____ is the process in which an institution voluntarily completes a process of determining whether the school meets or exceeds standards set forth by an accrediting body.

3. A(n) _____ is a required component of a student's education in which the student is scheduled to work unpaid in a physician's office, clinic, or possibly a hospital setting, under the direct supervision of a preceptor or supervisor.

4. _____ is awarded to candidates who pass the AMT certification examination.

5. The credential issued by the National Center for Competency Testing is the _____.

6. _____ means to assign work-related tasks.

APPLIED PRACTICE

Give two examples of each positive quality that a medical assistant should possess.

Quality	Examples
Integrity	
Empathy	
Discretion	
Confidentiality	
Thoroughness	
Punctuality	
Congeniality	
Proactivity	
Competence	

LEARNING ACTIVITY: TRUE/FALSE

Indicate whether the following statements are true or false by placing a T or an F on the line that precedes each statement.

_____ 1. Historically, medical assistants were trained on the job by physicians.

_____ 2. An externship is typically a paid position for a period of 160 hours.

_____ 3. A medical assistant can call herself a nurse only if certified by either an ABHES- or CAAHEP-accredited medical assisting program.

_____ 4. Membership in the AAMA is not necessary to take the AAMA certification examination.

_____ 5. For the CMA (AAMA) credential to remain current, it must be revalidated every 3 years.

_____ 6. The AMT is an accreditation body.

_____ 7. Entry-level medical assistants may find work as office managers, medical records managers, hospital unit secretaries, and instructors for medical assistant programs.

_____ 8. A rehabilitation center provides care to patients recovering from illness or injury.

_____ 9. As a medical assistant, if you witness behaviors that are unsafe to workers, you should notify OSHA.

_____ 10. As a medical assistant, it is a crime to perform procedures that only nurses or physicians are licensed to do.

CRITICAL THINKING

Answer the following questions to the best of your ability.

1. Sara Dunn is taking an administrative medical assisting class as part of her training toward earning a medical assisting certificate. She has been assigned the task of writing a paper that outlines the history of medical assisting. Part of the assignment is to include the milestones reached by this profession over the past 50 years. What important information might Sara include in her paper?

   _____

   _____

   _____

   _____

2. Diane Luder is a recent graduate of a medical assisting program. One of her fellow graduates has been talking with Diane about the importance of becoming certified in her field. She is considering becoming a CMA (AAMA). Why should Diane consider certification, and what specific requirement must Diane meet in regard to her schooling in order to be eligible to sit for the CMA (AAMA) exam?

   _____

   _____

   _____

   _____

   _____

RESEARCH ACTIVITY

Use Internet search engines to research the following topics and write a brief description of what you find. It is important to use reputable websites.

1. Research your state and local chapters of the American Association of Medical Assistants. What information is available? When and where are meetings held? If a chapter does not exist in your area, what are the requirements for starting a chapter?

   _____

   _____

   _____

   _____

CHAPTER 2
Medical Science: History and Practice

STUDENT STUDY GUIDE

Use the following guide to assist in your learning of the concepts from the chapter.

I. The History of Medicine

  1. Code of Hammurabi

    A. This code was used by _____ physicians in 3000 BC.

    B. Laws related to the _____ of _____ specified severe _____ for _____.

    C. Hammurabi was an early _____ of Babylon.

  2. Contributions of Ancient Civilizations

    A. Personal hygiene, the sanitary preparation of food, and other matters of public health were pioneered by the practices of the _____ culture.

    B. Some records of early _____ practitioners depict them using nonpoisonous snakes to treat the wounds of patients.

  3. Ancient Cures Are Today's Legacy

    A. _____ is used to treat heart patients.

    B. _____ from the foxglove plant is used to regulate and strengthen the heartbeat.

    C. _____ is used to treat urinary tract infections.

  4. Early Medicine

    A. Early medicine is considered to have begun in the _____ century BC.

    B. Advances in all branches of learning came to a near halt during _____ _____.

    C. Poor personal hygiene, _____ _____, and lack of sanitation led to many _____.

  5. Hippocrates

    A. Hippocrates is known as the _____ of _____ _____.

    B. He shifted medicine from _____ to science.

C. He stressed the body's healing _____, formed _____ _____ of diseases, and discovered the ability to _____some diseases by _____ to the chest.

D. The Hippocratic Oath serves as a widely used _____ guide for physicians.

E. When taking the oath, physicians pledge to work for the _____of patients, _____ no _____, _____ no deadly drugs, and give no _____ that could cause _____.

6. Galen

A. Galen stressed the value of_____.

B. He founded_____ _____.

C. He is known as the _____ of _____.

7. Other Influential Individuals of Early Medicine

A. _____ _____ first theorized about the circulation of blood in the human body.

B. _____ _____ invented the microscope.

C. _____ _____ is known as the first person to _____ and _____bacteria, which he referred to as "tiny little beasties."

8. Medicine During the Eighteenth Century

A. _____ _____ is noted as the Founder of Scientific Surgery.

B. _____ _____ invented the smallpox vaccine.

C. _____ _____ invented the stethoscope.

9. Medicine During the Nineteenth Century

A. The discovery of the _____ was one of the most enlightening discoveries of this era.

B. _____ _____ discovered that putrefaction, or decay, was caused by _____organisms known as _____.

C. _____ _____ introduced the _____system in surgery.

D. _____ _____ found that handwashing decreased the incidence of disease between _____.

E. _____ _____ was a pioneer in immunology,
_____, and the use of _____.

F. _____ _____ discovered X-rays.

G. _____ and _____ _____ discovered radium.

H. _____ _____ and _____
first demonstrated the use of _____ as a general anesthetic.

10. Medicine During the Twentieth Century

A. _____ _____ accidentally discovered
_____, an antibiotic.

B. Jonas Salk and Albert Sabin developed the vaccine for _____.

11. Women in Medicine

A. _____ _____ was the first female physician in the
United States.

B. Florence Nightingale is considered the founder of modern _____.

C. Clara Barton established the _____ _____.

12. Medical Firsts

A. Brigham Hospital in _____ performed the first
successful _____ transplant in 1954.

B. _____ invented a heart pump that made
_____ _____ surgery possible.

C. _____ engineering was a major medical breakthrough in the
_____.

II. Medical Practitioners

1. The Title Doctor

A. The title doctor designates a person who holds a(n) _____ degree.

B. Practicing medicine requires a minimum of _____ to _____ years of education
and training.

2. Others with the Title Doctor

A. The doctor of osteopathy (DO) degree has educational requirements similar to those for
a(n) _____ _____.

B. DOs learn the skill of _____ _____.

C. A DO places greater emphasis on the relationship between the _____
_____ and the _____ of the body.

D. A(n)_____ is trained in manipulation of the _____ _____ and other areas of the body.

E. A(n)_____ focuses on holistic, _____ prevention and comprehensive diagnosis and _____.

III. Medical Practice Acts

   1. Ways a Medical License May Be Granted (List three.)

     A. _____

     B. _____

     C. _____

   2. Causes for Revocation of a Medical License (List three.)

     A. _____

     B. _____

     C. _____

IV. Types of Medical Practices

   1. Types of Medical Practices (List six.)

     A. _____

     B. _____

     C. _____

     D. _____

     E. _____

     F. _____

V. Medical and Surgical Specialties

   1. Dermatologists specialize in diseases and problems of the _____.

   2. Physicians who specialize in bariatrics treat patients who are _____.

   3. _____ treat diseases and disorders of the heart and blood vessels.

   4. _____ _____ physicians treat individuals regardless of age or gender.

   5. A(n)_____treats diseases and disorders of the kidneys.

   6. A(n)_____ specializes in the diagnosis and treatment of patients with mental, behavioral, or emotional disorders.

VI. Health Care Institutions

   1. Categories of Hospitals (List four.)

     A. _____

     B. _____

C. _____

D. _____

2. Outpatient Surgical Centers

    A. _____ surgical procedures are performed in these facilities.

    B. Surgeries typically require _____ _____ recovery time.

3. Urgent Care Centers

    A. These facilities offer quick care for non-_____ situations.

    B. In some managed care systems, an urgent care center may be designated as a(n) _____ _____ facility.

4. Patient-Centered Medical Homes

    A. These homes provide a(n) _____ team of health care specialists in one _____ location.

    B. The focus is to provide _____, effective, and _____ care to patients.

    C. These homes _____ patients' participation in their _____ _____.

5. Nursing Homes

    A. The majority of nursing homes are _____ establishments run by nursing-home _____.

    B. Stricter regulations have been established by _____ public health departments and _____.

6. Types of Long-Term Care Institutions (List four.)

    A. _____

    B. _____

    C. _____

    D. _____

7. Hospice

    A. Hospice care emphasizes improved quality of care for _____ _____ patients.

    B. Hospice is provided in the _____ _____ or in a(n) _____ _____.

VII. Allied Health Professions

1. Education and Credentials

    A. Issuing of a certificate and credentials by a professional organization is called _____.

    B. _____ means that a professional organization in a specific health care field administers examinations, maintains a(n) _____ of qualified individuals, or _____.

C. _____ means that a government agency authorizes individuals to work in a given occupation.

2. Therapeutic Cluster Careers

   A. Careers in this cluster include those that relate to the _____ _____ status of patients, including treatment, _____, collection of patient data, and evaluation of patient _____.

3. Diagnostic Cluster Careers

   A. Careers in this cluster are involved with _____ that create a picture of the patient's health status at a specific point in time.

   B. These careers involve _____, _____, and reporting patient information.

4. Information Service Cluster Careers

   A. Careers in this cluster are involved with _____ client information, including managing, _____, _____, maintaining, and retrieving information.

KEY TERMINOLOGY REVIEW

Complete the following sentences using the correct key terms found at the beginning of the chapter.

1. _____ shows that an individual has met the educational and experience standards in his or her profession by passing an examination.

2. A dead human body is a(n)_____.

3. _____ provides proof that an individual has been authorized by a government agency to perform work in his or her profession.

4. The symbol for medicine that shows two snakes coiled around a healing staff is known as a(n) _____.

5. Rates of disease or illness are called _____ rates.

APPLIED PRACTICE

Match each of the following early contributors to medicine with the correct accomplishment.

a. Hippocrates		f. Leeuwenhoek
b. Galen		g. Fleming
c. Laennec		h. Roentgen
d. Long		i. Semmelweis
e. Salk		j. Blackwell

1. _____This was one of two individuals who discovered ether could be used as an anesthetic.

2. _____This person was the first to study bacteria and protozoa using a microscope.

3. _____This person conducted experiments with handwashing that led to reductions in the death rates of women giving birth in hospitals.

4. _____This person practiced and taught medicine on the Greek island of Kos and is known as the Father of Western Medicine.

5. _____This person discovered penicillin.

6. _____This person invented the stethoscope.

7. _____This person discovered the vaccine for polio.

8. _____This person discovered X-rays.

9. _____This person founded experimental physiology.

10. _____She was the first female physician in the United States.

LEARNING ACTIVITY: TRUE/FALSE

Indicate whether the following statements are true or false by placing a T or an F on the line that precedes each statement.

_____ 1. The Hippocratic Oath is no longer used, but it was used for nearly 2,000 years.

_____ 2. During the early part of the twentieth century, the main form of medical practice was solo practice.

_____ 3. In a partnership practice, each partner is responsible for the actions of all partners.

_____ 4. Many early and historic plant remedies are still used today for heart conditions, indigestion, bleeding, and urinary tract infections.

_____ 5. An associate practice consists of three or more physicians who share the same facility and practice medicine together.

_____ 6. A corporation is managed by a board of directors.

_____ 7. Reciprocity is granted to applicants who have successfully passed the National Board of Medical Examiners (NBME) exam.

_____ 8. Registered nurses have more training than nurse practitioners.

_____ 9. An EMT has obtained the most advanced emergency medical service training.

_____ 10. In nearly every state, a physician's assistant can prescribe medications.

CRITICAL THINKING

Answer the following questions to the best of your ability. Use the textbook as a reference.

1. Robert Bautista is taking an administrative medical assisting course as part of his training to earn a certificate in medical assisting. He has been asked to write a paragraph outlining the contributions the Greek physician Galen made to medicine. What information might Robert want to include?

_____

_____

_____

_____

_____

2. Who was Joseph Lister, and why is his contribution to medicine important?

_____

_____

_____

_____

3. Discuss early anesthesia. What is it, who discovered it, how was it used, and what compound was first used extensively?

_____

_____

_____

_____

_____

RESEARCH ACTIVITY

Use Internet search engines to research the following topics and write a brief description of what you find. It is important to use reputable websites.

1. Choose and research one of the early contributors to medicine and write a summary regarding your findings.

_____

_____

_____

_____

_____

CHAPTER 3
Medical Law and Ethics

STUDENT STUDY GUIDE

Use the following guide to assist in your learning of the concepts from the chapter.

I. Classifications of the Law

1. Law Classifications (List four classifications.)

   A. _____

   B. _____

   C. _____

   D. _____

2. Criminal Law

   A. The two categories of criminal law are _____ and _____.

   B. The punishment for committing a felony is _____.

   C. _____ and imprisonment for up to _____ year(s) are both punishments for misdemeanors.

3. Civil Law

   A. _____ law falls under civil law and covers acts that result in harm to another person or her property.

   B. _____ law includes enforceable promises and agreements between two or more persons.

   C. _____ law covers regulations that are set by government agencies.

4. Tort Law

   A. A tortfeasor is one who _____ a tort.

   B. Classifications of torts are _____ and _____.

   C. _____ occurs when a patient is injured as a result of a health care professional not exercising the reasonable person standard.

   D. Negligence is often a key factor in medical _____ _____.

   E. List the four *D*s of negligence.

      i. _____

      ii. _____

      iii. _____

      iv. _____

  F. A _____ is the person who files a lawsuit, and the _____ is charged with wrongdoing.

  G. If a patient contributed to his injury, it is termed _____ _____.

5. Contract Law

  A. List the four components of a contract between two parties.

      i. _____

      ii. _____

      iii. _____

      iv. _____

  B. A physician who has agreed to take care of a patient but improperly terminates the contract could be charged with _____.

  C. Both physicians and patients have the right to _____ a contractual relationship.

II. Professional Liability

1. *Respondeat Superior*

  A. Translated from Latin, *respondeat superior* means "let the _____ _____."

  B. A physician is _____ for _____ actions committed by his or her employees.

2. Physician's Standard of Care

  A. This standard asserts that the physician must provide the same _____, _____, and _____ that a similarly trained physician would provide under the same circumstances in the same locality.

  B. If the physician violates the standard of care, he or she is liable for _____.

3. Medical Assistant's Standard of Care

  A. A medical assistant may be _____ for working outside the _____ of _____ as identified by state laws.

  B. Many _____ performed by medical assistants could result in harm to the patient if not done _____.

  C. A(n) _____ can be found guilty of _____ for the improper performance of his or her medical assistant.

4. Malpractice

  A. List the three categories of malpractice.

      i. _____

ii. _____

iii. _____

B. List the four main types of malpractice insurance often purchased by physicians.

  i. _____

  ii. _____

  iii. _____

  iv. _____

5. *Res Ipsa Loquitur*

  A. This doctrine, translated from Latin, means "the _____ _____ for itself."

  B. Under *res ipsa loquitur*, the _____ of duty is so obvious that it does not need further _____.

6. Statute of Limitations

  A. The statute of limitations defines the period of time during which a(n) _____ may file a(n) _____.

  B. Statutes of limitations vary from one _____ to another.

  C. The period of time may begin when the problem is _____. This is known as the _____ of _____.

7. Good Samaritan Acts

  A. _____ laws help protect a health care professional from _____ while that professional is giving _____ _____ to an accident victim.

8. Defamation of Character

  A. Defamation of character is a(n) _____ statement about someone that can injure the person's _____.

III. Patient–Physician Relationship

  1. Physician Rights (List five rights.)

  A. _____

  B. _____

  C. _____

  D. _____

  E. _____

  2. Patient Rights

  A. The patient has the right to give _____, or permission, for all procedures and treatments.

  B. Consent can be either _____ or _____.

C. Patients expect that all information and records about their cases will be kept

_____.

3. Patient Obligations (List two.)

   A. _____

   B. _____

4. Right to Refuse Treatment

   A. _____ have the right to refuse treatment.

   B. Different _____ and _____ groups must be
   accommodated.

   C. If a patient leaves the hospital against _____ _____, the
   patient is considered to be leaving against _____ _____.

5. The Patient Care Partnership

   A. List six patient expectations.

      i. _____

      ii. _____

      iii. _____

      iv. _____

      v. _____

      vi. _____

6. Informed Consent

   A. Patients must be instructed about the possible _____ of having and of not
   having certain _____ and _____.

   B. List five components of the doctrine of informed consent.

      i. _____

      ii. _____

      iii. _____

      iv. _____

      v. _____

   C. A physician cannot _____ the duty of obtaining informed consent to
   another person except in _____ situations.

   D. A medical assistant must make sure that a(n) _____ informed consent form
   is obtained and placed in the patient's _____ _____.

7. Rights of Minors

   A. Most states consider _____ years to be the age of majority.

   B. Two types of minors who can provide consent for their treatment are _____
   _____ and _____ _____.

C. List the three legal implications to consider when treating a minor.

    i. _____

    ii. _____

    iii. _____

8. Patient Self-Determination Act

A. Health care institutions must encourage patients to make advance _____ regarding the type of _____ and _____ they wish to have or deny if they are unable to make their own decisions.

9. Living Will

A. A living will is made in advance by a patient and states which forms of _____ and _____ support intended to _____ the patient's life can or cannot be used.

B. A living will provides _____ for physicians and hospitals when they follow the patient's wishes.

10. Durable Power of Attorney (DPOA)

A. A DPOA allows an agent or a(n) _____ to act on behalf of the patient.

B. An agent may be a(n) _____, _____, _____ or _____.

C. A DPOA is used when a patient becomes physically or mentally _____

11. Uniform Anatomical Gift Act

A. This act allows a person _____ years or older and of sound mind to make a gift of any or all parts of his body for the purposes of organ transplantation or medical research.

B. The physician performing the _____ operation cannot be the same physician to determine _____ or the time of death.

C. No _____ is allowed to change hands for organ donations.

IV. Documentation

1. Use of Records in Litigation

A. An order to appear in court and to bring along certain medical records or materials for trial is termed _____ _____ _____.

B. Only the records specifically stated in the _____ are required.

2. Court Testimony

A. List six pointers for giving testimony in court.

    i. _____

    ii. _____

    iii. _____

    iv. _____

v. _____

vi. _____

V. Public Duties of Physicians

1. Duties of the physician include reporting _____, stillbirths,

_____, communicable illnesses or diseases, _____

_____, certain injuries, abuse of children or older adults,

_____ and _____ wounds, and animal

_____.

2. Compliance Reporting and Communicable Diseases

A. Federal, state, and local government agencies require _____ laboratories

and _____ to report when certain _____ are made.

B. This reporting helps in the identification of _____ and possible disease

_____ in specific _____.

C. Exact reporting requirements vary from one _____ to another.

VI. Risk Management in the Medical Office

1. _____ _____ refers to planning and implementing strategies

for reducing the physician's risk of _____ in the medical setting.

2. Office Management

A. Summarize five guidelines for office management related to risk management.

i. _____

ii. _____

iii. _____

iv. _____

v. _____

3. Documentation

A. Summarize six guidelines for documentation related to risk management.

i. _____

ii. _____

iii. _____

iv. _____

v. _____

vi. _____

4. Certification and Licensing

A. Summarize four guidelines for certification and licensing related to risk management.

i. _____

ii. _____

      iii. _____

      iv. _____

5. Safety

  A. Summarize four guidelines for safety related to risk management.

      i. _____

      ii. _____

      iii. _____

      iv. _____

6. Compliance Reporting

  A. Compliance reporting involves conforming to a specific rule or acting in

  _____ with established _____ to ensure that specific

  _____ are performed correctly.

  B. Errors may occur in patient care.

      i. Safeguard any patient whose _____ and _____ are

      affected by the _____ action of someone else.

      ii. Follow the _____ of _____ and report to your

      immediate supervisor any negligent action you observe.

  C. List four unsafe or illegal activities.

      i. _____

      ii. _____

      iii. _____

      iv. _____

VII. Code of Ethics

1. Medical Ethics

  A. Ethics is a branch of philosophy related to _____ or _____ principles.

  B. Medical ethics refers to the _____ conduct of people in medical professions.

  C. Every medical profession has a(n) _____ of _____ that sets the _____ _____ to which members of that profession are expected to adhere.

2. Ethical Standards of Behavior

  A. Ethical standards are more demanding than the _____.

  B. The AMA does not have authority to bring _____ action against _____ for unethical conduct.

  C. A(n) _____ _____ board may limit a physician's practice or _____ the license altogether for ethical _____.

3. AMA Principles of Medical Ethics (List seven.)

A. _____

B. _____

C. _____

D. _____

E. _____

F. _____

G. _____

VIII. Medical Assistant's Principles of Personal and Professional Ethics

1. The Blanchard and Peale Ethical Model (List four questions.)

A. _____

B. _____

C. _____

D. _____

2. Ethics, Morals, and Your Profession

A. A medical assistant may have a personal, moral, _____, or

_____ reason for wishing not to be involved in _____

_____.

B. Preferences should be stated to the employer _____ _____.

C. An individual should request to be _____ from participating in any

procedures about which he or she has _____ _____.

3. Scientific Discovery and Ethical Issues

A. New scientific discoveries are resulting in complicated _____

_____ that need to be addressed before choices can be made.

4. AAMA Code of Ethics

A. List the five sections in the AAMA Code of Ethics.

i. _____

ii. _____

iii. _____

iv. _____

v. _____

5. AAMA Creed

A. A medical assistant must know about the _____ _____ a

patient faces and be _____ to treat the patient with respectful care.

6. AMT Standards of Practice

A. These standards of practice reflect the ethical expectations for those with the _____

_____ credential.

B. Members of the AMT must recognize their responsibilities not only to their patients but also to society, to other health care professionals, and to _____.

IX. HIPAA

1. No information can be told to another _____ without the patient's _____.

2. The Health Insurance Portability and Accountability Act was passed in the year _____.

3. Medical practices are required to notify _____ about the uses, _____, and rights related to their protected _____.

4. Complaints related to HIPAA should be addressed to the U.S. Department of _____ and _____.

5. HIPAA's Parts (List the three parts.)

A. _____

B. _____

C. _____

KEY TERMINOLOGY REVIEW

Write a sentence using the selected key terms in the correct context.

1. *Bioethics:*

_____

_____

2. *Contributory negligence:*

_____

_____

3. *Informed consent:*

_____

_____

4. *Living will:*

_____

_____

5. *Practice of medicine:*

_____

_____

APPLIED PRACTICE

Provide answers to the following questions.

1. Considering the Latin terms discussed throughout the text, identify which Latin term pertains to each of the following situations and then translate each term.

   A. A physician is sued because he amputates the wrong leg during surgery.

   _____

   _____

   _____

   B. Dr. Lin is sued because his medical assistant injured a patient while suturing a 3 mm incision on the patient's lower leg, a procedure that is clearly outside the MA's scope of practice.

   _____

   _____

   _____

   C. Due to possible negligence by a physician, a child has been injured. When the case goes to court, an individual is appointed to represent the child.

   _____

   _____

   _____

2. Provide an example of an intentional tort and an example of an unintentional tort. Explain which type of tort is more common in medical malpractice lawsuits.

   _____

   _____

   _____

   _____

LEARNING ACTIVITY: TRUE/FALSE

Indicate whether the following statements are true or false by placing a T or an F on the line that precedes each statement.

_____ 1. Although they are less serious in nature, felonies may carry a punishment of fines.

_____ 2. Medical malpractice may be caused by medical errors, but not every error is considered medical malpractice.

_____ 3. Dereliction is one of the four *D*s of negligence.

_____ 4. Physicians have a duty to report gunshot wounds and insect stings.

_____ 5. In regard to a contract, the exchange of something valuable is the consideration.

_____ 6. Performing a lawful act in an improper way is called malfeasance.

_____ 7. Prior acts coverage covers any claims made prior to the time that a physician had a claims-made policy.

_____ 8. The statute of limitations varies from state to state.

_____ 9. An example of an emancipated minor is a married 17-year-old female.

_____ 10. A written statement of an oral testimony is termed a *subpoena duces tecum*.

CRITICAL THINKING

Answer the following questions to the best of your ability. Use the textbook as a reference.

1. A patient is planning to refuse the chemotherapy treatment that her physician recommended for her breast cancer. She is choosing to pursue a holistic and natural medicine approach. The physician is not happy with the patient's decision and has asked Julie Brown, a medical assistant, to try to convince the patient to change her mind and have chemotherapy. Considering the patient care partnership, how should Julie respond to the physician's request?

   _____

   _____

   _____

   _____

   _____

2. Create a medical malpractice scenario in which the statute of limitations defense would apply.

   _____

   _____

   _____

   _____

3. Jared Hernandez is an MA. Describe a scenario in which his personal morals could conflict and interfere with his duties as a medical assistant. Identify how he could overcome this issue without compromising patient care or personal integrity.

   _____

   _____

   _____

   _____

   _____

RESEARCH ACTIVITY

Use Internet search engines to research the following topic and write a brief description of what is found. It is important to use reputable websites.

1. Search for a medical malpractice case in your city or state. Describe the case, including whether the patient or the physician won the case. Did you feel that the case was decided fairly? Why or why not?

   _____

   _____

   _____

   _____

CHAPTER 4
Medical Terminology

STUDENT STUDY GUIDE

Use the following guide to assist in your learning of the concepts from the chapter.

I. The Structure of Medical Terms

    1. Medical terms are made up of _____ _____, each of which has a specific purpose.

        A. A(n) _____ _____ is the word part that carries the main meaning.

        B. A(n) _____ appears before a word root to modify its meaning.

        C. A(n) _____ appears after a word root to describe the type of condition or procedure of the root.

        D. A(n) _____ _____ is usually added _____ the root when joining it to a(n) _____ or combining it with another _____.

    2. Roots and Combining Forms

        A. When a word root has a(n) _____ attached so it can be combined with another _____, the root + vowel is termed a combining _____.

        B. If a suffix begins with a(n) _____, drop the combining vowel from the combining form and add the _____.

        C. If a suffix begins with a(n) _____, keep the _____ _____ when you add the suffix.

    3. Prefixes

        A. Prefixes are placed at the _____ of words to alter, or _____, their meanings or to create new _____.

        B. Some prefixes can have several _____.

    4. Suffixes

        A. A suffix is a syllable or group of syllables attached to the _____ of a word to alter, or modify, its meaning or to create a(n) _____ _____.

5. Taking Words Apart

    A. List six steps to follow in taking apart words.

      i. _____

      ii. _____

      iii. _____

      iv. _____

      v. _____

      vi. _____

6. Rules for Plurals

    A. Plurals are formed in a(n) _____ of ways.

    B. Some medical terms do not end in the letter _____ because they are based on _____ and _____, not English.

7. Writing and Pronouncing Medical Terms

    A. Careful _____ and _____ accuracy are important for identifying the correct meaning of a word part.

    B. Sometimes one different _____ can result in a word having a different _____.

    C. Knowing how to pronounce medical terms is important to ensure clear _____.

II. Medical Abbreviations

    1. Health care professionals must share a(n) _____ _____ of the meanings of abbreviations.

    2. Do not _____ _____ your own abbreviations.

    3. The _____ _____ has created a list of abbreviations that should be _____ in order to reduce the risk of _____ _____.

III. Gross Anatomy

    1. Directions and Body Planes

      A. Directional terms describe the location of a(n) _____ _____ or a(n) _____ in relation to the center of the body.

      B. Considering the coronal or frontal plane, the front is referred to as _____ or _____; the back is referred to as _____ or _____.

      Considering a transverse plane, the area above the plane is referred to as _____ or _____ or _____, and the area below the plane is termed _____ or _____.

C. Areas farther from the medial or midsagittal plane are _____; those closer to the plane are _____.

D. When referring to points relative to where the arms and legs attach to the body, those farther away are _____; those closer are proximal.

2. Body Cavities (Explain each one.)

   A. The body's _____ _____ are contained in cavities.

   B. The cranial cavity houses the _____.

   C. The _____ _____ is in the spinal cavity.

   D. The chest, or _____, cavity holds the lungs and heart.

   E. The _____ cavity holds the intestines, stomach, and reproductive organs.

3. Abdominal Regions and Quadrants

   A. In anatomy, "right" and "left" refer to the _____ right and left, not right and left as you _____ at the person.

   B. Identify the nine regions of the abdomen in Figure A below.

   C. Identify the four quadrants of the abdomen in Figure B below.

IV. Body Systems and Medical Specialties

   1. Integumentary System

      A. This system includes the largest organ of the body: the _____.

      B. It also includes hair, _____, _____, sweat glands, fat cells, and other _____.

      C. A physician who specializes in treating the skin is a(n) _____.

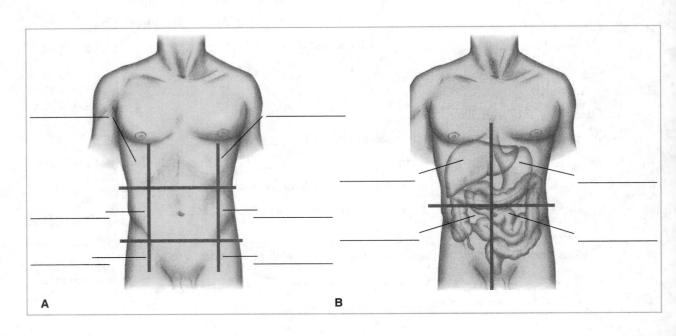

A   B

2. The Skeletal System

   A. The skeletal system consists of _____ and _____.

   B. A physician who specializes in treating the bones is a(n) _____.

   C. The combining form for the word *bone* is _____, and the combining form for the word *joint* is _____.

   D. _____ means inflammation of the bones and joints.

3. The Muscular System

   A. The muscular system includes _____, _____, _____, and _____.

   B. Muscles help _____ and move the _____ system.

   C. The combining forms used for muscles are _____ and _____.

4. The Nervous System

   A. The nervous system helps the body sense changes in the _____ and _____ environments and experience _____.

   B. Pain is referred to with the suffixes _____ and _____.

   C. The _____ is an organ of the nervous system.

5. Special Senses

   A. Special senses include _____, _____, taste, touch, and _____.

   B. A physician who specializes in the treatment of the eye is a(n) _____.

   C. A(n) _____ is a nonphysician health care provider who specializes in the care of the eye.

6. The Circulatory System

   A. The circulatory system consists of the heart, the blood vessels, the blood, and the structures that make up the _____ system.

   B. The cardiovascular system is a subsystem of the _____ system and is composed of the heart and its vessels.

   C. The _____ _____ helps ensure the body's fluid balance by gathering fluids that have leaked out of the _____ _____ and transporting them back into the _____ _____.

7. The Immune System

   A. The immune system protects the body from _____.

   B. Cells in the immune system are sometimes named for their _____ or the color they become when _____.

8. The Respiratory System
    A. The respiratory system exchanges oxygen (O_2) in the environment for _____ _____ in the body.
    B. The main organs of respiration are the _____.
    C. _____ is a combining form that means "lung."
9. The Digestive System
    A. The digestive system either _____ or _____ food and drugs for the body.
    B. The digestive tract begins with the _____.
10. The Urinary System
    A. The urinary system rids the body of excess _____ and the toxic by-products of _____.
    B. The combining form for the word *kidney* is _____.
    C. A physician with specialized training related to the kidney is a(n) _____.
11. The Endocrine System
    A. The endocrine system is the ductless glandular system that controls other body systems by secreting _____ into the bloodstream.
    B. *Endo–* means _____, and *–crine* means to _____.
    C. _____ glands secrete hormones into a system of ducts that lead to the outside of the _____.
12. The Reproductive System
    A. A physician with specialized training in women's health is a(n) _____.
    B. Female reproductive organs include the _____ and _____.
    C. Male reproductive organs include the _____ and _____.
V. Building Diagnostic and Procedural Terms
    1. Diagnostic terms and procedural terms are both usually built around a(n) _____ that identifies the _____ site involved.
    2. The _____ describes the type of condition or procedure.
    3. Most procedural terms end with the letter _____, which denotes a(n) _____.

KEY TERMINOLOGY REVIEW

Define the following key terms.

1. *anatomy:*

    _____

    _____

2. *combining vowel:*

_____

_____

3. *prefix:*

_____

_____

4. *suffix:*

_____

_____

5. *word root:*

_____

_____

APPLIED PRACTICE

1. Define each prefix.
   A. *bi–:* _____
   B. *eu–:* _____
   C. *peri–:* _____
   D. *hemi–:* _____
   E. *tachy–:* _____

2. Define each suffix.
   A. *–graphy:* _____
   B. *–megaly:* _____
   C. *–rrhea:* _____
   D. *–stomy:* _____
   E. *–tomy:* _____

3. Use a slash mark (/) to separate the word parts of the medical terms below.
   A. Melanoma _____
   B. Costectomy _____
   C. Caudal _____
   D. Phlebostasis _____
   E. Gastroenteritis _____

4. Write the plural form of each medical word listed below.
   A. Bursa _____
   B. Artery _____
   C. Ovum _____
   D. Phalanx _____
   E. Nucleus _____

CRITICAL THINKING

Answer the following questions to the best of your ability.

1. Dr. Smith uses electronic medical record (EMR) software in his office. While examining a patient, the EMR software freezes and then eventually crashes throughout the office. As a result, Dr. Smith must handwrite his examination findings and instructions for the patient. He asks his medical assistant, Andrea, who has been assisting him during the examination, to review the instructions with the patient. Dr. Smith leaves the examination room, and Andrea begins to review his written notes and instructions. She discovers that she is unable to decipher some of the information. How should Andrea handle this situation? Identify things she both should and shouldn't do.

   _____

   _____

   _____

   _____

   _____

2. Andrea is working with a patient who is new to the medical practice. She has completed a brief patient history and medication review and has obtained the patient's chief complaint. The patient has a history of high blood pressure and high cholesterol, and she had her gallbladder removed 2 years ago. She is being seen today because of painful urination and blood in her urine. When she is finished with the patient, Andrea informs the doctor that the patient is ready for examination. Dr. Smith asks Andrea to provide him with a brief overview of the patient. Using correct medical terminology, how can Andrea accurately provide the patient information to Dr. Smith?

   _____

   _____

   _____

   _____

   _____

   _____

RESEARCH ACTIVITY

Use Internet search engines to research the following topic and write a brief description of what you find. It is important to use reputable websites.

1. Select one of the systems of the body described in your textbook. Using information obtained on the Internet, conduct research on the various conditions and diseases that can affect this system. Write a few short paragraphs about your findings. Be sure to cite the websites you used.

   _____

   _____

   _____

   _____

   _____

CHAPTER 5
Communication: Verbal and Nonverbal

STUDENT STUDY GUIDE

Use the following guide to assist in your learning of the concepts from the chapter.

I. Interpersonal Dynamics

   1. To communicate effectively in the delivery of _____ _____, you must have a basic understanding of _____.

   2. Self-Awareness

      A. Self-awareness is understanding _____ and understanding the _____ among others.

      B. This understanding leads to more effective _____.

      C. List five key terms to understand regarding self-awareness.

         i. _____

         ii. _____

         iii. _____

         iv. _____

         v. _____

   3. The Learning Styles (List and explain three styles.)

      A. _____

      B. _____

      C. _____

II. The Communication Process

   1. SMCR (Write out the acronym components and explain each one.)

      A. _____

      B. _____

      C. _____

      D. _____

   2. Channels of Communication

      A. Channels of communication are various means by which the _____ or _____ word is communicated from one person to another.

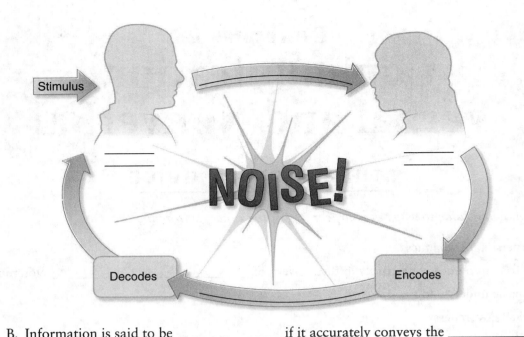

Stimulus

NOISE!

Decodes

Encodes

B. Information is said to be _____ if it accurately conveys the _____ of the speaker.

C. Fill in the blanks in the figure above for face-to-face communication.

III. Verbal and Nonverbal Communication

1. Verbal Communication

A. Verbal communication involves spoken words, _____, and _____ of voice.

B. Always communicate in a(n) _____ _____ if the message includes a patient's protected health information.

C. It is important to speak _____ and use correct _____.

2. Word Selection

A. Promote an open, _____ _____ for the patient.

B. Take care not to be rude or _____.

C. Don't use technical words or _____ _____ that the patient might not understand.

3. Positive Attitude

A. Always involve the _____ in your conversation.

B. It is disrespectful to talk in a manner that is _____.

C. Demonstrate empathy and _____ but be careful not to convey an attitude of _____.

4. Self-Boundaries

A. Self-boundaries help you be aware of topics you _____ _____ discuss with _____.

B. Sharing personal information can make patients _____.

    C. Introducing too much _____ to the relationship with a patient can be viewed as a violation of _____ and trust.

  5. Behaviors of Nonverbal Communication (List the eight behaviors.)

    A. _____

    B. _____

    C. _____

    D. _____

    E. _____

    F. _____

    G. _____

    H. _____

IV. Communication Techniques

  1. Questions About the Communication Process

    A. What is the _____ of this communication?

    B. What _____ do you want to send?

    C. What channel will be used to _____ the message?

    D. How will you _____ to the response?

    E. How will you get clarification and _____?

    F. Did you meet your goal, or do you need to _____ the _____?

  2. Listening Skill

    A. Listening is either _____ or _____.

    B. List three aspects of active listening.

      i. _____

      ii. _____

      iii. _____

    C. _____ _____ is listening to someone without having to _____ or respond in any way.

  3. Directive Communication Techniques (List the four types of questions.)

    A. _____

    B. _____

    C. _____

    D. _____

  4. Feedback

    A. Feedback is any _____ to a communication.

    B. List the three common forms of feedback.

      i. _____

ii. _____

iii. _____

5. Empathetic Listening

   A. _____ is the ability to understand what a patient is feeling because you have experienced the _____ feelings.

   B. _____ is taking positive _____ based on the empathy you feel.

   C. _____ is acknowledging the patient's feelings and difficulties even though you _____ _____ had the same experience.

   D. Pity is feeling _____ for a person.

6. Discussing Sensitive Issues

   A. Examples of sensitive issues include the patient's bill and _____ _____responsibility.

   B. Review HIPAA and HIPAA guidelines at the patient's _____ _____.

V. Developing Assertive Behaviors

1. Understanding Assertive Behaviors

   A. Being assertive means making a point in a(n) _____ _____.

   B. Being _____ is trying to impose your point of view on others or trying to manipulate them.

   C. Passive behavior is compliant or _____ behavior in which people do not let their needs and _____ be known.

   D. List five assertive behaviors.

      i. _____

      ii. _____

      iii. _____

      iv. _____

      v. _____

2. Communicating with Other Practices and Facilities

   A. Using your skills of _____ _____ is important when you are dealing with professionals outside your practice.

   B. Your instructions need to be _____ and _____ and also polite.

   C. You also need to be _____ and understanding of information others share about _____ _____.

3. Creating a Customer-Friendly Environment

   A. Medical assistants should view the patient as a(n) _____ of health care.

   B. Using good _____ skills in the health care setting generates a(n) _____-_____ atmosphere and a comfortable _____.

C. A patient should be greeted within _____ minute(s) of entering the office.

D. Knowing and _____ information about your patients will help you build a climate of _____ and _____.

VI. Communication Barriers

   1. Internal Communication Barriers (List seven barriers.)

      A. _____

      B. _____

      C. _____

      D. _____

      E. _____

      F. _____

      G. _____

   2. External Communication Barriers (List seven barriers.)

      A. _____

      B. _____

      C. _____

      D. _____

      E. _____

      F. _____

      G. _____

   3. Emotions

      A. Emotions can vary because of the person's general _____ _____ or because of that person's past _____.

   4. Stress

      A. Stress can be emotional, _____, or physical. It can also be spiritual, _____, or _____.

      B. A(n) _____ is a real or imaginary event that causes stress.

      C. Do not to let _____ stress affect your job performance.

      D. _____ of stress vary from person to person.

   5. Use of Medical Language

      A. Most patients have little understanding of _____ _____.

      B. Make an effort to avoid using medical terminology or _____ when speaking with patients.

      C. Failure to inform patients in terms they are able to understand could be construed as _____ and could increase the risk of a(n) _____.

6. Coping Mechanisms/Defensive Behaviors

   A. Adaptive coping mechanisms are _____ and _____.

   B. Nonadaptive coping mechanisms are _____ and _____.

   C. Defense mechanisms operate at a(n) _____ level to manage stress and anxiety by denying, _____, or distorting _____.

7. Responding to an Angry Patient

   A. What causes patients to be fearful? (List four examples.)

      i. _____

      ii. _____

      iii. _____

      iv. _____

   B. It is important to remain calm and use positive _____ and professional _____.

   C. With an angry caller, remain calm and speak to the patient in a(n) _____, calm _____ of voice, projecting your _____ for the patient.

8. Responding to an Anxious Patient

   A. "White coat" syndrome refers to patients being fearful when encountering _____ _____.

   B. List five methods for dealing with anxious patients.

      i. _____

      ii. _____

      iii. _____

      iv. _____

      v. _____

VII. Communication and Diversity

1. Sensory Impairment (List two types.)

   A. _____

   B. _____

2. Mentally/Emotional Impaired Patients

   A. In most cases, speak slowly and clearly to mentally/emotional impaired patients, stay _____, and keep your messages _____.

   B. Before _____ a mentally/emotional impaired patient for a procedure, explain what you are going to do.

3. Physically Challenged Patients

   A. Allow a physically challenged patient to _____ and _____ on his own.

B. When it appears necessary, offer the physically challenged patient _____.

C. Allow extra time with the patient and do not appear to be _____ or rushed.

4. Illiterate Patients

   A. Illiteracy is the inability to _____ and write.

   B. Discreetly ask patients if they need _____.

   C. It might be appropriate to move an illiterate patient to a(n) _____ _____ assist her by reading the _____ and _____ her answers.

5. Seriously/Terminally Ill Patients

   A. What four factors influence how a patient deals with the thought of his own death?

      i. _____

      ii. _____

      iii. _____

      iv. _____

   B. List the stages of grief, according to Dr. Elizabeth Kubler-Ross.

      i. _____

      ii. _____

      iii. _____

      iv. _____

      v. _____

6. Diverse Patient Populations

   A. Culture consists of the values, _____, _____, and customs shared by a group of people.

   B. Facial _____ and hand _____ vary from culture to culture.

7. Bias, Prejudice, and Stereotyping (List seven ways to avoid these negative behaviors.)

   A. _____

   B. _____

   C. _____

   D. _____

   E. _____

   F. _____

   G. _____

8. Language

   A. _____ is the second-most-common language spoken in the United States.

   B. Whenever possible, get someone to _____ for a patient who doesn't speak English.

C. When English is not the primary language, use simple and _____ words, avoid _____ terms, don't use _____, and determine if the patient _____ you.

9. Other Forms of Diversity (List other forms of diversity, not already listed here, that are discussed in the textbook.)

A. _____

B. _____

C. _____

D. _____

E. _____

VIII. Intraoffice Communication

1. Establishing Trust

A. Integrity means being _____ and demonstrating _____ principles.

B. Good staff communication depends on _____ and _____ interactions.

2. Rapport and Team Building

A. A work group must become a(n) _____ team.

B. Discussions about hobbies, _____, _____, _____, and friends help to establish trust and understanding.

C. _____ is unnecessary and unprofessional, and it often results in a negative conversation.

3. Conflict Resolution

A. Conflicts occur with miscommunication or _____ of a(n) _____.

B. When offered feedback/criticism, do not _____ with the person or become defensive.

C. Conflict also can stem from _____ or preconceived ideas.

4. Elements of Critical Thinking

A. _____ questions.

B. _____ the problem.

C. _____ the evidence.

D. _____ emotional reasoning.

E. _____ assumptions and bias.

F. _____ oversimplification.

G. _____ other interpretations.

H. _____ ambiguity.

I. _____ about one's own thinking.

5. Communicating with Superiors
   A. When a conflict needs to be discussed, choose an appropriate _____ or ask for a(n) _____.
   B. Ask _____ if tasks are unclear.
   C. Show _____.

6. Loyalty to Your Employer
   A. Support the physician and her _____ in every instance.
   B. Never share or discuss _____ _____ about your employer.
   C. A loyal employee protects and _____ an employer when other employees engage in _____ conversation.

IX. Communication and Patient Rights
   1. Privacy
      A. The HIPPA privacy rule provides for the _____ protection of health information.
      B. It allows patients to have better access to their _____ _____.
      C. It provides patients with _____ control over who can release medical information and how it will be done.
      D. PHI stands for _____ _____ _____.

   2. Advising Patients
      A. Medical assistants are not permitted to offer opinions about the _____ _____, discuss the course of _____ the physician has set forth, or tell the patient what they would do in the patient's _____.
      B. Advising patients is _____ the _____ of practice of a medical assistant.

   3. Patient Decision Making
      A. _____ empathetically to the patient.
      B. Ask _____ or clarifying questions.
      C. Clarify the information the _____ related to the patient regarding the course of _____.

KEY TERMINOLOGY REVIEW

Match each of the following terms with the correct definition.

a. sympathy
b. bias
c. active listening

d. leading questions
e. empathy

1. _____ Identification with another person's feelings.
2. _____ Questions that contain part of the answer.

3. _____ Unfair preference or dislike of something.

4. _____ Completely paying attention to the speaker, concentrating on the verbal message, watching for nonverbal cues, and offering a response.

5. _____ Feeling sorry for or pitying someone.

APPLIED PRACTICE

1. After reading the scenario below, give examples of how you can provide feedback to the patient using restatement, reflection, and clarification.

Scenario:

Julia Walton is a patient who is calling to make an appointment to see the doctor because she believes she has a new allergy to shellfish. She explains that her lips became swollen and itchy after eating crab legs last evening. She tells the MA on the phone that she is available for an appointment any day of the week before 11:45 a.m. because she works in the afternoon.

a. Restatement:

_____

_____

b. Reflection:

_____

_____

c. Clarification:

_____

_____

2. Place the following steps for problem solving in order.

a. _____ Identify alternative methods of resolving the problem.

b. _____ Recognize that a problem exists.

c. _____ Choose the best method for resolving the problem and implement it.

d. _____ Describe the problem and clarify the basic issue.

e. _____ Consider how the solution will affect those involved.

f. _____ Evaluate the results as the plan is being placed into effect.

3. Write a brief scenario or provide an example explaining how the following communication techniques could be displayed:

a. Empathy

_____

_____

_____

_____

b. Nonverbal communication

_____

_____

_____

_____

LEARNING ACTIVITY: MULTIPLE CHOICE

Circle the correct answer to each of the following questions.

1. Assertive behavior

   a. is imposing one's viewpoint on another.
   b. can result in resentment by others.
   c. is trusting one's own ideas or instincts.
   d. all of the above.

2. Which of the following is an open-ended question?

   a. "Mrs. Knight, would you explain to me how you are feeling today?"
   b. "Mrs. Knight, how are you feeling today?"
   c. "Mrs. Knight, do you need help?"
   d. None of the above

3. Which of the following can be a barrier to communication?

   a. Eye contact
   b. Use of meaningful statements
   c. Noise
   d. None of the above

4. Which of the following is *not* an example of a probing question?

   a. "Does your head hurt?"
   b. "Where does your head hurt?"
   c. "How long has your head hurt?"
   d. All of the above

5. Angela Mackie is 19 years old and recently found out she is pregnant. She asks Stacy, a medical assistant, for her personal cell phone number so she can call her if she has questions about her pregnancy after office hours. Which of the following is an appropriate response?

   a. Stacy provides Angela with her personal cell phone number.
   b. Stacey states she doesn't feel it is appropriate to give her personal number to patients.
   c. Stacey provides Angela with the direct number to the on-call physician for after-hours questions.
   d. None of the above

CRITICAL THINKING

Answer the following questions to the best of your ability. Use the textbook as a reference.

1. Mrs. Jean Smith has come into the office to address a concern she has. How can you make sure that you are actively listening to what Mrs. Smith is saying?

   _____

   _____

   _____

   _____

   _____

2. A patient has just walked into the office and begins to yell at Kevin, the medical assistant working at the front desk, about her bill. What should Kevin do when dealing with this angry patient?

_____

_____

_____

_____

3. Kristoff is reviewing medications with Datu Ocampo, a 27-year-old Filipino man who lives with his grandparents, who have emigrated from the Philippines. He reveals to Kristoff that he doesn't take the prescribed medication for his depression and anxiety because his family feels his diagnosis is a disgrace. What might Kristoff say to encourage Mr. Ocampo regarding his situation while being sensitive to his culture?

_____

_____

_____

_____

4. Consider the following biases: gender, race, religion, age, economic status, and appearance. Choose three of these biases and explain how a biased attitude could interfere with patient care.

_____

_____

_____

_____

_____

RESEARCH ACTIVITY

Use Internet search engines to research the following topic. It is important to use reputable websites.

1. Conduct a search regarding how to help pediatric patients with autism or other disorders on the autism spectrum. List some specific techniques and guidelines that could be implemented to help such a patient have a productive and enjoyable experience in the medical office. Be sure to cite the websites you've used to find your information.

_____

_____

_____

_____

_____

_____

_____

_____

Chapter 6
The Office Environment

STUDENT STUDY GUIDE

Use the following guide to assist in your learning of the concepts from the chapter.

I. General Safety Measures

  1. Occupational Safety and Health Administration (OSHA)

    A. OSHA is concerned with any _____ hazard.

    B. OSHA ensures safety by _____ and _____ standards; providing training, outreach, and _____; establishing _____; and encouraging continual _____ in workplace safety and health.

    C. _____ are levied against employers who fail to comply with regulations.

  2. General Safety Guidelines

    A. _____, don't run, during an emergency.

    B. Walk on the _____ side of the hallway.

    C. Use _____ when using stairways.

    D. Never carry _____ syringes or sharp objects.

    E. Report any unsafe conditions_____.

    F. Use different _____ for lab specimens and medications.

    G. Store _____ substances in locked cabinets.

  3. Planning for Office Safety

    A. List six types of disasters that may occur.

      i. _____

      ii. _____

      iii. _____

      iv. _____

      v. _____

      vi. _____

    B. All _____ _____ employees should be trained in all emergency steps within the _____ day of employment.

4. Evacuation Plans

   A. An evacuation plan outlines how to safely remove _____ and _____ from the building during a(n) _____.

   B. Evacuation plans should comply with _____'s emergency standards.

5. Safety Hazards

   A. List four hazards that are common to medical offices.

      i. _____

      ii. _____

      iii. _____

      iv. _____

6. Guidelines for Fire Safety

   A. Fire extinguishers should be placed no more than _____ feet from any employee area.

   B. Fire drills should be conducted at least _____ a year.

   C. RACE stands for _____, _____, _____, _____.

7. Electrical Safety

   A. _____ equipment should be grounded.

   B. _____ protectors should be used for all electronic equipment.

   C. Use _____ outlets for "wet" areas.

8. Mechanical Safety

   A. Equipment that could cause harm includes the centrifuge, _____, _____, and oxygen equipment.

   B. Read the entire _____ _____ before installing any equipment.

9. Chemical Safety

   A. _____ materials can cause serious illness or death when there is _____ through skin contact, ingestion, or _____.

   B. OSHA has established the _____ _____ Standard (HCS), which requires employers to disclose toxic and _____ substances in the workplace.

10. Safety Data Sheets (SDSs)

   A. SDSs are documents that contain printed information about potentially harmful _____ used in the _____.

   B. An SDS provides the following information

      i. Hazards of using the _____

     ii. Protecting oneself from injury by using the appropriate personal _____

        _____

     iii. Actions to take if an accidental _____ or other exposure occurs

II. Safety Signs, Symbols, and Labels

   1. _____ should be large enough to be recognized from a distance.

   2. _____ are adhesive-backed paper applied to bottles, boxes, or other containers.

   3. _____ are graphic images that make it easier to identify a message.

   4. Color Schemes for Signs and Labels

     A. _____ signs warn of an immediate _____, action that must be taken, or activity to be avoided.

     B. _____ or amber signs warn of precautionary steps that should be taken.

     C. _____ signs are mandatory _____.

     D. _____ signs promote _____ in a positive manner.

III. Employee Safety

   1. Medical Waste (List the four types.)

     A. _____

     B. _____

     C. _____

     D. _____

   2. Disposal of Medical Waste

     A. Sharps must be placed in _____-proof and _____-proof containers.

     B. Medical offices must follow _____ and _____ laws regarding disposal of medical waste.

   3. OSHA Bloodborne Pathogen Standards and Standard Precautions

     A. _____ _____ is a reasonable anticipation that the employee's duties may result in skin, mucous membrane, eye, or parenteral contact with _____ material.

     B. Each at-risk employee must be offered the _____ _____ (HBV) vaccine series within the first _____ days of employment and at the expense of the _____.

     C. OSHA requires each medical office to have a written _____ _____ _____ to assist in minimizing employee exposure.

   4. Universal Precautions and Standard Precautions

     A. Universal precautions are issued by the _____ for _____ _____ and _____.

B. These standards treat all blood and body fluids as if they are contaminated with

_____ pathogens.

C. Guidelines regarding the use of PPE

   i. The employer must supply the PPE and provide _____ or

   _____.

   ii. PPE must be of a strength to act as a(n) _____ to infectious materials.

   iii. _____ gloves may not be reused.

   iv. Protective eye equipment must have _____ sides to prevent infectious

   material from entering the area.

   v. All PPE must be _____ and placed in a(n) _____

   container before the employee leaves the office.

D. _____ _____ are CDC-issued guidelines that are more

complete than the universal precautions.

5. Preventing and Responding to Needlestick Injuries

A. Needlestick injuries can lead to serious or _____ infections with

_____ pathogens.

B. When exposed, follow these steps

   i. Wash needlesticks and cuts with _____ and _____.

   ii. Use water to _____ splashes to the nose, mouth, or skin.

   iii. _____ eyes with clean water, _____, or sterile irrigants.

   iv. Report the incident to the _____.

   v. Immediately seek _____ _____.

6. Responding to Spills

A. A sample spill kit would include plain clay _____ _____, a

small _____ pan, and a(n) _____ bag.

B. Cat litter is used as a(n) _____ _____ to allow sweep-up of the

material.

7. Responding to Eye Contamination

A. A(n) _____ _____ is used in the event that harmful materials

enter the eyes.

B. It should be checked each _____ to ensure that it is working properly.

8. Housekeeping Safety

A. Housekeeping personnel should not empty _____ waste and

_____ containers.

B. A(n) _____ with an outside housekeeping agency should state that all

personnel must be trained in bloodborne pathogen standards and standard precautions.

IV. Proper Body Mechanics

   1. Correct methods of standing and lifting objects will help prevent _____ and

      _____.

   2. _____ _____ is coordination of body alignment, balance, and

      movement.

   3. Ergonomics

     A. OSHA _____ _____ provides regulations for ergonomics.

     B. The _____ workstation is a common problematic area.

V. Office Security

   1. Ensure that doors and windows have _____ _____.

   2. Change _____ _____ if a key is missing.

   3. A(n) _____ _____ activates and deactivates an electronic security

      system.

   4. Any suspicious concerns should immediately be reported to the _____ or

      _____ _____.

VI. Incident Reports

   1. Incidents (List three types and give one example of each.)

     A. _____

     B. _____

     C. _____

   2. Incident reports should be completed in _____ _____ or using a

      computer-based _____.

   3. Incident reports protect both the employer and the medical assistant against

      _____ _____.

VII. Quality Medical Care

   1. Quality medical care is a(n) _____ of all patients.

   2. Major Areas of Health Care Regularly Examined to Determine Quality (List five areas.)

     A. _____

     B. _____

     C. _____

     D. _____

     E. _____

   3. The AMA's Eight Essentials of Quality Care

     A. Emphasize _____ detection and treatment.

     B. Encourage the patient's _____ in the decision-making process regarding his or

      her treatment.

C. Demonstrate _____ for the patient and the patient's family.

D. Achieve the _____ goal through the wise use of technology and other resources.

E. Provide adequate _____ in the patient's medical record to facilitate _____ evaluation and _____ of care.

VIII. Quality Assurance

1. Quality assurance (QA) is the process of _____ and _____ information about the services provided.

2. Formal Quality Assurance Programs (QAPs)

   A. A QAP includes _____ and educational components to identify and _____ problems.

   B. Basic components of a QAP

      i. Establish a QA _____.

      ii. Review all clinical and administrative _____ and _____.

      iii. Set up a(n) _____ for identifying items to review.

      iv. _____ all issues.

      v. _____ the number of issues.

      vi. Maintain careful _____.

3. Implementing a QAP

   A. The goal of a QAP is to improve the quality of care so that there is no _____ between what _____ be done and what is _____ being done.

   B. Implementing a QAP requires the development of patient-centered _____ based on acceptable _____ of care.

4. Medical Assistant's Role in Quality Assurance

   A. _____ patient complaints.

   B. _____ patient education.

   C. _____ telephone follow-up regarding a patient's _____.

   D. _____ laboratory tests done in the _____.

   E. _____ the results of laboratory tests given over the _____.

   F. _____ patient _____ to the attention of the physician.

5. Health Plan Employer Data and Information Set

   A. Categories of Performance (List eight.)

      i. _____

      ii. _____

      iii. _____

      iv. _____

v. _____

vi. _____

vii. _____

viii. _____

6. CLIA

   A. All clinical laboratories that test _____ _____ must be controlled.

   B. CLIA stands for _____ _____ _____ _____.

   C. List the three categories of testing.

      i. _____

      ii. _____

      iii. _____

7. The Joint Commission

   A. This organization was formerly known as the Joint Commission on _____ of Healthcare _____.

   B. The Joint Commission establishes guidelines for _____ and other health care agencies to follow regarding _____ of care.

   C. Surveyors visit a health care facility and review patient _____ _____, medical _____ organizations, and the _____ _____ of the facility.

KEY TERMINOLOGY REVIEW

Match each of the following terms with the correct definition.

a. incident

b. ergonomics

c. personal protective equipment (PPE)

d. OSHA

e. biohazards

1. _____ Examples include gloves, fluid-resistant lab coats, safety glasses, and a surgical mask, shield, or respirator.

2. _____ Responsible for the safety of all employees of companies operating in the United States.

3. _____ A prescription pad is missing.

4. _____ Biological substances, such as medical waste and samples of a virus or bacterium, that pose a threat to human beings and are potentially infectious.

5. _____ Applies scientific information and data regarding human body mechanics to the design of objects and the overall environment for human use.

APPLIED PRACTICE

1. Consider the following clinical activities and select the appropriate PPE that would be required for each.

   a. Performing a capillary stick

   _____

   _____

   _____

   _____

   b. Performing a blood smear

   _____

   _____

   _____

   _____

2. Match the label with the correct hazardous warning.

HAZARD CLASS	

   1. _____ Corrosive
   2. _____ Reactive
   3. _____ Compressed gas
   4. _____ Other toxic
   5. _____ Seriously toxic
   6. _____ Biohazardous/infectious
   7. _____ Oxidizing
   8. _____ Flammable/combustible

   A

   B

   C

   D

   E

   F

   G

   H

CRITICAL THINKING

Answer the following questions to the best of your ability. Use the textbook as a reference.

1. Tammy, a certified medical assistant, is in a rush and doesn't wear gloves or a lab coat while she performs wound care for a patient. During the dressing change, blood and pus from the patient's wound came into direct contact with Tammy's hands and scrub top. To make matters worse, Tammy's left hand had a small paper cut near her index finger. Her actions are a direct violation of the Centers for Disease Control and Prevention's universal precautions. What are the consequences for both Tammy and her patient?

   _____

   _____

   _____

   _____

   _____

2. Consider safety in the medical office. What items might be included on a checklist used to evaluate a workplace for safety every day?

   _____

   _____

   _____

   _____

   _____

RESEARCH ACTIVITY

Use Internet search engines to research the following topic and write a brief description of what you find. It is important to use reputable websites.

1. Research the website for the Occupational Safety and Health Administration (OSHA), www.osha.gov. What information can you find for health care facilities? List some facts you find at the OSHA website.

   _____

   _____

   _____

   _____

   _____

CHAPTER 7
Telephone Techniques

STUDENT STUDY GUIDE

Use the following guide to assist in your learning of the concepts from the chapter.

I. Telephone Techniques

1. Answering the Telephone

   A. Answer the telephone with a(n) _____.

   B. Answer the telephone by the _____ ring.

   C. An appropriate greeting includes the name of the office, _____

   _____, and asking how you can be of _____.

   D. List four elements of speech when speaking on the phone.

   i. _____

   ii. _____

   iii. _____

   iv. _____

   E. _____ the caller helps to _____ the patient's confidential information.

   F. Take time to _____ to the caller rather than attempt to multitask.

2. Business Telephone Systems

   A. Many phone systems answer the initial call with a(n) _____ and then direct the call to the appropriate person after the caller chooses a(n) _____.

   B. Telephone calls made in the office should be limited to _____ calls.

   C. Never put a call on hold before you have given the _____ a chance to say whether it is a(n) _____.

   D. When a caller is waiting on hold, check on him or her approximately every _____ _____.

   E. Summarize the five steps for transferring a call.

   i. _____

   ii. _____

   iii. _____

iv. _____

v. _____

3. Taking a Message

A. Electronic medical records allow messages to be entered _____ into the patient's medical record.

B. _____ telephone messages or _____ can be used for recording telephone messages for offices that don't use electronic medical records.

C. List five important components of a message.

i. _____

ii. _____

iii. _____

iv. _____

v. _____

D. Voice messaging systems may be used for both _____ and _____ calls.

E. _____ _____ is used to forward incoming calls to another telephone.

F. A medical office may need to block the office number from showing up on the patient's _____ _____.

G. When calling a number with _____ _____ attached, you must state from where you are calling.

H. _____ are ergonomically correct and allow for your hands to be free while talking on the telephone.

I. When pagers are used, some offices use _____ message systems.

J. _____ _____ can interfere with electronic monitors.

II. HIPAA Compliance

1. Return Calls and Callbacks

A. Before calling a patient, review his _____ _____ to establish who has been given permission to receive information about the patient.

B. Do not indicate why you are calling until you have the _____ on the phone.

C. When leaving a message

i. State your _____.

ii. State the name of the patient's doctor for whom you work, *not* the _____ of the _____.

iii. State the _____ _____ where you can be reached.

iv. Do not leave any additional information as doing so could breach _____ _____.

2. Test Results
   A. Results may not be divulged until the _____ has reviewed the results and given verbal or written permission to share the results with the patient.
   B. Never leave a message that includes test _____.
3. Appointment Reminders
   A. An appointment reminder should be given at least the _____ _____ an appointment.
   B. Some offices call to remind patients a(n) _____ in advance.
   C. Authorization forms must be signed prior to using _____ or _____ reminders for patients.
4. Documentation
   A. _____ telephone interactions must be documented in the patient's medical record, especially when _____ a(n) _____ for the patient.
   B. Document the _____, the _____, and the name of the person who was given the message for the patient.

III. Typical Incoming Calls
1. Patient Calls (List five common types of patient calls.)
   A. _____
   B. _____
   C. _____
   D. _____
   E. _____
2. Nonpatient Calls (List four common types of nonpatient calls.)
   A. _____
   B. _____
   C. _____
   D. _____

IV. Prescription Refill Requests
1. Due to a high volume of calls, _____ _____ systems are often used for refill requests.
2. The MA should check for refill messages at least _____ time(s) a day.
3. The _____ must sign off on all refill requests and may need to review the patient's _____ _____.
4. Calling the Pharmacy with a Refill Request
   A. Medical assistants are often responsible for calling the pharmacy with refill requests.

B. Computerized _____ _____ has decreased the number of times the MA has to call the pharmacy.

V. Telephone Triage

1. The _____ of a patient's illness or injury determines the order of treatment.

2. A(n) _____ and procedure _____ should explain the office's preferred method of screening telephone calls.

3. Handling an Emergency Call

A. Written _____ should be established for handling emergency calls.

B. Your voice should remain _____ and reassuring.

C. _____ hang up the phone on a patient.

D. Have a coworker call _____ on behalf of a patient.

VI. Handling Difficult Calls

1. Do not to lose your _____.

2. Patients may have displaced _____ and may be frustrated with _____.

3. Be _____ while remaining in control of the situation.

VII. Using Telephone Directories

1. Pay close attention to the _____ that are offered.

2. Often, you can dial _____ to speak with an operator.

3. Telephone companies provide directories that contain _____ and _____ pages.

A. _____ pages are for telephone service customers.

B. _____ pages are for businesses.

4. Long-Distance and Conference Calls

A. Long-distance calls are made to anywhere outside your _____ _____.

B. Long-distance _____ may be implemented to reduce potential abuse of long-distance calls.

5. Telephone logs keep track of _____ _____ calls being made.

6. Conference Calls

A. A conference call is used when several people from _____ _____ wish to have a joint discussion by phone.

B. If your telephone system doesn't allow for conference calls to be placed, the _____ can place these calls.

7. Keep in mind _____ _____ when making long-distance and conference calls.

 A. The four main time zones in the United States are _____,

 _____, _____, and _____.

8. Answering Services

 A. List the three common designated times for using an answering service.

 i. _____

 ii. _____

 iii. _____

 B. Although an answering service is considered a necessary service, there are often

 _____ attached to using such services.

KEY TERMINOLOGY REVIEW

Complete the following sentences using the correct key terms found at the beginning of the chapter. Key terms may be more than one word in length.

1. Mrs. Smith has been told that before seeing a specialist, she must get a(n) _____.

2. When the office is closed, the _____ typically handles all emergency calls.

3. _____ refers to the quality or state of being understandable.

4. When calling a patient, it is important for a medical office to set up a system to block the office number from showing up on the patient's _____.

5. A medical assistant is on the phone with a patient; the process she uses to determine the order in which patient calls should be handled is called _____.

APPLIED PRACTICE

Using your textbook, complete the following activities and answer the following questions.

1. With a classmate, role-play a telephone call from a patient to the medical office. Role-play a scenario in which a message must be taken, such as a patient calling in with a prescription refill or a question to the billing department about a bill. Use the message pad template opposite to document the message accurately.

Caller Name: _____	Dr. _____
Date of Birth: _____	Pharmacy Name: _____
Telephone Number: _____	Pharmacy Phone: _____

Message: _____

_____

_____

_____

☐ Return Call   ☐ Will Call Back

Date: _____ Time: _____

Message Taken By: _____

_____

2. Tyler works as a medical assistant for Pearson Heights Family Medicine. What would be an appropriate greeting for Tyler to use when he answers the medical office telephone?

_____

_____

_____

LEARNING ACTIVITY: MULTIPLE CHOICE

Circle the correct answer to each of the following questions.

1. Which of the following would be appropriate to play for callers who are on hold?
   a. A local radio station
   b. Prerecorded music
   c. A message about seasonal allergies
   d. All of the above

2. Which of the following might be offensive or irritating for callers to listen to while they are on hold?
   a. Religious music
   b. Prerecorded music
   c. A message about seasonal allergies
   d. A local radio station

3. How long is an acceptable period of time to leave a caller on hold?
   a. 3 minutes
   b. 20–30 seconds
   c. 45–60 seconds
   d. 1–2 minutes

4. What items should a medical assistant have available before answering the office telephone?
   a. Pen or pencil
   b. Paper
   c. Telephone message pad
   d. All of the above

5. The medical office telephone should be answered within how many rings?

    a. On the first ring
    b. By the second ring
    c. By the third ring
    d. After more than five rings

6. What rule are you violating if a patient's private information is thrown into the trash?

    a. OSHA's privacy rule
    b. A HIPAA privacy rule
    c. The AAMA's privacy rule
    d. The AMA's privacy rule

7. Which of the following telephone calls should be taken care of first?

    a. A patient who says she needs to schedule her yearly mammogram
    b. An angry patient who is calling about her bill
    c. A patient who says he is having chest pains
    d. A patient who is calling to find out his laboratory results

8. What information would you expect to find in a telephone triage notebook?

    a. Driving directions to the medical office
    b. The hours the clinic is open
    c. The questions to ask a patient who complains of chest pains
    d. All of the above

9. In the event of a medical emergency in the office, what information should the medical assistant have available before calling for emergency services?

    a. The patient's name
    b. The patient's age
    c. The patient's sex
    d. All of the above

10. Which of the following emergency telephone numbers should the medical assistant have readily available at the front desk?

    a. Poison control
    b. The local police department
    c. The local fire department
    d. All of the above

CRITICAL THINKING

Answer the following questions to the best of your ability. Use the textbook and other resources such as the Internet in considering your answers.

1. Rosie Sanchez, CMA (AAMA), has been working as an administrative medical assistant in an internal medicine clinic for the past year. A large part of her day is spent answering the office telephone and scheduling appointments. She would like the office to provide her with a hands-free headset for the telephone system. The clinic director has asked Rosie to create a list that outlines the benefits of having a hands-free headset over a conventional telephone headset. What should Rosie list?

_____

_____

_____

_____

2. Dr. Ahlberstat has reviewed the results of Alexis Huntley's pregnancy test. Her blood test reveals that she is approximately 8 weeks pregnant. When you call Alexis with the results, as directed by Dr. Ahlberstat, a man answers Alexis's home telephone, identifying himself as her husband, and he states that Alexis isn't home. What type of message would you leave for Alexis?

_____

_____

_____

_____

RESEARCH ACTIVITY

Use Internet search engines to research the following topic and write a brief description of what you find. It is important to use reputable websites.

1. Search for on-call, after-hours answering services that are available for medical offices in your area. What types of services are offered by these companies? What is the general cost for on-call answering services?

_____

_____

_____

_____

_____

CHAPTER 8
Patient Reception

STUDENT STUDY GUIDE

Use the following guide to assist in your learning of the concepts from the chapter.

I. Duties of the Receptionist

  1. The Duties of a Receptionist

    A. _____ patients upon arrival

    B. Assisting new patients with _____ of proper forms

    C. _____ copayments

    D. Maintaining a(n) _____ and _____ environment in the reception area

    E. _____ any disturbances in the reception room

    F. _____ incoming telephone calls

    G. _____ return appointments

    H. Making _____ calls for upcoming appointments

  2. Personal Characteristics

    A. Looking people in the _____, speaking _____, smiling, and exercising basic _____ have a great impact by helping people feel welcomed and cared for.

    B. Paying attention to _____ and _____ are also paramount.

  3. Physical Appearance

    A. Careful _____, good hygiene, and _____ dress are important.

    B. Accessories should be _____ and minimal.

    C. Name pins or tags should be _____ at all times.

  4. Communication Skills

    A. Good communication requires

      i. _____ to what others are saying

      ii. Understanding their _____

      iii. Responding in a(n) _____ and nondefensive manner

II. Maintaining the Reception Area

1. The term _____ area is more positive than the outdated term _____ room.

2. Neatness

    A. The receptionist must monitor the _____ and _____ of the room.

    B. It might be most convenient to check the reception room when returning from _____ and _____.

3. Cleaning

    A. The reception room should be _____, _____, and dusted every day.

    B. _____ should be emptied.

    C. Glass should be polished and kept free of _____ and smudges.

    D. Don't use commercial _____ _____ or fragrances because patients may have allergies to them.

4. Furniture Placement

    A. Furniture should be placed to allow access and movement for _____.

    B. A relatively straight traffic path should be approximately ____ to ____ inches wide.

    C. The furniture should be appropriate for the _____ population.

5. Children's Areas

    A. Children's areas should be furnished with toys, _____, and appropriately sized _____.

    B. Toys should be _____ daily.

6. Television

    A. Content on the TV should be appropriate for all _____.

    B. Keep the volume relatively _____.

III. Daily Workflow

1. Opening the Office

    A. Arrive _____ minutes before office hours begin.

    B. Disengage the security system and turn on _____.

    C. Prepare patient medical records and _____ slips.

    D. Count the _____ box.

    E. Print out a master list of the daily _____.

    F. Check with the _____ _____ or voice mail and distribute messages to the appropriate individuals.

2. Preparing Office Equipment

   A. All office machines should be turned on and made _____ for _____.

   B. Fill _____ bins.

3. Managing Patient Records

   A. A medical record is either _____ or paper based.

   B. Making charts available for the physician can be done by either _____ _____ electronic charts or _____ paper-based charts.

   C. _____ is filing all information and test results for a patient into that patient's medical record.

4. Checking In Patients (List five components of the check-in process.)

   A. _____

   B. _____

   C. _____

   D. _____

   E. _____

5. Greeting Patients

   A. Patients should be able to conduct their business in _____.

   B. Contagious patients should be immediately placed in _____ _____ in order to limit exposure to others.

   C. Patients take precedence over other office _____.

6. Signing In

   A. The sign-in sheet or patient register must be _____ compliant.

   B. Sign-in sheets may be _____ or paper based.

7. Preventing Identity Theft

   A. Ask the patient to state her demographic information when checking in, such as _____ and _____.

   B. Obtain a copy of the patient's driver's license or state ID at his _____ _____.

   C. Some offices take a(n) _____ of each patient at the first visit and make it part of the patient's medical _____.

8. Tracking Appointment Status

   A. Patients who do not keep their appointment and do not call to reschedule are marked as _____.

   B. Electronic scheduling programs generate reports to help the office identify _____ and _____.

C. In the event of a rescheduled appointment or no-show, make a notation in the patient's record indicating

    i. _____

    ii. _____

    iii. _____

    iv. _____

9. Registering New Patients

  A. New patients must fill out the following information

    i. _____

    ii. _____

    iii. _____

    iv. _____

  B. Provide the patient with clear _____ and explain the purpose of each _____.

10. Updating Established Patients

  A. At every visit, ask patients to verbally confirm their current _____, telephone number, and _____ information.

11. Explaining Payment Policies

  A. A(n) _____ of _____ form authorizes the insurance company to send payments directly to the physician.

  B. Check the insurance card to determine whether a(n) _____ is required from the patient.

  C. It may be necessary to call the insurance company to verify a patient's _____ and the participation _____ of the physician the patient is scheduled to see.

12. Collecting Copayments

  A. Copayments help establish patient _____ responsibility.

  B. Copayments are usually paid at the _____ of _____.

  C. A patients should receive a(n) _____ for a payment.

13. Initialing Encounter Forms

  A. Encounter forms contain common _____ and _____ codes.

  B. These forms may be printed out or handled completely _____.

14. Completing the Check-in Process
    A. Do not assume that patients _____ what to _____ when the check-in process is complete.
    B. Tell the patients _____ what to do next.

15. Consideration of the Patient's Time
    A. Excessive wait time is one of the most common _____

      _____.

    B. _____ should not be behind in schedule due to scheduling errors.
    C. Be aware of patient _____ times and periodically check on them.
    D. If the expected wait time exceeds _____ minutes, the receptionist should inform the _____ as soon as possible after check-in.

16. Escorting the Patient into the Examination Room
    A. Escorting is usually done by the _____ _____who is assigned to patient care rather than by the _____.
    B. To verify that you have the correct medical record, ask the patient to state his or her name and _____ of _____.
    C. _____ at the patient's speed and offer assistance as needed.
    D. In the examination room, clearly explain whether the patient should remove any articles of _____ and provide a(n) _____ if necessary.
    E. Never leave the patient alone with his or her _____.

17. Completing the Patient Visit
    A. Patient _____ are provided after the physician has completed the _____.

    B. The physician should indicate what treatment was given, the supporting _____, and the charge on a(n) _____ form.
    C. Patients should receive a copy of the _____ _____.
    D. _____ regulations require privacy for discussions involving protected health information; such discussions with patients must not take place in any area where another patient may overhear.

18. Patient Education
    A. Most patient education is completed by _____

      _____.

    B. Basic education that may be conducted at the reception desk includes
      i. _____
      ii. _____

iii. _____

iv. _____

C. Ensure that patient communication is provided at a(n) _____ the patient understands.

19. Closing the Office

A. The purposes of closing procedures are to ensure the _____ of the premises and to prepare for the _____ _____.

B. Compile a list of all _____ appointments.

C. Count and balance the _____ _____ in the presence of another staff member.

D. Prepare medical records for patients scheduled for the _____ _____.

E. Turn off all _____ and _____ and secure the _____.

KEY TERMINOLOGY REVIEW

Match each of the following terms with the correct definition.

a. copayments

b. demographic

c. collate

d. queuing up

e. no-show

1. _____ Activating or displaying a computerized list.

2. _____ Designated amounts that some medical insurance plans require patients to pay for medical services.

3. _____ Information, such as age, gender, ethnic background, education, and Social Security number.

4. _____ Filing and sorting information in a medical record.

5. _____ Patient failure to keep an appointment or call to cancel.

APPLIED PRACTICE

Using information from your textbook and other sources you may find on the topic, complete the following activity.

1. Aubrey Cody is a CMA (AAMA) who has been hired as a medical assistant for a new pediatric practice that is being built. How could Aubrey design the medical office reception area? What theme, toys, and reading materials would be appropriate for the reception area? Explain your answers.

_____

_____

_____

_____

_____

LEARNING ACTIVITY: TRUE/FALSE

Indicate whether the following statements are true or false by placing a T or an F on the line that precedes each statement.

_____ 1. The medical assistant who opens the office should arrive 30 minutes before the start of office hours.

_____ 2. Receptionists usually are responsible for escorting patients to examination rooms.

_____ 3. Open-toed shoes are acceptable footwear for a receptionist.

_____ 4. Encounter forms authorize insurance companies to send payments directly to the physician.

_____ 5. A 20-minute wait time is usually accepted by most patients.

_____ 6. Counting the cash box at the end of the day should be done privately in a closed room.

_____ 7. Patients with a medical emergency should be taken directly to an examination room.

_____ 8. Patient sign-in sheets must be HIPAA compliant.

_____ 9. Receipts are not required when patients pay a copayment.

_____ 10. IDC-10 codes and CPT codes are listed on the patient demographic form.

CRITICAL THINKING

Answer the following questions to the best of your ability. Use the textbook as a reference.

1. Marcus Winston, RMA, has been hired to work as an administrative medical assistant at the front desk in a small, one-physician medical office. Dr. Quan has been using a paper sign-in sheet for his patients for many years. Marcus has recently completed his medical assisting education and remembers learning that sign-in sheets must be HIPAA compliant. What can Marcus tell Dr. Quan about the paper sign-in system that he is currently using?

   _____

   _____

   _____

   _____

   _____

2. Sara Womack, CMA (AAMA), is the medical office manager in a women's clinic. She has two employees, Aaron and Michael, who share the job of front desk receptionist. Aaron is often short with the patients, some of whom have complained to the physician about his attitude. Michael has a sunny personality and thoroughly enjoys the fast pace at the front desk. What would you do about Aaron and Michael if you were Sara? What sort of ramifications might occur if Sara allows Aaron to continue working at the front desk?

   _____

   _____

   _____

   _____

   _____

3. Marjorie Sorensen, CMA (AAMA), has just been hired to work as the office manager for Dr. Rodriguez. The doctor tells Marjorie that she has noticed that many tasks aren't being completed at the beginning of the day, when the office opens. This has resulted in disorganization and delays in

the schedule. Dr. Rodriguez would like Marjorie to come up with a solution to this problem. What might Marjorie suggest?

_____

_____

_____

_____

_____

RESEARCH ACTIVITY

Use Internet search engines to research the following topic and write a brief description of what you find. It is important to use reputable websites.

1. Using the information and decor theme of the reception area that you designed in the Applied Practice activity, search the Internet and obtain figures and estimates regarding the cost of decorating a reception area. Take into consideration paint, accessories, seating, tables, and so forth. Be sure to cite the websites you use to find this information.

_____

_____

_____

_____

_____

Chapter 9
Appointment Scheduling

STUDENT STUDY GUIDE

Use the following guide to assist in your learning of the concepts from the chapter.

I. Appointment Scheduling Methods

   1. Factors to Be Considered in Selecting a Scheduling System (List seven factors.)

      A. _____

      B. _____

      C. _____

      D. _____

      E. _____

      F. _____

      G. _____

   2. Specified Times

      A. Each patient has a(n) _____ _____ slot.

      B. Appointment length is based on the _____ for the office visit.

      C. This method leads to long _____ times.

   3. Wave Scheduling

      A. All the patients are told to come in at the _____ of the hour in which they are to be seen.

      B. Patients are seen in the _____ in which they arrive.

      C. Each hour is divided into _____ amounts of time.

      D. Three _____-minute or four _____-minute appointments could be seen in an hour.

   4. Modified Wave Scheduling

      A. There are many _____ with modified wave scheduling.

      B. Patients are scheduled within the _____ half of an hour block.

   5. Scheduling by Grouping Procedures

      A. Patients requiring the same type of examination are scheduled during a particular _____ of _____.

6. Double-Booking Scheduling

   A. _____ patients are scheduled to be seen during the same time slot.

   B. This type of scheduling is considered ineffective but sometimes _____ in order to accommodate patients.

7. Open Hours Scheduling

   A. This is least _____ of all the systems.

   B. Generally patients are seen in the order of their _____.

   C. This type of scheduling is commonly used in _____ _____ clinics.

II. Types of Scheduling Systems

1. Computerized Systems

   A. These systems may be purchased based on the medical practice's _____

      _____.

   B. _____ guidelines must be followed when using computerized systems, including compliance issues such as _____ _____,

      _____, and _____.

   C. These appointment systems help to _____ workflow and ensure that scheduling _____ are followed.

   D. Advantages

      i. The ability to _____ and _____ patient appointments with a click or touch of a button

      ii. The ability to track regular _____ in the medical practice

      iii. _____ scheduling and completion of forms

   E. Disadvantages (List two.)

      i. _____

      ii. _____

2. Manual Systems

   A. These systems involve a hard-copy schedule _____ and a(n)

      _____.

   B. The appointment book and schedule must protect _____ _____ at all times.

   C. Advantages (List two.)

      i. _____

      ii. _____

   D. Disadvantages

      i. _____ due to frequent changes

      ii. Lack of _____ _____ to data and statistics

      iii. Usable by only _____ _____ at a time

III. Patient Scheduling Process

    1. Steps for Patient Scheduling (Summarize the steps.)

      A. Form an appointment _____.

      B. Identify the _____ and the need.

      C. Determine the patient _____, which can be either _____ patient or _____ patient.

      D. _____ an appointment time.

      E. Confirm the appointment _____.

    2. Communication Skills for Scheduling

      A. The medical assistant must apply professional, _____, and _____ communication skills when scheduling patients.

    3. Responding to Urgent and Emergency Situations

      A. _____ _____ are illnesses or injuries that patients suddenly experience and that require treatment but are not life threatening.

      B. The _____ should always be informed immediately regarding a potential emergency.

      C. Generally, sudden _____ of _____ must be considered an emergency until otherwise determined by the physician.

      D. List five items that need to be documented after a patient calls with an emergent medical situation.

         i. _____

        ii. _____

       iii. _____

       iv. _____

        v. _____

IV. Maintaining the Schedule

    1. Changes such as _____ appointments, _____, or cancellations occur daily.

    2. Rescheduling Appointments

      A. A patient should ideally call to reschedule _____ to _____ hours in advance.

      B. Office scheduling _____ should define acceptable rescheduling _____ _____ for various types of appointments.

      C. When using a manual scheduling system, note the rescheduled appointment in both the appointment book and the patient's _____.

3. Patient Cancellations

   A. Cancellations should be documented in the patient _____ and should include as much information discussed with the patient as possible.

   B. The _____ should be notified of any cancellations that could endanger the patient's _____.

   C. With a manual system, the notation "_____" indicates a cancelled appointment.

4. No-Shows

   A. When no-shows occur, the medical assistant should

      i. Contact the _____.

      ii. Offer to _____ the appointment.

      iii. Mention any extra _____.

      iv. _____ it in the medical record.

   B. Careful, legible documentation is needed to legally protect the physician from a claim of _____ _____.

   C. Some medical practices charge patients for _____ appointments.

   D. Information regarding fees is often posted in the reception area near the _____ _____.

5. Future Appointments

   A. A patient scheduling her next appointment before leaving the office is called _____ _____.

   B. Regularly scheduled checkups and required _____ appointments are often scheduled this way.

   C. A patient should be given a(n) _____ _____ card with all the office information as well as the date and time of his next appointment.

6. Follow-Up

   A. A(n) _____ _____ notifies the office of certain tasks to be performed, such as appointment reminders.

   B. Electronic reminders can be sent using secure _____ or _____ messages if approved in advance by the patient.

   C. Telephone call appointment reminders may be performed personally by an individual or using a(n) _____ _____ that announces the appointment details.

7. Buffer Time

   A. Small blocks of _____ _____ can be built into the schedule to help compensate for extra time that may be needed throughout the day.

B. Open time is often scheduled at the end of the _____ and again at the end of the _____.

V. Arranging Outside Appointments

1. List three examples of outside appointments that are often scheduled.

A. _____

B. _____

C. _____

VI. Scheduling Nonpatient Appointments

1. Examples of nonpatient appointment types include sales representatives selling office _____, pharmaceuticals, and _____.

A. Office _____ are usually in place for handling nonpatient visitors and vendor representatives.

B. These appointments should _____ take priority over patient appointments.

KEY TERMINOLOGY REVIEW

Match each of the following terms with the correct definition.

a. archived
b. cycle time
c. double-booking

d. matrix
e. triage

1. _____ Sorting or grouping according to the seriousness of the patient's condition.
2. _____ Stored.
3. _____ A grid that shows the availability of each physician, as well as periods of time that are not available for appointments.
4. _____ The length of time the average patient spends in the medical office.
5. _____ Scheduling more than one patient for the same appointment time.

APPLIED PRACTICE

Follow the directions for each assignment.

1. Using the following information and the manual schedule on the following pages, create a matrix for the medical office. (*Remember to use a pencil.*)

   a. The medical offices open at 8:30 A.M. every day.
   b. The last appointment of the day is scheduled no later than 3:30 P.M.
   c. The office is closed for appointments for lunch starting at 12:00 P.M.; it reopens at 1:15 P.M.
   d. Dr. Cho has hospital rounds every Wednesday from 7:30 A.M. to 10:00 A.M.
   e. Dr. Jackson has hospital rounds every Thursday from 7:45 A.M. to 10:15 A.M.
   f. On February 3, Dr. Cho has a meeting at Alliance Assisted Living that starts at 3:30 P.M.
   g. On February 2, Dr. Jackson has a meeting with a pharmaceutical representative that is scheduled for 12:45 to 1:30 P.M.

Pearson Family Clinic

Wednesday, February 2, 20xx

	Dr. S. Cho	Dr. A. Jackson
7:30		
7:45		
8:00		
8:15		
8:30		
8:45		
9:00		
9:15		
9:30		
9:45		
10:00		
10:15		
10:30		
10:45		
11:00		
11:15		
11:30		
11:45		
12:00		
12:15		
12:30		
12:45		
1:00		
1:15		
1:30		
1:45		
2:00		
2:15		
2:30		
2:45		
3:00		
3:15		
3:30		
3:45		
4:00		

Thursday, February 3, 20xx

	Dr. S. Cho	Dr. A. Jackson
7:30		
7:45		
8:00		
8:15		
8:30		
8:45		
9:00		
9:15		
9:30		
9:45		
10:00		
10:15		
10:30		
10:45		
11:00		
11:15		
11:30		
11:45		
12:00		
12:15		
12:30		
12:45		
1:00		
1:15		
1:30		
1:45		
2:00		
2:15		
2:30		
2:45		
3:00		
3:15		
3:30		
3:45		
4:00		

2. Schedule the following patients on the appointment schedule.

   a. LaToya Atwater is a new patient to see Dr. Cho. Wednesdays work best for LaToya. (45-minute appointment)

   b. Sujin Dalywhal wants to see Dr. Jackson on Thursday afternoon for an abdominal suture removal. (15-minute appointment)

   c. Jose Alvarez calls on Wednesday morning because he has had a terrible headache for the past 2 days and needs to be seen as soon as possible. (30-minute appointment)

   d. Anna Maria DeCamillo is a diabetic patient who wants to see Dr. Jackson for her 3-month diabetic checkup on Wednesday afternoon. (30-minute appointment)

   e. Mark Tomlinson wants to see Dr. Cho for his annual checkup on Thursday. (30-minute appointment)

   f. Aiden Taylor needs to be seen on Thursday morning for his 3-year well-child visit with Dr. Jackson. (30-minute appointment)

   g. Dr. Cho requests that an appointment be made on Wednesday morning with her patient, Lydia Pazmino, regarding her blood test results.

LEARNING ACTIVITY: MULTIPLE CHOICE

Circle the correct answer to each of the following questions.

1. How many minutes do most patients consider to be an acceptable wait time prior to seeing a doctor?

   a. 10
   b. 15
   c. 20
   d. 35

2. Which of the following is an acceptable way to note a missed appointment using a manual appointment system?

   a. Use white correction fluid to cover the patient's name.
   b. Use a black marker to obliterate the patient's name.
   c. Use an eraser to remove the patient's name.
   d. Write no-show (NS) next to the patient's name on the appointment schedule and in her medical record.

3. What is one way to remind patients of an upcoming appointment in the medical office?

   a. Send out a reminder card to the patient just prior to the appointment.
   b. Call the patient to remind him or her of the appointment.
   c. Send an e-mail to the patient to remind him or her of the appointment.
   d. All of the above

4. Which method of scheduling involves scheduling three patients at the beginning of each hour?

   a. Wave
   b. Modified wave
   c. Open hours
   d. Fixed appointment

5. In which method of scheduling are patients scheduled only for the first half of each hour and seen in the order in which they arrive?

   a. Wave
   b. Modified wave
   c. Open hours
   d. Fixed appointment

6. Which method of scheduling is most commonly used in walk-in clinics, laboratories, and X-ray facilities where patients are typically seen on a first-come, first-served basis?

   a. Wave
   b. Modified wave
   c. Open hours
   d. Fixed appointment

7. To eliminate the need to "squeeze in" an emergency or unscheduled appointment, a medical assistant should integrate _____ into the office schedule, if office policy allows.

   a. more time
   b. time patterns
   c. wave scheduling
   d. none of the above

8. Examples of emergency conditions that require patients to be seen immediately include

   a. skin rash.
   b. pain or burning on urination.
   c. severe dizziness.
   d. all of the above.

9. When confirming an appointment with a patient on the telephone, the patient should be asked to repeat which of the following information?

   a. Name of the person helping them
   b. Date and time of the appointment
   c. Insurance information
   d. All of the above

10. Which of the following is true of triage?

    a. It becomes necessary when more than one seriously ill patient is waiting to see the physician.
    b. It takes place each time a patient visits the office.
    c. It is done only in a hospital setting.
    d. It is a skill performed only by the physician.

CRITICAL THINKING

Answer the following questions to the best of your ability. Use the textbook as a reference.

1. Dylan Reilly, CMA (AAMA), is working in a busy family practice office. The physicians and staff all agree that the appointment-scheduling system is not working, and patients are frequently waiting long periods of time for appointments. How should Dylan go about creating a new scheduling procedure for this office?

   _____

   _____

   _____

   _____

2. Anna Simonenko, CMA (AAMA), is working at the front desk in a family practice clinic. She has been asked to schedule Roger Edetsberger for a procedure to be performed in the hospital. Anna tells Roger that she will need to call his insurance company before she can schedule the procedure.

Roger asks, "Why do you need to do that? Can't you just schedule the procedure now and call the insurance company some other time?" What can Anna say to Roger?

_____

_____

_____

_____

3. Darnell Troutman, RMA, is working with Winston Humphry, a patient of Dr. Jackson. Mr. Humphry has just been informed that the results from his colonoscopy were abnormal, and he needs to see a specialist and have another colonoscopy performed. What type of communication skills should Darnell display while he is working with Mr. Humphry to get his appointments scheduled?

_____

_____

_____

_____

_____

RESEARCH ACTIVITY

Use Internet search engines to research the following topic and write a brief description of what you find. It is important to use reputable websites.

1. Research various appointment-scheduling software programs for medical offices. What products are available? What must be considered prior to purchasing medical office software? What type of technical support is available?

_____

_____

_____

_____

Chapter 10
Office Facilities, Equipment, and Supplies

STUDENT STUDY GUIDE

Use the following guide to assist in your learning of the concepts from the chapter.

I. Facilities Planning

   1. The Americans with Disabilities Act

     A. List six protections the ADA affords to disabled individuals.

       i. _____

       ii. _____

       iii. _____

       iv. _____

       v. _____

       vi. _____

     B. Accessibility for disabled individuals includes _____ hallways, elevators or _____, and accessible _____ facilities.

   2. Reception rooms should be comfortable and _____.

II. Office Layout

   1. Medical Office Layout and Design (List four factors.)

     A. _____

     B. _____

     C. _____

     D. _____

   2. The medical office is divided into _____ and _____ areas.

   3. Office Flow

     A. A well-_____ office area lends itself to smooth office flow.

     B. List six features that office entranceways should include.

       i. _____

       ii. _____

       iii. _____

       iv. _____

     v. _____

    vi. _____

4. Reception Area

  A. The reception desk should be neat and should not have any confidential

    _____ _____ visible.

  B. HIPAA states that the medical records area should not be accessible to

    _____.

  C. Seating should provide good _____ and be easy to

    _____.

  D. List three forms of media patient education may include.

    i. _____

    ii. _____

    iii. _____

  E. All toys should be disinfected _____.

  F. _____ is not allowed in medical facilities.

  G. Proper _____ helps patients get around the medical office.

5. Examination Rooms

  A. Examination rooms should contain only _____ and

    _____ needed to examine a patient.

  B. The temperature in examination rooms should be maintained around ____°F.

  C. At least one examination room should be configured to accommodate a(n)

    _____-bound patient.

  D. Examination rooms should be _____ so that conversations cannot be

    heard from one room to another.

6. Bathrooms

  A. Bathrooms should be kept clean and free of _____.

  B. At least one bathroom must meet _____ guidelines for accessible restroom

    facilities.

  C. Patient bathrooms need a(n) _____ or other designated area for urine

    _____.

7. Housekeeping

  A. Housekeeping services are often contracted to clean the front office area,

    _____ _____, and _____ rooms every

    night.

B. Staff are responsible for disposing of _____ waste.

C. Cleaning services often sign a HIPAA _____ _____ agreement, stating that they will adhere to HIPAA patient _____ laws.

III. Office Equipment

   1. Essential Office Equipment

      A. List nine examples of essential administrative equipment.

         i. _____

         ii. _____

         iii. _____

         iv. _____

         v. _____

         vi. _____

         vii. _____

         viii. _____

         ix. _____

      B. Attempt to _____ equipment before calling for service as doing so may prevent expensive _____ calls.

   2. Capital Equipment

      A. The purchase of capital equipment requires a(n) _____ dollar amount, and this type of equipment has a(n) _____ life expectancy.

      B. _____ is a loss in value of a product resulting from normal aging, use, or deterioration.

      C. List six examples of administrative capital equipment.

         i. _____

         ii. _____

         iii. _____

         iv. _____

         v. _____

         vi. _____

   3. Purchasing Equipment

      A. It is important to compare and research equipment based on

         i. _____

         ii. _____

         iii. _____

         iv. _____

    v. _____

   vi. _____

  B. It is important to identify _____ to _____ possible vendors to research for comparison.

4. Warranties

  A. A warranty provides for replacement of _____ _____ at no charge within a certain period of _____.

  B. Many warranties cover only certain kinds of _____ or part _____.

  C. Heavily used equipment might be covered by a(n) _____ _____ for preventive maintenance.

5. Equipment Life and Safety

  A. Life and safety information related to equipment is available in a manufacturer's _____ _____.

  B. The manual provides _____, maintenance, and _____ directions.

  C. If a manual is lost or extra copies are needed, it may be possible to _____ it from the manufacturer's website.

6. Equipment Records

  A. List four examples of records to keep and file.

    i. _____

    ii. _____

   iii. _____

   iv. _____

  B. A comprehensive master list of all equipment owned by the office is maintained on a(n) _____ _____ _____.

  C. A maintenance log includes when regular maintenance is _____, when the maintenance _____, and who provided the service.

IV. Clinical Equipment

1. Examples of Clinical Equipment (List eight examples.)

  A. _____

  B. _____

  C. _____

  D. _____

E. _____

F. _____

G. _____

H. _____

2. _____ _____ Improvement Amendments (_____)

   regulates laboratory testing and equipment.

3. Authorized and trained staff members should perform _____ and

   _____ on clinical equipment.

V. Supplies

   1. Medical Assistant Responsibilities Related to Supplies (List four.)

      A. _____

      B. _____

      C. _____

      D. _____

   2. Business Vendors

      A. List four factors to consider when selecting a product vendor.

         i. _____

         ii. _____

         iii. _____

         iv. _____

      B. _____ _____ assist with company products and are

         often assigned to geographic regions.

      C. _____ _____ supply drug samples to the medical office

         and often schedule lunches with offices to showcase new products.

   3. HIPAA Business Associates

      A. List four examples of business associates.

         i. _____

         ii. _____

         iii. _____

         iv. _____

      B. Business vendors must appropriately safeguard personal _____

         _____ (_____).

   4. Inventory Management

      A. Inventory is best tracked using a spreadsheet or _____

         _____ software.

B. List six options for reordering supplies.

    i. _____

    ii. _____

   iii. _____

   iv. _____

    v. _____

   vi. _____

C. _____ points must be established for all inventory items.

5. Ordering Systems

  A. Compare the total cost of the delivered product, which includes the product _____, shipping and handling costs, _____ _____ costs, and sales _____.

  B. Basic math skills are used to convert all prices to the same _____ for product comparison.

  C. Discounts are often available for _____ quantities, but _____ can be problematic.

6. Placing an Order

  A. Orders may be placed using a(n) _____ or a(n) _____ order form.

  B. Accounts may be opened and _____ may be established with frequently used vendors.

  C. Office policy may require a formal _____ _____ for ordering items.

7. Receiving an Order

  A. Compare all items received against the _____ _____ that are included with shipment.

  B. Check for notations that indicate whether certain items are _____ or shipping separately.

  C. Place the newer supplies on the _____ of the shelf so that older supplies are used _____.

8. Drug Samples

  A. The _____ _____ Agency (_____) requires that a list of all drug samples be maintained.

  B. A medical office must secure and organize the samples in a(n) _____ supply cabinet or drawer.

C. Expired samples should be discarded following office policies and procedures and in accordance with _____, _____, and DEA regulations.

9. Postage

A. Postage _____ replace postage stamps, which are often cumbersome and inefficient.

B. A(n) _____ can be used to weigh items in order to determine exact postage.

C. _____ _____ involves using a computer that interfaces with the postal system to print postage.

KEY TERMINOLOGY REVIEW

Complete the following sentences using the correct key terms found at the beginning of the chapter.

1. The _____ is legislation that protects the rights of disabled individuals regarding access to employment, public buildings, transportation, housing, schools, and health care facilities.

2. Supplies that are used up quickly and have a relatively inexpensive unit cost are called _____ supplies.

3. _____ equipment refers to items whose purchase price is large (generally more than $500) and that have a relatively long life.

4. A medical facility generally has a flow that lends itself easily to teamwork, time management, organized and efficient office equipment usage, and patient flow. This is known as _____.

5. _____ refers to the positive or negative state of mind of employees with regard to their work or work environment.

APPLIED PRACTICE

Read the scenario and answer the questions that follow.

Scenario

Javier Gomez, CMA (AAMA), is working in the front office of a busy family practice. His manager, Chris, has asked him to create a detailed inventory list of all the supplies needed for his station at the patient check-out desk. Here is the list that Javier has started:

Name	Company	Amount on Hand
Pens	Office Supplies R Us	14
Message pad	Office Supplies R Us	2 tablets
Receipt booklet	Office Supplies R Us	2 booklets

1. Based on the inventory list, what additional important information should Javier include before submitting his list to Chris?

   _____

   _____

   _____

2. Considering that Javier is working at a patient check-out desk, where patients pay copayments and schedule follow-up appointments as needed, what additional items would Javier be likely to add to his inventory list? Name at least five additional items.

   _____

   _____

   _____

LEARNING ACTIVITY: MULTIPLE CHOICE

Circle the correct answer to each of the following questions.

1. ADA regulations ensure that every public facility

   a. is made easily accessible to disabled individuals.
   b. provides unrestricted hallways.
   c. has elevators or ramps available.
   d. all of the above.

2. When addressing safety issues in a medical office, concerns noted may include

   a. the use of throw rugs.
   b. the culture of the office.
   c. the tone of the office.
   d. all of the above.

3. Issues to be considered when setting up a medical office include

   a. the employees who work in the office.
   b. the office design and layout.
   c. other offices in the building.
   d. none of the above.

4. Which of the following is the first element of office flow?

   a. Restrooms
   b. Patient entrance
   c. Placement of examination rooms
   d. Staff offices

5. Which of the following is considered capital equipment?

   a. Copy machine
   b. EKG paper
   c. Medications
   d. All of the above

6. Uses and advantages of using a postal meter include which of the following?

   a. Metered mail does not have to be stamped when it arrives at the post office.
   b. A postal meter uses a scale to calculate the exact postage required for all items.

c. A postal meter allows for postage to be printed directly onto an envelope or onto an adhesive-backed strip that is placed directly on an envelope or package.

d. All of the above are correct.

7. Which of the following are examples of expendable supplies?

a. Scanners
b. Telephones
c. Clinical supplies such as syringes
d. All of the above

8. An inventory list of all sample drugs must be maintained to adhere to _____ regulations.

a. Drug Enforcement Administration (DEA)
b. Americans with Disabilities Act (ADA)
c. Food and Drug Administration (FDA)
d. None of the above

9. Which of the following guidelines should be followed with regard to drug samples?

a. They must be placed in a secure and locked location.
b. They should be organized according to category.
c. All samples should be rotated like other supplies, with newer samples placed in the back, behind samples of the same medication and strength with earlier expiration dates.
d. All of the above are correct.

10. Which of the following is true of a warranty?

a. It is a manufacturer's guarantee in writing that the product will perform correctly under normal conditions.
b. It can be purchased to cover a period of time after the original warranty has expired.
c. It states in detail what is actually covered by the contract.
d. None of the above is correct.

CRITICAL THINKING

Answer the following questions to the best of your ability. Use the textbook as a reference.

1. Corey Steinberg, CMA (AAMA), has recently been hired to work as an administrative medical assistant in a busy cardiology practice. Corey has been given the task of creating a manual that outlines the warranty information as well as the maintenance schedule for each piece of medical office equipment. How should Corey go about beginning this task?

_____

_____

_____

_____

2. Monte Beaton, RMA, is the office manager in a gastroenterology practice. Monte has recently hired three new medical assistants and wants to ensure that they are properly trained to use each piece of equipment in the medical office. How can Monte ensure that the training is done properly?

_____

_____

_____

_____

3. Joanne Felmer, CMA (AAMA), works in a walk-in clinic. At the weekly office staff meeting, the office manager mentioned the need for purchasing a new EKG machine. The office manager has asked Joanne to research the various options available. How should Joanne handle this task?

_____

_____

_____

_____

_____

RESEARCH ACTIVITY

Use Internet search engines to research the following topic and write a brief description of what you find. It is important to use reputable websites.

1. Conduct an Internet search for office and medical supply companies in your area and outside your area. Compare prices. Which companies supply products at competitive prices? What are the shipping charges? Which company seems to have the best variety of products? How could this information be useful for medical offices?

_____

_____

_____

_____

_____

CHAPTER 11
Written Communication

STUDENT STUDY GUIDE

Use the following guide to assist in your learning of the concepts from the chapter.

I. Tone of Letter Writing

1. Medical office letters should be _____, courteous, businesslike, _____ in tone, and protective of the _____ of the physician and the patient.

II. Grammar and Word Choice

1. Using _____ _____ is appropriate when writing to other medical professionals but not when writing to patients.

2. Written correspondence must reflect a(n) _____ bias toward the genders.

3. Short, _____ sentences and paragraphs are preferred in medical writing.

4. Avoid the use of the personal pronoun _____ in professional writing.

5. Redundancy is repeating the same idea in similar _____, _____, or statements.

6. The _____ voice is considered more effective because it is simpler, more _____, and less wordy.

7. _____ are words that sound alike but have different meanings.

   A. _____ _____ are not commonly recognized by spellcheck software.

8. In general, plurals of nouns are formed by adding _____ or _____.

9. The numbers _____ to _____ are spelled out in writing; other numbers are written using numerals.

10. Parts of Speech (List eight.)

   A. _____

   B. _____

   C. _____

   D. _____

   E. _____

F. _____

G. _____

H. _____

11. Generally, spell out _____ abbreviations in correspondence for clarity.

12. Because correspondence reflects on the _____ of the entire medical office, it should be error free.

13. References in Office Libraries (List five.)

A. _____

B. _____

C. _____

D. _____

E. _____

III. Formatting Correspondence

1. Standard Components of the Business Letter (List nine components.)

A. _____

B. _____

C. _____

D. _____

E. _____

F. _____

G. _____

H. _____

I. _____

2. The _____ _____ and any pages following must begin with the date and subject line of the letter.

3. Form Letters

A. A form letter contains standard content that is used _____.

B. The body of the letter is the _____ _____.

C. Areas of the letter that require personalization are called the _____.

4. Letter Styles (List four.)

A. _____

B. _____

C. _____

D. _____

5. Interoffice memorandums, also called _____, are sent to people within the office or _____.

6. Items Generally Included on Medical Reports (List eight.)

A. _____

B. _____

C. _____

D. _____

E. _____

F. _____

G. _____

H. _____

IV. Editing and Proofreading

1. Editing

A. Editing involves checking for _____ and clarity.

B. Medical reports cannot be _____ to change the meaning. Check with the _____ of a report before making content changes.

2. Proofreading

A. Proofreading is checking for errors in _____ and _____.

B. Do not accept the _____'s recommendations blindly.

C. After _____, reread the document carefully to catch content and keying errors.

V. Preparing Outgoing Mail

1. Common sizes for letterhead include standard, _____ or executive, and _____.

2. Letters should be folded so that information remains _____ and the letter is easy to open.

3. Addressing Envelopes

A. OCR equipment used by the U.S. Postal Service _____, _____, and _____ envelopes.

B. Envelopes should be addressed using _____ letters and no _____.

C. The city, two-letter state abbreviation, and zip code cannot exceed _____ characters.

4. Every piece of outgoing mail should have a(n) _____- or _____-digit zip code.

VI. Classes of Mail

1. Common Classes of Mail (List four.)

A. _____

B. _____

C. _____

D. _____

2. USPS Extra Services (List seven.)

    A. _____

    B. _____

    C. _____

    D. _____

    E. _____

    F. _____

    G. _____

3. Ancillary Services Commonly Used by a Medical Office (List four.)

    A. _____

    B. _____

    C. _____

    D. _____

VII. Size Requirements for Mail

1. The USPS standardizes _____ sizes for machine-sorted mail.

2. Guidelines for Preparing Mail to Be Metered

    A. Separate _____ mail from _____ mail.

    B. Face all letter-size envelopes in the same _____.

    C. Try not to overstuff _____-size envelopes.

    D. Seal all envelopes larger than No. _____ before sending them.

    E. Keep the top-_____ _____ of each mailing piece free of markings for the postmark.

VIII. Incoming Correspondence

1. MA's Responsibilities Related to Incoming Correspondence

    A. _____ the incoming mail.

    B. _____ each piece.

    C. _____ it to the appropriate person.

IX. Electronic Technology

1. Forms of Electronic Technology Used in a Medical Office (List four.)

    A. _____

    B. _____

    C. _____

    D. _____

KEY TERMINOLOGY REVIEW

Without using your textbook, write a sentence using each selected key term in the correct context.

1. *active voice*
   _____
   _____

2. *electronic mail*
   _____
   _____

3. *homophones*
   _____
   _____

4. *letterhead*
   _____
   _____

5. *reference initials*
   _____
   _____

APPLIED PRACTICE

Follow the directions for each assignment.

1. Proofread the following entry in a patient's medical record. Make the necessary corrections.

   Mrs. SUSAN Rowe (8-12-1877 was seen in my office today. She presents with complaints of upper right quadrant pain times too weeks. Mrs. Rowe states that along with the pain, she is experiencing nausea and vomiting. Upon palpation the abdomin appears bloated and is sensitive to the touch.

2. Using word processing software, create an interoffice memo. Andrew Edwards, CMA (AAMA), is the sender of the memo, and all clinical staff members are intended to be the recipients. The purpose of the memo is to inform the clinical staff that a pharmaceutical sales representative will be presenting information on a new cardiac drug that Dr. Sheila Tyrone is considering using for patient therapy. The presentation will occur on Friday during the lunch hour.

LEARNING ACTIVITY: MULTIPLE CHOICE

Circle the correct answer to each of the following questions.

1. Which of the following is the size of a standard business envelope?
   a. 3½" × 8½"
   b. 4⅛" × 9½"
   c. 4¼" × 9¼"
   d. None of the above

2. How much postage is required to mail an interoffice memo?
   a. $0.49
   b. $0.35
   c. $0.55
   d. None of the above

3. In order to catch all the errors in a written document, how many times should a medical assistant read a letter before sending it out?
   a. Once
   b. Twice
   c. Three times
   d. Four times

4. The _____ of a professional letter typically appears two lines below the inside address.
   a. closing
   b. subject line
   c. salutation
   d. letterhead

5. Which of the following pieces of information is typically included in the office letterhead?
   a. Office name
   b. Office address
   c. Office e-mail address
   d. All of the above

6. Which of the following statements is written correctly?
   a. Patients use their canes to assist with balance.
   b. Patients use there canes to assist with balance.
   c. Patients use they're canes to assist with balance.
   d. None of the above are correct.

7. Which of the following words is misspelled?
   a. aerosol
   b. palliative
   c. pyrexia
   d. occlushion

8. The closing appears _____ lines below the end of the body of the letter.
   a. one
   b. two
   c. three
   d. four

9. Which of the following parts of speech modifies a noun or a pronoun?

   a. Verb
   b. Adverb
   c. Adjective
   d. Preposition

10. Which of the following styles of letters is spaced with all lines flush with the left margin except for the first line of each paragraph?

    a. Modified block
    b. Simplified letter block
    c. Semi-simplified letter block
    d. None of the above

CRITICAL THINKING

Answer the following questions to the best of your ability. Use the textbook as a reference.

1. Henry Connelly, CMA (AAMA), has just been hired to work at the front desk in a family practice. Part of his job is to open and sort the mail. No written office policy about this task is currently on file in the office, so Henry decides to create one. What might Harry's new office policy entail?

   _____

   _____

   _____

   _____

2. Dr. Stuart asked Willie Pachinko, CMA (AAMA), to contact Mr. Becker regarding the results of his lab work. Willie wasn't able to reach Mr. Becker by telephone, and instead of leaving a voice mail message asking the patient to return his call, Willie e-mailed the patient his lab results. Later that day, Mr. Becker called the office very upset and told Willie that his boss intercepted the e-mail and now knows that he was screened for a possible sexually transmitted disease. What did Willie do wrong?

   _____

   _____

   _____

   _____

3. Mallory Valdez is taking an administrative medical assisting class. She has been given the assignment of writing a short paper that outlines the various mailing services offered by the U.S. Postal Service. What should Mallory include in her paper?

   _____

   _____

   _____

   _____

   _____

RESEARCH ACTIVITY

Use Internet search engines to research the following topic and write a brief description of what you find. It is important to use reputable websites.

1. Visit www.usps.com and research information regarding certified mail, rates, and extra services available. When might some of the extra services be useful in dealing with written correspondence between a medical office and patients?

   _____

   _____

   _____

   _____

   _____

CHAPTER 12
Computers in the Medical Office

STUDENT STUDY GUIDE

Use the following guide to assist in your learning of the concepts from the chapter.

I. Use of Computers in Medicine

    1. Medical Assistant Responsibilities

        A. Making entries in electronic _____ _____

        B. Electronic _____

        C. Billing and _____ processing

        D. _____ scheduling

        E. _____ data tracking

II. Types of Computers

    1. List six types of computers used in a medical office. (Refer to Table 12-1 in your textbook.)

        A. _____

        B. _____

        C. _____

        D. _____

        E. _____

        F. _____

III. Computer Hardware

    1. Required Hardware

        A. The central processing unit (CPU) is the _____ of the computer.

        B. Memory provides the capacity to store _____.

        C. Storage devices permanently retain large amounts of _____ when the computer is _____ _____.

        D. Input devices feed data and _____ into a computer.

        E. Output devices allow users to see what the _____ has accomplished.

    2. Central Processing Unit

        A. The amount of time it takes for electrical signals to come and go is measured in _____.

        B. The heart of the CPU is the _____.

3. Memory
   A. A computer's memory is measured and stored in _____,
      _____, or _____.
   B. There are two types of memory: _____ memory and
      _____ memory.
4. Storage Devices
   A. Common types of storage devices include _____ disks, CDs and DVDs, and
      _____ drives.
   B. Devices that contain _____ _____ _____
      must be safeguarded and transported in a secure manner.
5. Input Devices (List seven common types.)
   A. _____
   B. _____
   C. _____
   D. _____
   E. _____
   F. _____
   G. _____
6. Output Devices (List three common types.)
   A. _____
   B. _____
   C. _____
7. Installing Computer Hardware
   A. A(n) _____ _____ installs hardware in order to control the
      operation of the hardware component.
IV. Computer Software
   1. Operating System
      A. The operating system allows the computer to _____.
      B. It manages computer _____ resources.
      C. It enables _____ software to function.
   2. General-Purpose Applications (List five types.)
      A. _____
      B. _____
      C. _____
      D. _____
      E. _____

3. Specialized Medical Office Applications
   A. Practice _____ software is a comprehensive software program that manages many of the _____ and _____ functions of a medical practice.
   B. A(n) _____ _____ record is a computerized version of a patient's medical history.
   C. Typical accounting software functions include _____ ledger, accounts _____, accounts receivable, _____, and budgeting.
4. Installing Computer Software
   A. Installation steps vary for each software program, so reading _____ and following onscreen _____ is very important.
5. Troubleshooting Computer Problems
   A. Close all open _____ and windows.
   B. Check for obvious _____ issues.
   C. _____ the application.
   D. Press the _____ key to access the Help window.
   E. Write down any _____ messages.
   F. _____ the computer.
   G. Reopen the _____ in which the issue occurred.
   H. Shut _____ the computer and turn off the _____.
   I. Restart the computer and _____ the application.
   J. Conduct a(n) _____ search for solutions to the problem.
   K. Check the _____ website to ensure that the most recent _____ of the software is installed.
   L. If the problem persists, contact your system administrator or _____.

V. Computer System Security
   1. HIPAA Security Rule
      A. Required safeguards for covered entities are _____, _____, and _____.
   2. Security Practices
      A. Passwords protect against _____ accessing the medical office software and limit access to _____ _____.
      B. Access logs are required as part of the _____ Act and keep track of the date and _____ of access, the _____ accessing the record, the information accessed, and any _____ performed by the user.

C. Data _____ involves copying all files from the computer to a(n) _____ medium.

D. System maintenance includes _____ protection, firewalls, and file _____.

VI. Electronic Communication

1. The Internet

A. The World Wide Web

i. Many medical offices have _____ that provide information about the practice and various types of patient interaction.

ii. The Web is a convenient and user-friendly _____ for patients to research _____.

B. Social Media (List five common social media sites.)

i. _____

ii. _____

iii. _____

iv. _____

v. _____

C. Several medical associations have published _____ for maintaining a medical office's social media presence.

D. Cloud computing provides constant availability of _____ and applications, wherever _____ access is available.

E. Medical assistants may need to use the Internet to access information related to _____ _____.

2. E-mail sent on behalf of a(n) _____ _____ should follow business standards for use of proper English, _____, spelling, and _____.

3. EHR uses _____ _____ to identify who entered each piece of information into the patient's chart.

VII. Selecting a Computer System

1. The first phase of selecting a computer is to determine what _____ will be used.

2. After application selections and determining how the computer will be used, it is necessary to consider the _____ requirements.

3. _____ _____ requirements are an important consideration and are determined based on the type of applications used and the amount of data stored.

4. Questions to Consider When Comparing Products

    A. Do some manufacturers have a better _____ _____ than others?

    B. What happens if the computer system _____?

    C. Who _____ to have the computer system fixed?

    D. Is a(n) _____ provided?

    E. How will users be _____ and supported?

VIII. Computer Ergonomics

    1. Extended use of a computer with improper ergonomics can lead to _____ _____.

    2. Ergonomic tips to consider in order to promote safety include proper use of your _____, _____, _____, and _____.

KEY TERMINOLOGY REVIEW

Match each of the following terms with the correct definition.

    a. central processing unit (CPU)

    b. Internet service provider (ISP)

    c. output devices

    d. universal serial bus (USB) drive

    e. input devices

1. _____ Provides access to the Internet.

2. _____ Allow the user to see what the computer has accomplished.

3. _____ Acts as a traffic controller, directing the computer's activities and sending electronic signals to the right place at the right time.

4. _____ Feed data and instructions into a computer.

5. _____ A small portable storage device that can hold up to 64 GB or more of data.

APPLIED PRACTICE

Read the scenario and answer the questions that follow.

Scenario

Shane Eiler, RMA, is an office manager for Inner Harbor Sports Medicine. His office computer has recently sustained an attack from a malware program, and the attack has left his computer unusable.

1. Shane has been asked to research the cost of purchasing a new computer for the medical office. What are some considerations Shane should take into account as he thinks about the computer purchase?

   _____

   _____

   _____

   _____

   _____

2. The physicians have asked Shane to create a list of suggestions for securing the office computers against unauthorized access. What suggestions should Shane make?

   _____

   _____

   _____

   _____

   _____

   _____

LEARNING ACTIVITY: MULTIPLE CHOICE

Circle the correct answer to each of the following questions.

1. A(n) _____ creates a digital image of printed paper records and converts them into a format the computer can read, using optical character recognition.

   a. thumb drive
   b. personal digital assistant
   c. printer
   d. page scanner

2. The _____ is the computer equipment.

   a. hardware
   b. software
   c. peripheral
   d. USB

3. The computer's CPU is considered to be the computer's

   a. brain.
   b. memory.
   c. keyboard.
   d. mouse.

4. _____ makes it possible for a computer to temporarily store data and programs.

   a. A mass storage device
   b. Memory
   c. Software
   d. The CPU

5. _____ save time, improve the accuracy of information, and save paper.

   a. USB devices
   b. Touch screens
   c. Card scanners
   d. Digital cameras

CRITICAL THINKING

Answer the following questions to the best of your ability. Use the textbook and other resources such as the Internet in considering the following questions.

1. Marcia Dukat is taking a computer applications class in a medical assisting program. She has been given an assignment to create a list of steps that medical office staff can take to protect the office computers from viruses. What should Marcia's list include?

   _____

   _____

   _____

   _____

2. Rolf Schneider, RMA, is discussing the need for a new computer system with the physician. Dr. Nyrse has asked Rolf to describe the difference between the hardware, the software, and the peripherals that go with various computer systems. How might Rolf define these three components?

   _____

   _____

   _____

   _____

3. Riley Gaddum is taking a computer class as part of his medical assistant training. He has been given an assignment to describe the difference between ROM and RAM. What might Riley write for this assignment?

   _____

   _____

   _____

   _____

   _____

RESEARCH ACTIVITY

Use Internet search engines to research the following topic and write a brief description of what you find. It is important to use reputable websites.

1. Use the Internet to research practice management software programs. What software program do you like the most? What features does it have that appeal to you? Why would you recommend its use?

   _____

   _____

   _____

   _____

CHAPTER 13
The Medical Record

STUDENT STUDY GUIDE

Use the following guide to assist in your learning of the concepts from the chapter.

I. Introduction

   1. EMR stands for electronic _____ _____.

   2. EHR stands for electronic _____ _____.

   3. EMR refers to a digital version of a patient chart kept in a(n) _____ _____'s office.

   4. An EHR shares information across all _____ and _____ involved in a patient's medical care.

II. Purpose and History of Electronic Health Records

   1. EHRs allow access to patient information by multiple physicians and hospitals through the use of _____ _____ and _____.

   2. Appropriate Use of Terminology

     A. _____ was chosen as the preferred and exclusive term to describe all types of computerized medical records.

     B. The _____ Act, which provides incentive payments for implementing EHRs, uses the term electronic health record.

   3. Personal Health Records (PHRs)

     A. A PHR is maintained by a(n) _____ _____, whereas an EHR is maintained by health care providers.

     B. A tethered PHR is a function of _____-based EHRs that allows patients to access their EHRs _____.

   4. History and Legislation

     A. Presidents _____ _____, _____ _____, and _____ _____ helped advance EHRs through their administrations.

B. The HITECH Act provides _____ incentives for providers who adopt EHRs and demonstrate related improvements in _____, safety, and _____ of care.

    i. Eligible _____ providers can receive as much as $44,000 over a(n) _____-year period.

    ii. Eligible _____ providers can receive as much as $63,750 over _____ years.

C. To receive incentive payments, providers must meet _____ _____ criteria for how EHRs are used.

D. Certified EHR technology

    i. Includes patient _____ and clinical _____ information.

    ii. Provides _____ decision support.

    iii. Supports physician _____ _____.

    iv. Captures and queries information relevant to health care _____.

    v. _____ electronic health information and _____ information with other sources.

E. The _____ _____ Office estimates that billions of dollars will be saved by using comprehensive electronic health records.

5. Differences Between Electronic and Paper-Based Records

A. Differences between the two record systems include _____ formats, medical record _____, and _____ and storage requirements.

B. _____ paper-based medical records is eliminated when using an EHR because a queue provides an automatic list of patient reports that are automatically filed to patient records after review by physicians.

6. Difference Between EHR and Practice Management Software

A. An EHR system manages medical records of _____ _____.

B. PMS manages _____ and _____ functions of a medical practice.

III. Benefits of EHR Systems

  1. Benefits of EHRs

    A. Reviewing _____ _____ by other providers to avoid
duplication or medication interactions

    B. Accessing a patient's medical history to more quickly identify a(n) _____
or risk _____

    C. Viewing _____ _____ electronically to better
understand the progression of a patient's condition

  2. Improved Diagnostics and Patient Outcomes

    A. Improved _____

    B. Improved care _____

    C. Avoidance of _____ errors

  3. Improved Patient Participation

    A. Online _____ access

    B. Health _____

  4. Improved Efficiency and Cost Savings

    A. Multi-user _____

    B. _____ signatures

    C. Staff _____

IV. Ownership of the Medical Record

  1. The Medical Record as a Legal Document

    A. A common saying in health care is "If it wasn't _____, it wasn't
_____."

    B. Documentation should be _____.

    C. Entries in paper records

      i. Write them in _____ ink.

      ii. Handwriting should be _____ and easy to read.

      iii. _____ and date all entries.

  2. Ownership of the Medical Record

    A. Patients own the _____ in their medical records.

    B. The facility that _____ the information owns the _____
or _____ record.

    C. A(n) _____ _____ should always be present when a
patient reviews his record.

3. Ownership of Radiology Images
    A. The original image is almost always the property of the medical facility
       _____ the X-ray.
    B. Many physician offices are _____ _____ to large
       radiology centers or hospitals.
    C. Patients are often provided with a(n) _____ or _____ containing the
       image.
4. HIPAA and Confidentiality of Medical Records
    A. The Office for _____ _____ is responsible for
       implementing and enforcing the privacy regulation.
    B. Privacy and security rules for covered entities
        i. Provide reasonable and appropriate _____ to protect the
           _____ and confidentiality of health care information.
        ii. Train _____ to protect confidentiality of health care information.
        iii. Provide _____ and _____ on security and
           confidentiality protective measures within the medical office.
5. Transporting Medical Records
    A. Medical records should never be _____ from a medical office.
    B. Clearances must be obtained from a(n) _____ or _____
       to physically transport medical records.
    C. Medical records must be transported in a locked _____ or box with no
       _____ visible from the outside.
    D. Medical records that are lost outside the office must be reported as a(n)
       _____ breach.
6. Releasing Medical Records
    A. Signing the _____ of _____ _____
       gives permission for a patient's PHI to be released for treatment, payment, and operations,
       as defined by HIPAA.
    B. Patients must explicitly _____ _____ of their records in
       writing for all other purposes.
    C. List those who, in addition to the patient, are able to sign for an authorization release of
       medical records.
        i. _____
        ii. _____
        iii. _____

D. List specially protected health information.

    i. _____ _____ treatment records

    ii. _____ notes

    iii. _____ and AIDS information

    iv. _____ health records

E. Sometimes medical records can be released _____ the patient's

_____; however, strict _____ apply to those who receive

the information.

7. The Role of the Medical Assistant Regarding Medical Records

A. MAs should adhere to four standards in regard to the use of medical records:

_____, _____, _____, and

_____.

8. Making Corrections in the Medical Record

A. Correcting electronic records

    i. The user marks the erroneous information for _____ and enters the

correct information.

    ii. The correction may be viewed on a(n) _____

_____ or may appear with a(n) _____

_____ through the entry.

B. Correcting paper records

    i. Draw a(n) _____ _____ through an error

    ii. Enter your _____ and _____ above the single line.

    iii. Write the word "_____."

V. Privacy and Security of EHRs

1. Logins

A. A login is the combination of a(n) _____ and _____.

B. Each person has _____ login information so the software can

_____ activity within the EHR system.

C. Each station must be _____ _____ when the user is away from

the desk.

D. _____ _____ must not be viewable by other patients.

2. Laptops and Mobile Devices

    A. Special _____ measures are required when _____ is stored on portable or mobile devices.

    B. List three levels of security measures.

        i. _____

        ii. _____

        iii. _____

    C. Backing up electronic health records is usually _____ executed on a(n) _____ basis.

VI. Documentation Formats

    1. Common Documentation Formats (List four formats.)

        A. _____

        B. _____

        C. _____

        D. _____

    2. Chronological Medical Record

        A. This record follows a patient over a period of _____.

        B. Each visit has a new entry by date rather than by _____ or _____.

    3. Problem-Oriented Medical Record (List the four parts.)

        A. _____

        B. _____

        C. _____

        D. _____

    4. SOAP Charting

        A. S stands for _____.

        B. O stands for _____.

        C. A stands for _____.

        D. P stands for _____.

    5. Source-Oriented Medical Record

        A. Patient information is organized in _____.

        B. Information in each section is maintained in _____ _____ order.

        C. _____ _____ are included with each patient encounter.

VII. Components of a Medical Record

   1. List the components of a medical record.

     A. Patient _____

     B. Family and medical _____

     C. _____ examination results

     D. _____ test results

     E. Informed _____ forms

     F. Diagnosis and _____ plan

     G. Patient correspondence and _____ care

     H. Clinical _____ note

     I. _____ sheet

     J. _____ report

     K. _____ report

     L. _____ report

     M. _____ report

     N. _____ summary

     O. _____, tables, and graphs

     P. Additional _____

     Q. Medical _____

VIII. Implementing an EHR System

   1. List the steps in implementing an EHR system.

     A. _____ the practice readiness.

     B. _____ a plan.

     C. Select or _____ to a certified EHR.

     D. Conduct _____ and implement an EHR system.

     E. Achieve _____ _____.

     F. Continue _____ improvement.

IX. Filing, Storage, and Retention of Medical Records

   1. Three Categories for Patients

     A. _____ records are records of patients who have been seen within the past 3 years and are currently being treated.

     B. _____ records are records of patients who have not been seen within the past 3 years or another time period determined by office policy.

     C. _____ records are records of patients who have actively terminated their contact with the physician.

2. File Storage
   A. List three types of file storage systems.
      i. _____
      ii. _____
      iii. _____
   B. File folders and guides are designed to meet the _____
      _____ of the office.
   C. Labels are primarily used to identify the patient's _____ or
      _____ _____ number.
   D. _____ file labels are often used to aid in filing.
3. Rules for Filing
   A. List three common systems for filing.
      i. _____
      ii. _____
      iii. _____
   B. _____ is placing an informational message in the file to alert
      the health worker that a file can be found under another name.
   C. Locating _____ _____ is time-consuming and
      frustrating, and it requires a thorough search of the office.
4. Tickler Files
   A. These files are used to remind medical assistants of a(n) _____ or a(n)
      _____ that will take place at a(n) _____ date.
   B. Tickler files should be reviewed _____.
5. Collating Paper Records
   A. This process involves _____ and organizing information.
   B. All _____ should be collected on patients before they are seen by
      physicians for scheduled appointments.
   C. Follow-up is required for information that has not been _____.
   D. Reports should be organized, _____, and _____ as they
      come in.
6. Long-Term Storage
   A. All files must be kept safe from _____, flood, or other
      _____.

B. List three storage media options, other than hard copy.

    i. _____

    ii. _____

    iii. _____

7. Retention of Electronic Records

    A. EHRs are more _____ and less _____ to store than paper records.

    B. A large amount of data can be stored on the main _____ system.

    C. Data can be archived so it does not take up unnecessary _____ space.

    D. Most software has a built-in function that removes _____ _____ from the program and saves them in a(n) _____ format.

X. Office Flow with Electronic and Paper Medical Records

1. Point of Care Documentation

    A. Physicians can enter information into a computer while the _____ is _____ rather than try to remember and document the visit later.

    B. Many medical practices have computer terminals in each _____ _____.

    C. Sometimes it is possible to automatically enter _____ _____ and diagnostic test results from the equipment directly into the EHR.

2. Computerized Physician Order Entry

    A. Providers are able to order tests, _____, lab work, and _____ using the computer.

    B. Orders are generated and sent electronically and also saved in the _____'s _____.

    C. Only _____ health care professionals, including credentialed _____ _____, are allowed to enter orders into the CPOE system for it to count toward _____ use.

KEY TERMINOLOGY REVIEW

Match each of the following terms with the correct definition.

a. active records
b. inactive records
c. medical record

d. POMR
e. SOAP

1. _____ The source of all documentation related to the patient.

2. _____ A charting method used to identify patient problems and chart based on those problems.

3. _____ Patients who have been seen within the past 3 years and are currently being treated.

4. _____ A charting method that is distinct because of its four-part approach.

5. _____ Patients who have not been seen within the past 3 years or another period determined by office policy.

APPLIED PRACTICE

Follow the instructions for each question.

1. Indicate whether the following would be considered active, inactive, or closed patient files.

   a. Lori Hughes, a patient who has moved out of the state

      Patient file status: _____

   b. Quin Tao, a patient who has not been seen in the office for 5 years

      Patient file status: _____

   c. Gloria Sanchez, a patient who was in the office for care last week

      Patient file status: _____

   d. Sara Womack, a patient who died last year

      Patient file status: _____

2. Accurately place the statements below into SOAP format on the accompanying Progress Note form. Mario Reynolds, born August 12, 1990, presents to the office with the following:

   - T: 100.3°
   - Positive Rapid Strep Test
   - "My throat is sore."
   - Pharyngitis and Strep Throat
   - Throat appears red, and white spots present on tonsils.
   - Penicillin V 250mg BID × 10 days
   - BP: 118/86
   - Wt: 192#
   - Patient has been sick with a fever for 3 days.

PROGRESS NOTE

Patient: _____ DOB: _____

	S	O	A	P

LEARNING ACTIVITY: MULTIPLE CHOICE

Circle the correct answer to each of the following questions.

1. Under which of the following circumstances can the patient's medical record be copied and released?
   a. When the patient's spouse comes to the office to request a copy
   b. When the patient's employer calls the office to request a copy
   c. When the patient has signed a release form
   d. When the patient's brother sends a signed letter, asking for a copy

2. Filing medical folders according to the last two digits of the patients medical ID is termed
   a. straight numeric filing.
   b. terminal-digit filing.
   c. middle-digit filing.
   d. subject matter filing.

3. With _____, a physician can order prescriptions and lab work directly from a computer rather than writing the orders.
   a. meaningful use
   b. collated practice order entry
   c. HITECH measures
   d. computerized physician order entry (CPOE)

4. The simplest numerical method of filing is
   a. straight numerical filing.
   b. terminal-digit filing.
   c. middle-digit filing.
   d. unit-number filing.

5. The cheapest and most convenient form of long-term medical record storage is
   a. electronic health records.
   b. microfiche.
   c. microfilm.
   d. off-site storage of hard copies.

CRITICAL THINKING

Answer the following questions to the best of your ability. Use the textbook and other resources such as the Internet in considering the following questions.

1. Chris Nichols, CMA (AAMA), answers a telephone call from Marguerite Kessler, inquiring about lab work results for her 21-year-old son, Edward. When Chris reviews Edward's medical record, he sees that Edward has not given permission for anyone to receive his medical information. Considering HIPAA rules, how should Chris proceed?

   _____

   _____

   _____

   _____

2. Sara Hernandez, RMA, is escorting a patient to an examination room from the reception area. As she and the patient are walking by the counter in the clinical area, she notices that her coworker, Sasha, has left her laptop unattended and open, with a patient's electronic health record visible on the screen. What might Sara say to Sasha about this situation and the importance of protecting the integrity of medical records?

   _____

   _____

   _____

   _____

3. The physicians of Pearson Medical Associates have asked their office manager, Leslie, to ensure that their electronic health record software is compliant with the HITECH Act in regard to certified EHR technology. Why is it important for Leslie to research this, and how would she determine if the software the office uses is compliant?

   _____

   _____

   _____

   _____

RESEARCH ACTIVITY

Use Internet search engines to research the following topic and write a brief description of what you find. It is important to use reputable websites.

1. Research the types of filing systems that may be found in a medical setting. Describe the advantages and disadvantages of each system.

   _____

   _____

   _____

   _____

   _____

CHAPTER 14
Medical Insurance

STUDENT STUDY GUIDE

I. Health Insurance Policies

1. The History and Purpose of Health Insurance

    A. In the United States health insurance began in the mid-_____ as _____ income insurance.

    B. Hospital insurance began in _____.

    C. Medicare and Medicaid were enacted in _____.

    D. Health care costs rapidly increased in the _____ and _____.

    E. During the _____, most Americans with health insurance were enrolled in managed _____ plans.

    F. In _____, the health insurance exchange debuted as a part of the Patient _____and Affordable _____Act.

        i. The individual mandate requires those without health insurance to pay a(n)_____ penalty.

2. The Role of the Medical Assistant in Health Insurance Claims

    A. List MA duties related to health insurance.

        i. Gather _____information.

        ii. _____ patient questions related to health insurance.

        iii. _____patient insurance coverage.

        iv. _____ insurance coverage.

        v. Prepare health insurance _____.

        vi. _____ on past-due claims.

        vii. Pursue _____amounts.

3. Policy Provisions and Terminology

    A. The person who owns an insurance policy is called the _____, subscriber, insured, or _____.

    B. Those covered by government insurance programs are known as _____.

    C. Dependents are _____ _____also covered on commercial insurance plans.

D. A monthly payment made to the insurance carrier for coverage is called a(n)_____.

E. A list of charges for services offered by health care providers is called a(n)_____ _____, and the amount considered to be an appropriate fee is the _____ amount.

F. List three common types of out-of-pocket expenses.

    i. _____

    ii. _____

    iii. _____

G. As a result of PPACA, all group insurance policies must offer coverage to everyone, regardless of preexisting _____.

H. As a result of HIPAA, no _____ _____exists for a preexisting condition if the patient was continuously covered by health insurance for the past _____ months.

I. According to GINA, it is illegal for health plans to deny individuals health care coverage because they may have a(n) _____ _____to developing a disease in the future.

J. _____ _____is one of several criteria payers use to determine if and how much they will pay for a particular service.

4. Types of Insurance Plans

A. _____, or fee-for services, plans

B. _____ care plans, including health _____ organizations, _____ provider organizations, and point of _____ plans

5. Types of Service Coverage

A. Insurance policies include the benefits that are most _____and most _____ for each group or individual.

B. The _____ is a list of drugs approved for coverage by an insurance plan.

II. Health Insurance Payers

1. Private Health Insurance

A. Commercial health insurance is coverage for health care services offered by private _____.

B. Laws that govern private health insurance are established by _____ legislature and implemented by the state Department of _____.

C. Group insurance

    i. Group insurance is usually the _____ expensive type of private health insurance.

    ii. Commonly those who have group insurance are employees and _____ members.

    iii. If a patient has recently changed jobs, it is important to determine when _____ begins.

D. Blue Cross/Blue Shield plans

    i. Blue Cross/Blue Shield offers both group and _____ insurance plans.

    ii. Each BCBS plan is separate and unique regarding _____, cost sharing, and other requirements.

    iii. Member ID numbers begin with three _____ that are a code indicating the member's home plan.

E. A(n)_____plan sets aside money in a reserve fund and pays for employees' medical expenses from the fund.

F. The federal Consolidated _____ _____ _____Act requires employers to extend health insurance coverage at group rates to any employees who are no longer employed due to certain circumstances.

G. _____health insurance policies are usually the most expensive.

H. The purpose of the _____ _____ _____ is to create an organized and competitive market for buying health insurance.

I. Complaints regarding health insurance issues can be filed with the state's _____ _____.

2. Government Insurance

A. List the groups of people eligible for government health insurance.

    i. _____

    ii. _____

    iii. _____

    iv. _____

B. Medicare

    i. Medicare insures people aged _____ and older, patients who have been disabled for more than _____ month(s), and patients with end-stage _____ _____.

    ii. Medicare is _____ by the Centers for Medicare & Medicaid Services.

  iii. Claims must be submitted within _____ days, with some exceptions.

  iv. Participating providers are required to become _____ in order to participate in the health insurance programs.

  v. Medicare Part A covers _____ services, and there is _____ premium.

  vi. Medicare Part B covers _____ care, therapy, and _____testing, and members must pay _____-based premiums because Part B is a voluntary program.

  vii. If a service may be denied by Medicare, members must sign _____ _____ _____, informing them that they may be obligated to pay.

  viii. Medicare Part C is known as the _____ _____ and is often sold by private insurance companies offering all parts of Medicare coverage.

  ix. Medicare Part D covers _____ _____through private companies contracted with Medicare.

  x. _____ plans supplement Medicare coverage to fill the gaps in Part A and Part B coverage.

  xi. _____ _____Payer rules determine whether Medicare is the primary or secondary payer when a patient has both Medicare and other health insurance.

  xii. One physician filling in for another is called _____ _____, and when it occurs, specific criteria must be met in order to bill for Medicare services.

C. Medicaid

  i. Medicaid covers _____-_____ patients.

  ii. _____ determine Medicaid eligibility and coverage rules.

  iii. Medicaid coverage must be verified every _____ a patient is seen.

  iv. Low-income elderly and disabled individuals may have both Medicaid and _____.

D. TRICARE

  i. TRICARE was formerly known as _____.

  ii. TRICARE provides health insurance benefits for _____ _____and _____ military personnel.

  iii. Three plans are offered: TRICARE _____, TRICARE _____, and TRICARE _____.

E. CHAMPVA

    i. CHAMPVA covers health care expenses for families of _____ with total, permanent, service-related covered disabilities; it also covers the _____ and dependent _____ of veterans who _____ in the line of duty.

    ii. Patients may use any civilian health care provider, without _____.

F. Third-party liability insurance

    i. _____ _____ insurance covers workers who have been injured in the workplace or as a result of a workplace-related _____.

    ii. There are three types of claims with workers' compensation insurance: _____ claims, _____ disability claims, and _____ disability claims.

    iii. Property and casualty provides insurance on homes, _____, and _____.

    iv. Property insurance is regulated by each state's_____ of _____.

    v. Disability income insurance reimburses a patient for lost wages because of a(n)_____-_____-_____ disability that prevents the individual from _____.

    vi. Disability income insurance is either _____ term or _____ term.

    vii. The Family _____ _____Act allows employees to take unpaid leave for specified family and medical reasons, while protecting their jobs.

G. Working with fee schedules

    i. Physician fee schedules are often established based on _____-based fee schedules and _____-based fee structures.

    ii. Medicare uses the _____-_____ _____ _____scale to determine Medicare's fee schedule, which is based on three components: _____ _____ value unit, geographic _____ _____, and _____ _____ conversion factor.

iii. Insurance companies establish their own _____ and don't have to pay what physicians _____.

    a. _____-based reimbursement is determined based on the usual, customary, and _____ fee.

    b. _____-based reimbursement has three forms: _____, per diem, and per _____.

III. Health Insurance Claims

1. Gathering Patient Information

    A. The first step in proper claims processing is obtaining accurate patient information or _____.

    B. New patients should complete a(n) _____ form that should be reviewed at each _____ and updated _____.

    C. Both sides of the patient's _____ _____ card should be photocopied.

2. Verification of Benefits

    A. The following information should be confirmed during a verification of benefits.

        i. What is the _____ _____ of the policy?

        ii. Who is the _____?

        iii. Is the type of _____ the patient is seeking covered?

        iv. What are the _____, copayment, and/or _____ amounts for this service?

        v. Is a referral or _____ required for this service?

        vi. Where should a(n)_____ claim be submitted? For electronic claims, what is the payer _____?

        vii. What are the _____ _____ and phone number of the person who verified the benefits?

3. Determining Coordination of Benefits

    A. When a patient has two insurance plans, it is necessary to determine the _____ of benefits.

    B. The policy billed first is considered _____.

    C. The policy billed second is considered _____.

    D. The birthday _____ is based on the month and _____ of the parent's birthday.

4. Obtaining Authorizations and Referrals

   A. Approvals that insurance companies often require before services and procedures are performed are _____ and _____.

   B. Preauthorization may also be called _____.

   C. _____ processes are required by law for the patient's use if a preauthorization is _____.

   D. In managed care, insurance carriers may _____ claims that were not properly authorized, and physicians are not able to bill the _____ for these services.

5. Documenting Insurance Company Calls

   A. Coverage information may be obtained _____, but a phone call is often required to clarify patient benefit information.

   B. List the information to document.

      i. _____

      ii. _____

      iii. _____

      iv. _____

      v. _____

6. Preparing Health Insurance Claims

   A. The _____ _____ _____ is a unique, _____-digit number assigned to health care providers by CMS.

   B. Most physicians submit _____ claims, but some may still use _____ claims.

   C. Paper claims are submitted using the _____ form.

      i. The form is divided into two sections: the _____ and _____ information and the _____ or _____ information.

      ii. Most information obtained to complete the CMS-1500 form is gathered from the patient _____ form, _____ card, _____ form, and medical _____.

      iii. Accuracy in identifying and _____ the data is essential.

7. Secondary Policies

   A. A secondary policy can be billed _____ the primary policy has _____.

   B. In addition to the CMS-1500 form, the _____ from the primary payer is also sent when billing secondary insurance.

8. Electronic Transactions

   A. Electronic transactions are also called electronic _____

   _____.

   B. The _____ is the standard format for electronic claims.

   C. In addition to claims submission, electronic transactions can be used for the following.

      i. Tracking claim _____

      ii. _____ RAs

      iii. _____ of benefits

      iv. _____ inquiries

      v. _____

      vi. Authorization_____

   D. List three ways electronic claims can be submitted.

      i. _____

      ii. _____

      iii. _____

9. Paper Claims

   A. Optical _____ _____ scanners read printed or typed

   text and convert it to data that a computer can process.

   B. The CMS-1500 form is printed in a specific color of _____ ink so that it

   is recognizable by OCR scanners.

10. Filing Timelines

   A. Insurance companies may accept claims for as long as up to _____

   _____ from the date of service or for as little as _____ days.

   B. It is best to submit a claim _____ _____ service is

   rendered to avoid rejection.

11. Supporting Documentation

   A. Supporting documentation is often required for _____-cost services.

   B. Determining whether supporting documentation is necessary with claims submission should

   be done when contacting customer service to obtain _____.

   C. Sending proper documentation with the_____ billing helps avoid

   _____ payment.

12. UB-04 Claim Form

   A. The UB-04 is used by _____ _____.

   B. The electronic format of inpatient services is the _____.

   C. The form contains _____ form locators that must be completed.

KEY TERMINOLOGY REVIEW

Match each of the following terms with the correct definition.

a. claim
b. deductible
c. formulary

d. premium
e. referral

1. _____ The portion the patient must pay before the insurance company will pay any benefits.
2. _____ An approved list of medications specific to each insurance carrier.
3. _____ Used to send a patient for treatment to another facility or physician.
4. _____ A fixed monthly fee or semimonthly fee for health insurance coverage.
5. _____ A written and documented request for reimbursement.

APPLIED PRACTICE

Select and complete Activity 1 if you currently have health insurance. Select and complete Activity 2 if you currently do not have health insurance. Answer the questions that accompany your activity.

1. If you have health insurance, do you know everything about your plan? Conduct research either through the Internet or by calling your insurance company to find out the following information:

   a. What are your deductible, coinsurance, or copayment amounts?

   _____
   _____
   _____
   _____
   _____

   b. Are there conditions that are not covered (sometimes called exclusions), and is it possible to receive coverage of these for an additional fee?

   _____
   _____
   _____
   _____

   c. When is preauthorization required, and who typically should perform this activity?

   _____
   _____
   _____
   _____
   _____

2. If you do not have health insurance, begin to research the types of health insurance plans that may be affordable for you in your area.

    a. Does your school offer health insurance for students? If so, what is the cost, and what type of coverage is offered?

_____

_____

_____

    b. List two other types of insurance plans you found in your area that may be affordable for you. If your school offers health insurance, what is the difference between these two other plans and the plan offered by the school?

_____

_____

_____

_____

    c. When is preauthorization required for the plans you researched, and who typically should perform this activity?

_____

_____

_____

_____

_____

CRITICAL THINKING

Answer the following questions to the best of your ability. Use the textbook and other resources such as the Internet in considering the following questions.

1. Monica Swinger is taking an administrative medical assisting course. She has been given the assignment of writing an essay describing how health insurance began in the United States. What information should Monica include?

_____

_____

_____

_____

2. Erica Owsley, CMA (AAMA), has just received a denial from Global Health Insurance regarding a preauthorization request for an MRI for patient, Kelley Fennel. Notation in the preauthorization denial indicated that medical necessity was not met due to a lack of documentation. Erica informs the ordering physician, Dr. Westing, by saying "*That MRI you ordered for Kelley Fennel wasn't authorized. You barely had any documentation and it was a long-shot at best. It was a waste of time to even attempt to get it approved with the notes we had to work with. Now we have to start all*

over again." Obviously, Erica needs to work on her communication skills with Dr. Westing. How might Erica better convey her message to Dr. Westing with more tactful communication?

_____

_____

_____

_____

3. Jameria Jackson, RMA, works in the medical billing department of Pearson Family Medicine. Henry O'Leary has called to talk with Jameria because he is confused about a bill he received from the office. It is the beginning of the year, and Mr. O'Leary has a $200 deductible that must be met before his insurance company will pay anything on his behalf. He doesn't understand why he must pay $89.15 for his office visit when he usually only has a $25 copayment for visits. What should Jameria say to Mr. O'Leary to help him understand the difference between his deductible and copayments on his insurance plan?

_____

_____

_____

_____

_____

RESEARCH ACTIVITY

Use Internet search engines to research the following topic and write a brief description of what you find. It is important to use reputable websites.

1. Using the Internet, find your state's Medicaid website and research the criteria for being covered under Medicaid in your state. What are the requirements to receive health care coverage?

_____

_____

_____

_____

_____

CHAPTER 15
Diagnosis Coding

STUDENT STUDY GUIDE

Use the following guide to assist in your learning of the concepts from the chapter.

I. Introduction to Medical Coding

1. _____ codes identify the reasons that health care services were provided.

2. _____ codes describe services performed for patients.

3. _____ are responsible for coding and billing for all the services they personally provide.

4. The Medical Assistant's Role in Coding

A. Most offices hire or contract with _____ _____

_____ who are trained in the details of assigning medical codes.

B. The MA's role regarding coding involves the following.

   i. Assisting in _____ between coders and _____ when a question arises

   ii. Providing appropriate _____ codes when an insurance preauthorization is required for a(n) _____ or when a patient is referred to another provider

   iii. Facilitating communication with _____ who may need information about medical codes related to _____ patients they represent

   iv. Answering patients' questions about the meanings of codes on their _____ _____ or other paperwork

   v. Reviewing or facilitating _____ _____ to help ensure that it provides adequate specificity (detail) for coding

5. History of Diagnosis Coding

A. The Bertillon Classification of Causes of Death was adopted in _____ by the American Public Health Association (APHA).

B. Coding was historically used to track the study of _____ and causes of death.

C. Now the highly classified coding system includes more than _____ codes.

6. Overview of ICD-10-CM

    A. The ICD-9-CM was used in the United States from 19____ to 20____.

    B. The expected benefits of using the ICD-10-CM include

       i. More accurate and detailed data about _____

        _____

       ii. Fewer _____ and _____ errors

       iii. Overall savings of _____ and _____

7. Compliance

    A. Compliance simply means _____ the _____.

    B. _____ is knowingly billing for services that were not provided or billing for a service that has a higher _____ than the service actually provided.

    C. _____ is mistakenly accepting payment for items or services that should not be paid as a result of improper _____ and _____ practices.

    D. The purpose of the Office of the Inspector General is to fight _____, fraud, and _____ in Medicare, _____, and more than _____ other HHS programs.

    E. The _____ _____ and _____ _____ Act mandates compliance programs for providers who contract with Medicare and Medicaid.

II. Organization of the ICD-10-CM Manual

  1. Introductory Material

    A. _____ are specialized rules, abbreviations, _____, and symbols that alert users to important _____.

    B. Certain conventions are universal to _____ ICD-10-CM manuals, and others are specific to _____ _____.

    C. _____ means that the condition represented by the code and the condition listed as excluded are mutually _____ and should not be coded _____.

    D. _____ means that the condition excluded is not part of the condition represented by the _____, but the patient may have both conditions at the same time, and they are not mutually _____.

    E. The _____ character of an ICD-10-CM code is reserved for special use.

    F. Placeholders are used in two ways: to reserve a position for _____ use and to fill in any _____ positions.

G. Official Guidelines for _____ and _____ are rules that provide _____ for how to code selected _____ and establish the rules for how to identify which diagnoses should be reported on a claim for any given patient.

2. Index to Diseases and Injuries
   A. Conditions, _____, and reasons for seeking medical care are listed alphabetically by _____ term and _____.
   B. List three additional references.
      i. _____
      ii. _____
      iii. _____

3. Tabular List
   A. This list is an alphanumerically sequenced list of all _____ codes, divided into _____ chapters based on cause, or _____, and body system.
   B. After locating a code in the _____, you can _____ it by referencing the tabular list.

III. How to Code Diagnoses
   1. List the three basic steps in diagnosis coding.
   A. Identify the diagnosis listed _____.
   B. Research the diagnosis in the _____.
   C. Verify the code(s) in the _____ _____.
   2. Abstract Diagnostic Information
   A. Information is abstracted from the medical record to identify the _____ necessary to code for _____ and the _____ they were provided.
   B. Look for a definitive _____ statement by the physician regarding the _____ for the visit.
   C. When a physician has not determined the root cause, an uncertain or _____ diagnosis is given.
      i. An uncertain diagnosis should not be used for _____ coding; rather, look for the patient's signs or _____ that are a part of the _____ complaint.

3. Research Codes in the Index

  A. List the three steps for using the index.

    i. _____

    ii. _____

    iii. _____

  B. List examples of main terms.

    i. A(n) _____

    ii. A(n) _____

    iii. The reason for a(n) _____

    iv. A(n) _____

    v. A(n) _____ or acronym

    vi. A nontechnical _____

    vii. A(n) _____

  C. List examples of subterms.

    i. _____

    ii. _____

    iii. _____

    iv. _____

4. Verify Codes in the Tabular List

  A. The tabular list contains 21 chapters based on _____ or the body system.

  B. Chapters are divided into sections with boldfaced or _____ headings.

  C. List the three tabulated levels within the sections.

    i. Category (_____-character entries)

    ii. _____ (four- and five-character entries)

    iii. _____ (the most specific entry that requires no additional characters)

  D. Before finalizing a code, the MA must interpret the _____ that appear with the code and its _____.

  E. ICD-10-CM codes can be between _____ and _____ characters in length.

5. Coding for Special Situations

  A. Many diagnoses require _____ coding skills to accurately capture the details of a specific patient's situation.

  B. It is important to show _____ by recognizing when additional expertise is required to assign codes.

  C. An MA who is unsure how to select a code should reach out to a supervisor or _____ _____.

KEY TERMINOLOGY REVIEW

Match each of the following terms with the correct definition.

a. ICD-10-CM
b. compliance
c. fraud

d. abuse
e. qualified diagnosis

1. _____ A resource that contains numeric and alphanumeric diagnostic codes.
2. _____ Uncertain diagnosis.
3. _____ Following the rules.
4. _____ Knowingly billing for services that were not provided.
5. _____ Mistakenly accepting payment for items or services that should not be paid as a result of improper billing and coding practices.

APPLIED PRACTICE: ICD-10-CM CODING EXERCISES

For each of the following, look up each condition in the ICD-10-CM index to diseases and then verify the code in the tabular list. Write the code on the line provided.

1. _____ Pain in the right shoulder
2. _____ Plantar wart
3. _____ Cluster headache syndrome, not intractable
4. _____ Encounter for routine child health examination, without abnormal findings
5. _____ Atypical atrial flutter
6. _____ Kidney stones (calculi)
7. _____ Addison anemia
8. _____ Open bite, right thigh, initial encounter
9. _____ Malignant neoplasm of the large intestine
10. _____ Paralytic lagophthalmos, left lower eyelid
11. _____ Diaper rash
12. _____ Celiac disease
13. _____ Congenital glaucoma
14. _____ Type 2 diabetes with diabetic nephropathy
15. _____ Chronic fatigue
16. _____ Acute bronchitis due to *Streptococcus*
17. _____ Incomplete spontaneous abortion, without complication
18. _____ Cannabis abuse with intoxication delirium
19. _____ First-degree burn, left shoulder, subsequent encounter
20. _____ Cholesteatoma of the tympanum, right ear

CRITICAL THINKING

Answer the following questions to the best of your ability. Use the textbook as a reference.

1. Teresa Clymer is taking a course in medical coding as part of her medical assistant training. She has been asked to write a paragraph describing how proper diagnostic coding is linked to proper reimbursement from insurance carriers. What information should Teresa include in her paragraph?

   _____

   _____

   _____

   _____

2. Mavis Raschenko, RMA, has received extensive training in medical coding. She works for Dr. Bajat, who specializes in podiatry. While working on claims submissions, Mavis identifies a diagnosis code that she believes to be inaccurate. How could she tactfully discuss this matter with Dr. Bajat, who originally assigned the diagnosis code?

   _____

   _____

   _____

   _____

   _____

RESEARCH ACTIVITY

Use Internet search engines to research the following topic and write a brief description of what you find. It is important to use reputable websites.

1. Go to your state's Department of Health website. Research the laws that apply to billing for medical services in your state. Create a list of the laws that are relevant to the issue of fraudulent practices in billing and coding.

   _____

   _____

   _____

   _____

CHAPTER 16
Procedural Coding

STUDENT STUDY GUIDE

Use the following guide to assist in your learning of the concepts from the chapter.

I. Overview and History of Procedure Coding

1. CPT stands for _____ _____ _____.

2. Five-character _____ codes and descriptions are used to report outpatient medical services and procedures.

3. The Role of the Medical Assistant in Procedure Coding

A. The extent to which a medical assistant is involved in procedure coding _____ from one office to another.

B. Patient care information must be properly _____ in the patient's chart.

C. MAs should understand the scope of their _____ and when it is necessary to reach out to a(n) _____ _____ for assistance.

4. The History of CPT Coding

A. The first edition of the CPT was published in _____ by the American _____ Association, and codes were _____ numbers long.

B. The second edition of the CPT, published in _____, expanded _____ procedures.

C. The fourth edition, which is used today, was published in _____.

D. HCPCS was adopted by the federal government in _____.

E. The CPT lists more than _____ procedure codes and is updated every _____.

5. Overview of CPT Coding

A. Procedure codes identify _____ services provided to _____.

B. Physicians are paid for _____ codes, and _____ codes explain the reasons services were provided.

C. On the CMS-1500 form, each _____ code must be linked to one or more _____ codes that identify _____ necessity.

D. _____ companies and other payers establish their own medical necessity guidelines.

E. Only _____ code is correct in any given situation.

6. Federal Compliance

   A. Fraudulent coding carries severe penalties, including _____ and possible _____.

   B. _____ created several programs to further control fraud and abuse in health care.

   C. _____ is billing for a higher level of service than was actually provided in order to gain higher _____.

   D. _____ is coding for a lower level of service than was actually provided.

   E. Fraud and abuse

      i. Examples of fraud

         a. Billing for services not _____

         b. Billing for services not _____

         c. Misrepresenting a diagnosis to justify _____

         d. Billing for _____ that the patient failed to keep

         e. Altering _____ to receive a higher payment amount

         f. Soliciting, offering, or receiving a(n) _____

         g. _____ (billing for separate services that are included in a single procedure code)

         h. Falsifying certificates of medical necessity, plans of _____, and medical records to justify _____

         i. _____ (billing for a service at a higher level than was actually provided)

         j. _____ (billing for a lesser service to gain partial reimbursement for a more complex procedure that is not covered)

      ii. Examples of abuse

         a. Charging excessively high fees for _____ or _____

         b. Billing for services that were provided but not _____ _____

         c. Routinely filing duplicate _____ for the same encounter

         d. Billing for _____ that were given to the patient but not medically necessary

      iii. The _____ website offers information to consumers and patients to encourage them to identify and _____ fraud.

II. Organization of the CPT Manual

   1. Introductory Matter

      A. This is found within the first several _____ of the CPT manual.

      B. Quick reference is made with lists of commonly used symbols, _____, and place-of-_____ codes.

      C. Medical abbreviations are found on the _____ of the _____ cover.

   2. Tabular List

      A. The tabular list is a(n) _____ listing of all CPT codes, divided into _____ categories.

      B. Category I codes describe widely used _____ and procedures approved by the _____ and _____ Administration.

      C. Category II codes are used to collect and track data for _____ measurement.

         i. _____ pays physicians a financial incentive for reporting Category II codes.

        ii. Category III codes are _____ codes used for collection of data and tracking the use of _____ technology, services, and procedures.

        iii. If available, a Category III code should be used in place of a Category _____ code.

   3. Appendices

      A. Appendices provide _____ information.

      B. Appendices used most often by MAs

         i. Appendix A: _____

        ii. Appendix B: Summary of _____

        iii. Appendix C: _____ Examples

   4. Index

      A. The index lists CPT codes alphabetically by _____ term and _____ terms.

      B. The coding process begins in the _____ but should be verified in the _____ _____.

III. How to Assign CPT Procedure Codes

   1. Tools for CPT Coding

      A. _____ coding manual

      B. _____ manual

      C. Medical _____

      D. Completed documentation in the _____ _____

2. Step 1. Abstract Procedures from the Patient's Medical Record

    A. Coding must be performed to the highest level of _____.

    B. Documents often needed for outpatient coding

        i. The _____ form

        ii. _____ notes

        iii. In-house lab and _____ reports

        iv. Operative reports or outpatient _____

    C. Documents used for inpatient coding

        i. Daily _____ sheet

        ii. Daily _____ notes

        iii. Operative reports for _____ procedures

    D. Three primary steps for abstracting procedures

        i. Identify the _____ service or procedure.

        ii. Identify _____ services or procedures.

        iii. Identify the _____ of each procedure.

3. Step 2. Look Up the Procedures in the Index

    A. Three steps in using the index

        i. Identify the _____ _____.

        ii. Review the _____ terms and/or instructional _____.

        iii. Identify the _____ code(s).

    B. Methods to locate a main term

        i. Look up the name of the _____ or _____.

        ii. Look up the name of the _____ or _____ site.

        iii. Look up the name of a(n) _____ or _____.

        iv. Look up the _____.

    C. Modifying terms are _____ words in the index that appear _____ under the main term to further describe the service or _____.

    D. Preliminary codes are printed immediately to the _____ of modifying terms.

4. Step 3. Verify the Code in the Tabular List

    A. Locate the preliminary codes in the _____ _____.

        i. Codes are listed in _____ order and divided into six sections.

    B. Interpret tabular list _____.

        i. Tabular list conventions include formatting, _____, verbal instructions, and _____.

ii. Information _____ a semicolon is a common descriptor that is shared with indented codes, and information _____ the semicolon is a unique descriptor that applies to only one code number.

iii. Three types of narratives are provided for proper coding

    a. _____

    b. _____

    c. _____

iv. Symbols alert the user to certain _____ that may affect use or _____ of codes.

C. Select the code with the highest level of _____ by carefully interpreting the conventions associated with each code, category, and section.

D. Review the code for appropriate _____, which are specific coding and billing criteria that are checked for accuracy based on _____ rules.

  i. Bundling edits refers to multiple _____ that are included in a single code.

  ii. Add-on codes are limited to a few codes that are listed in _____ notes and must be verified.

  iii. CPT codes differ regarding how to report the quantity of _____.

E. Append modifiers

  i. Modifiers are two-digit _____ that affect the complete description of a service and frequently have a significant impact on _____ and coding compliance.

  ii. Use of modifiers can be described in the _____ notes, special instructions, or _____.

F. Compare the final code with the _____ and verify that all conditions of the _____ agree with the medical record.

G. Assign the code and _____ the number as you wrote or keyed it to avoid transcription _____ that are easy to make.

IV. Coding for Evaluation and Management Services

1. E&M codes are the codes _____ _____ used in most medical office.

2. E&M codes begin with the numbers _____.

3. Physicians often mark E&M codes on the _____ form.

4. Auditing is a detailed process of verifying that every _____ of the E&M code is clearly _____.

5. Step 1. Identify the Type of Service

   A. Identify the category.

      i. Codes are selected based on the category of _____.

      ii. The category may describe the location or type of _____.

   B. Identify the subcategory.

      i. Patient status distinguishes between _____ and _____ patients.

      ii. Location establishes whether a patient is a(n) _____ or inpatient.

      iii. Frequency determines whether the encounter is initial or _____ hospital care.

   C. Read the reporting instructions.

      i. Definitions and instructions describe _____ terms, how codes are to be _____, and what may be bundled.

6. Step 2. Determine the Key Components and Contributing Factors

   A. History

      i. History describes the background, onset, and _____ of the current condition.

      ii. The complexity of the history can be classified as _____ focused, _____ problem focused, or _____.

   B. Examination

      i. Examination describes the complexity of the _____ _____ of the patient.

      ii. The complexity of the examination can be classified as _____ focused, _____ problem focused, _____, or _____.

      iii. Each level has specific _____ and official documentation _____.

   C. Medical decision making

      i. Medical decision making describes the complexity involved in establishing a _____ and selecting a management option.

      ii. Types of medical decision making include the following.

         a. _____

         b. _____ complexity

         c. _____ complexity

         d. _____ complexity

D. Contributing factors

    i. Counseling

    ii. _____ of care

    iii. The nature of the presenting problem may be any of the following

        a. Minimal

        b. Self-_____, or minor

        c. _____ severity

        d. _____ severity

        e. _____ severity

    iv. Face-to-face time is the time the _____ spends with the _____ and/or family.

7. Step 3. Verify the Final Code with Documentation

    A. Refer to the original documentation to verify that all _____ of the code agree with the _____ _____.

    B. Double-check the _____ of the code number.

8. Step 4. Identify Bundled and Separately Billable Services

    A. Services included in E&M codes

    i. _____ the current problem with patients and their families

    ii. Conducting a physical _____

    iii. Reviewing test results, reports from other _____, and records of outside _____

    iv. _____ tests and services

    v. Writing _____

    vi. _____ procedures

    vii. Obtaining _____ or preauthorization

    viii. Providing instructions and _____ to patients and their families

    B. List five services billed in addition to the E&M code.

    i. _____

    ii. _____

    iii. _____

    iv. _____

    v. _____

9. Step 5. Append Modifiers, if Needed

    A. Certain modifiers tell payers that an E&M service should be _____ rather than bundled with another _____.

V. Coding for Special Situations

1. Coding for Surgery

   A. The surgical section is the _____ section in the CPT manual.

   B. The _____ _____, also known as the global surgical concept, identifies bundled services.

   C. The _____ _____ refers to the number of days surrounding a surgical procedure during which all services related to that procedure are considered part of the surgical _____.

   D. Services available for reimbursement separate from the surgical package include

      i. Complications, exacerbations, and recurrences requiring _____

         _____

      ii. _____ care for the condition for which a procedure was performed

      iii. Care for _____ conditions or injuries

   E. CPT _____ notes and guidelines may indicate that a particular code includes certain related or supporting procedures.

      i. Separating procedures that should be included in a bundled code is called _____, and it is illegal.

2. Coding for Radiology

   A. Steps for providing a radiologic examination

      i. Order the _____.

         a. There is no _____ for ordering a radiologic examination.

      ii. Perform the _____ imaging.

         a. The provider or _____ providing the service reports the radiologic examination.

         b. The _____ component of a radiology code includes creating the image and involves personnel and equipment.

      iii. Analyze and _____ on the examination results.

         a. The _____ _____ of a radiology code is performed by a qualified physician who reviews the image results and writes a(n) _____ about the findings.

   B. _____ are not used when the physician provides both the technical and professional components of a radiology service.

   C. Some procedures are coded based on the number of _____ taken of the anatomic site.

3. Coding for Pathology and Laboratory

   A. Steps for performing a laboratory test

      i. _____ the test.

         a. Do not _____ for writing orders.

      ii. _____ and handle a _____.

         a. The collection method used to obtain the sample is coded _____.

      iii. _____ the actual test.

         a. Performing the test, including personnel and equipment, is the _____ _____ of a laboratory code.

      iv. _____ and report on the test results.

         a. The _____ _____ involves a qualified physician reviewing the test results and writing a report that details the findings.

   B. List five main terms for pathology or laboratory procedures and services.

      i. _____

      ii. _____

      iii. _____

      iv. _____

      v. _____

   C. When a(n) _____ is reported, all the listed tests must have been performed, with no substitution.

4. Coding for Medicine

   A. The _____ section of the CPT manual contains codes for reporting diagnostic testing and noninvasive or minimally invasive procedures.

   B. Codes are listed in the index, divided by medical _____, and can be located in the index by looking up the _____ or conditions for which they are provided.

   C. Immunizations require _____ codes: one for the _____ of the immunization and one for the particular _____ or toxoid.

      i. Add-on codes are provided when more than one _____ is administered at the same _____.

VI. The Healthcare Common Procedure Coding System

   1. Coders call these codes "hicks-_____."

   2. This code set reports

   A. Professional _____

   B. _____ services

   C. _____

D. _____ medical equipment

E. _____ drugs

3. CPT codes are HCPCS Level I codes for _____ services.

4. A Level II code begins with a(n) _____ followed by four

_____.

5. HCPCS Level II codes are mandated by _____ as a uniform code set for insurance carriers.

6. The HCPCS Level II coding manual contains a(n) _____ and a(n) _____ listing.

7. The modifier _____ indicates that a Medicare Advanced Beneficiary Notice form has been signed by the patient when a covered service is expected to be _____.

KEY TERMINOLOGY REVIEW

Match each of the following selected key terms with the correct definition.

a. edits

b. parent code

c. downcoding

d. symbols

e. upcoding

1. _____ Specific coding and billing criteria that are checked for accuracy based on predetermined rules.

2. _____ Alert the user to certain circumstances that may affect use or interpretation of codes.

3. _____ Often performed to prevent potential fraud and abuse and results in lower reimbursement.

4. _____ Also known as a standalone code.

5. _____ Billing for a higher level of service than what was actually provided.

APPLIED PRACTICE: CPT CODING EXERCISES

For each of the following, look up each procedure in the CPT index and then select and verify the code in the tabular list. Write the code on the line provided.

1. _____ Surgical laparoscopy with partial nephrectomy

2. _____ Allergy patch application test, 5 tests

3. _____ Repair of blood vessel, direct, right hand

4. _____ Evaluation and management of a new patient for an office visit that includes an expanded problem-focused history, an expanded problem-focused examination, and straightforward medical decision making

5. _____ Urinalysis, non-automated, without microscopy

6. _____ Gill operation

7. _____ Needle biopsy of cervical lymph node

8. _____ Anesthesia for an open total hip arthroplasty
9. _____ Diagnostic thyroid uptake scan, nuclear medicine
10. _____ Partial laryngectomy, laterovertical
11. _____ Nephrostomy with drainage
12. _____ X-ray of the cervical spine, 4 views
13. _____ Flexible colonoscopy, proximal to splenic flexure, diagnostic
14. _____ Excision of a malignant lesion from the skin of the right arm, excised diameter 1.1 to 2.0 cm
15. _____ Routine obstetric care, including antepartum care, vaginal delivery, and postpartum care
16. _____ Myringotomy, including aspiration
17. _____ Nissen fundoplasty (esophagogastroduodenoscopic) via laparotomy
18. _____ Routine ECG, 12 leads, with interpretation and report
19. _____ Incision and drainage of a bursa on the left foot
20. _____ Lipid panel laboratory test

LEARNING ACTIVITY: MULTIPLE CHOICE

Circle the correct answer for each of the following questions.

1. The tabular list is divided into _____ sections.
   a. three
   b. four
   c. five
   d. six

2. All CPT codes are _____ digits long.
   a. four
   b. five
   c. six
   d. seven

3. In the CPT manual, _____ indicate(s) a new code in the edition.
   a. a black circle
   b. a triangle
   c. two triangles
   d. a circle with a dot in it

4. In the CPT manual, _____ indicate(s) a revised code.
   a. a black circle
   b. a triangle
   c. two triangles
   d. a hashtag or pound sign

5. In the CPT manual, _____ indicate(s) a resequenced code.
   a. a black circle
   b. a triangle
   c. two triangles
   d. a hashtag or pound sign

CRITICAL THINKING

Answer the following questions to the best of your ability. Use the textbook as a reference.

1. Kira Stansfield, CMA (AAMA), is taking an online course to become a certified professional coder. One of her assignments is to write a paragraph about how E&M codes are used and selected. What information should Kira include in her assignment?

   _____

   _____

   _____

   _____

2. Gloria Heritage, RMA, is working in the billing office of a pediatric practice. One of the physicians in the practice frequently chooses a high-level E&M code when billing for his patients. When Gloria consults the patients' charts, she finds that there is not sufficient information to use the higher billing codes and determines that lower codes would be more appropriate. What can Gloria do in this situation?

   _____

   _____

   _____

   _____

RESEARCH ACTIVITY

Use Internet search engines to research the following topic and write a brief description of what you find. It is important to use reputable websites.

1. Using the Internet, research at least five changes that have been made to the current edition of the CPT manual. How do the changes make this edition different from the previous edition?

   _____

   _____

   _____

   _____

CHAPTER 17

Patient Billing and Collections

STUDENT STUDY GUIDE

Use the following guide to assist in your learning of the concepts from the chapter.

I. Overview of Patient Accounting

1. A record of charges and payments for a specific patient is known as a(n) _____ _____.

2. _____ _____ is money owed to the business by customers in exchange for goods and services.

3. The Medical Assistant's Role in Patient Accounting

   A. MAs are often the link between the billing office and the _____.

   B. MA involvement depends on the type and _____ of the medical practice and overall job description.

   C. An MA is a liaison and a(n) _____ for the patient.

4. Accounts Receivable Transactions

   A. Three types of AR transactions

      i. Charge: a(n) _____ that _____ the account balance

      ii. Payment: a(n) _____ that _____ the account balance

      iii. Adjustment: a positive or _____ change to a patient's account balance that does not involve the _____ of money or the addition of a charge for services

5. A day sheet records patient account transactions.

   A. List five common types of patient account transactions.

      i. _____

      ii. _____

      iii. _____

      iv. _____

      v. _____

B. List the items to which day sheets are reconciled at the end of each day.

    i. _____

    ii. _____

    iii. _____

6. Patient Billing Record

    A. The patient billing record includes patient _____ and the patient _____.

    B. The patient ledger is also referred to as the _____ _____.

    C. When posting transactions, it is important to be accurate when entering patient account _____ so that transactions are posted to the proper accounts.

7. Accounts Receivable Systems

    A. Separate accounts may be maintained for _____ compensation or third-_____ liability insurance.

    B. Patient accounting software

        i. Patient accounting software is also called a(n) _____ _____ _____.

        ii. Each employee has a login that consists of a(n) _____ and _____.

        iii. A user log identifies the following

            a. _____

            b. _____

            c. _____

    C. Pegboard system

        i. This is a(n) _____ bookkeeping system used for patient accounting.

        ii. It is also called the _____ method.

8. Accounts Receivable Analysis

    A. Days in AR

        i. Days in AR is the _____ number of days that money has been _____ to the practice.

        ii. Days in AR is calculated by _____ the total AR dollar amount by the average daily _____ of the practice.

        iii. When the practice collects payments rapidly, the number of days in AR is _____ than if the practice collects payments slowly.

    B. AR aging analysis

        i. This analysis categorizes AR according to the _____ of _____ since it has been billed.

      ii. Current accounts are less than _____ days old.

     iii. Accounts older than _____ days should be reviewed at least once a(n) _____.

II. Collecting Patient Payments

  1. Patient Financial Obligation

    A. An initial office visit should include information on _____, payments, and financial _____.

    B. Office brochures often address many financial _____ and procedures.

    C. It is important to inform patients who need surgery or other procedures about possible fees, insurance _____, and methods of _____.

  2. Professional Fees

    A. Considerations relating to fees include time, _____, and the prevailing _____ in the community.

    B. Prevailing fees are determined by two factors.

      i. _____ level of the community

      ii. Average fee charged by physicians in the same _____

    C. A schedule of fees is approved by the _____.

  3. Collecting Copayments

    A. A copayment is a(n) _____ amount of money that a(n) _____ policy says a patient must pay for certain types of visits.

    B. Copayments are deducted from the insurance company's _____ _____ when calculating benefits.

    C. Providers cannot waive _____ obligations.

    D. Managed care contracts often require that a copayment be paid at the time of a(n) _____.

  4. Accepting Copayments

    A. Be courteous and _____ when asking for payment.

    B. Generating a(n) _____ receipt for each payment is a form of internal _____.

    C. Thank the patient and then _____ the payment in the cash drawer.

  5. Security Precautions

    A. All forms of payment carry a small risk of being _____.

    B. If a medical office is not confident that a form of payment is _____, it has the right to refuse that form of payment.

    C. A check returned for _____ funds requires _____ action.

III. Collecting Insurance Payments

    1. Remittance Advice/Explanation of Benefits

        A. The remittance advice statement is also known as the _____ of

           _____.

        B. Items listed on the RA/EOB

           i. Name of the _____

          ii. Name of the _____

         iii. Date of _____

         iv. Amount _____

          v. Amount _____

         vi. Amount _____

        vii. Amount the _____ may bill the patient

        C. Reason codes identify reasons for _____ _____ and denials.

        D. Types of claim statuses

           i. _____ claims are awaiting additional _____.

          ii. _____ claims were received, but no _____ was made.

         iii. _____ claims were never accepted because of invalid information.

    2. Posting Insurance Payments

        A. _____ item posting occurs when payment is allocated to each

           _____ line on the claim.

        B. Providers who contract with insurance carriers must accept the _____

           _____ of the claim as payment in full.

        C. Providers not contracted with insurance companies are allowed to _____

           _____ patients, whereas contracted providers are not.

    3. Claims Follow-Up

        A. Medical assistants must determine the reason a(n) _____ is not

           _____ in full.

        B. Unpaid claims can be easily identified by running a report using _____

           _____ _____ software (PMS).

        C. _____ guidelines determine the time frame in which an insurance carrier must

           pay or _____ a claim.

        D. To _____ a claim is to investigate why payment has been denied.

        E. Tracing claims is most often done by _____ the insurance company.

4. Rejections, Denials, and Appeals
   A. Delayed insurance claim payment may be due to
      i. Incorrect _____ numbers
      ii. Incorrect _____ dates
      iii. Missing _____ codes
      iv. Missing _____ documentation
   B. A(n) _____ claim should be corrected and resubmitted as a new claim.
   C. A denied claim is not paid because of _____ or coverage issues.
   D. A(n) _____ is the amount of the charge that is above the maximum allowable fee.
   E. Contact the insurance company for specific _____ on how to resubmit a corrected claim.
   F. An appeal includes writing a letter or completing a form that clearly states why the _____ believes the denial is not _____.
   G. _____ should become involved in the appeal process because better results may occur when the patient _____ an appeal.
5. Balance Billing
   A. Balance billing is handled differently for _____ and nonparticipating providers.
   B. The _____ is viewed as misrepresenting the true fee if he or she does not bill the disallowance to the patient.

IV. Billing Patients
   1. Reasons a Patient May Owe Money
      A. The _____ was not collected at the time of service.
      B. The patient must pay a(n) _____ amount before the insurance _____ start.
      C. _____ is due on a portion of the service.
      D. The patient received _____ or _____ not covered under the insurance policy.
      E. The insurance policy has paid out the _____ _____ allowed by the policy.
      F. The provider is not _____ with the patient's insurance company, and the patient owes the _____ amounts.
   2. The Billing Cycle
      A. Billing methods depend on the _____ and policies of the _____ office.

B. Two types of billing cycles

    i. _____ billing: Patient statements are generated once a month.

    ii. _____ billing: Each week, _____ percent of patient accounts are billed.

3. Fee Adjustments

A. _____ fees are charged when patients do not pay their bills on time.

B. _____ _____ are offered to patients who do not have health insurance and pay in full at the time of service.

C. _____ _____ is a discount given to other physicians, staff, family members, or clergy.

D. Patients who are experiencing _____ _____ may receive free service or reduced charges.

E. List three reasons overpayments and refunds are issued.

    i. _____

    ii. _____

    iii. _____

4. Insurance Company Refunds

A. The medical office is _____ _____ to notify insurance companies of any overpayment that may have been made in error.

B. The practice is expected to keep adequate _____ in order to identify _____ on any specific claim.

C. The decision of how to handle a refund is up to the _____ _____, not the _____ _____.

5. Patient Refunds

A. A patient refund may occur because of

    i. _____ regarding the deductible, copayment, or coinsurance amount

    ii. The patient mistakenly paying the same bill _____

B. Payments made by cash or check should be refunded with a(n) _____.

C. Payments made by credit card should be refunded to the same _____ _____ used for the transaction.

6. Credit Policy

A. Credit arrangements are often made when a patient will have to pay a(n) _____ out-of-pocket amount due to a surgery or procedure.

B. If a payment schedule is set and the patient will make more than ____ payments, a(n) _____-in-lending form must be signed.

C. List the three items the truth-in-lending form must clearly state.

    i. _____

    ii. _____

    iii. _____

V. Collecting from Patients

  1. Delinquent Accounts

    A. Educate patients about _____ and collection _____ so they understand what is expected.

    B. Delinquent bills occur because the patient

      i. Believes that _____ will cover the bill

      ii. Is _____ to pay

      iii. Has a(n) _____ about the fee

      iv. Does not feel that the bill is _____

    C. An MA must determine the reason that payments are _____ and then implement the _____ _____.

    D. Medical offices might have a(n) _____ policy for small dollar amounts that are overdue.

  2. Collection Techniques

    A. Collection techniques may include

      i. _____ notices

      ii. _____ calls

      iii. _____ letters

      iv. A collection _____

  3. Regulations

    A. Several laws provide protection against unscrupulous _____ _____ that harm individuals.

    B. Become familiar with your particular _____ _____ when applying collection techniques.

  4. Telephone Calls

    A. Collection calls should be tactful, _____, and to the point.

    B. Only discuss the matter with the person _____ _____ for the payment.

  5. Collection Letters

    A. A letter should inquire why the _____ has not been paid.

    B. There should be an offer to assist the patient with making _____ _____.

C. Convey the message that action will be taken to _____ the payment _____.

6. Collection Agencies

    A. These are companies that collect payment for _____ bills.

    B. When an account is turned over to a collection agency, most offices _____ the physician–patient relationship.

7. Selecting a Collection Agency

    A. Reputable agencies have _____ that can be checked and readily discuss their collection _____ and HIPAA _____ practices.

    B. Usually a collection agency is paid only when a(n) _____ _____ is received.

8. Working with a Collection Agency

    A. When turning over an account for collection, include only the following information

        i. _____ due

        ii. Itemized _____

        iii. _____ information

    B. Never include a(n) _____ or other medical information.

    C. Medical practices may pay a flat fee or a(n) _____ fee, which may range from _____ to _____ percent of the amount collected.

9. Special Problems

    A. Special problems make collecting challenging.

        i. _____ _____: A patient moving and not providing a forwarding address.

        ii. _____: Court protection of the patient

        iii. _____ _____ _____: A patient dying, in which case bills should be sent to the estate of the deceased

        iv. _____ of _____: The amount of time a legal collection suit may be brought against a debtor

KEY TERMINOLOGY REVIEW

Match each of the following terms with the correct definition.

a. remittance advice

b. copayment

c. professional courtesy

d. statute of limitations

e. truth-in-lending form

1. _____ A physician opts to reduce the charges for other physicians, staff, family members, or clergy.
2. _____ Also known as an explanation of benefits.
3. _____ The amount of time a legal collection suit may be brought against a debtor.
4. _____ A document that a patient must sign if credit is extended and it is determined that the patient will make set payments to the physician over four or more installments.
5. _____ A predetermined amount of money that the patient must pay for medical services at every visit, as determined by the insurance company.

APPLIED PRACTICE

Complete the activities and answer the questions that follow.

1. Call a local medical office in your area and ask to speak to someone in the billing office. Interview this person about his job function. Ask the person the following questions:

   a. What type of system does your office use for billing (manual or computerized)?

   _____

   _____

   _____

   b. If the office uses a computer system for billing, what is the name of the software used?

   _____

   _____

   _____

   c. What functions of the computer system help the billing office staff better perform their jobs?

   _____

   _____

   _____

2. Read the following scenario and answer the accompanying questions.

Scenario

Kaley McManus, RMA, works for Havensburg Audiology. The payment policy for the audiology practice states that all copayments are expected at the time of service. A patient, Arturo Alamos, is responsible for paying 20 percent of all services, and his insurance company, Healthy Care, will reimburse the physician the remaining 80 percent.

Mr. Alamos has a $35 copayment for specialist visits, and the charges for his procedures today are as follows:

CPT CODE	Description of Service	Fee
92557	Comprehensive audiometry threshold evaluation and speech recognition	$65
92563	Tone decay test	$45

---

a. How much should Kaley collect from Mr. Alamos today?

_____

_____

_____

b. How much will Healthy Care be billed for the services provided to Mr. Alamos?

_____

_____

_____

c. As Mr. Alamos gets ready to pay for his office visit, he realizes that he has only a $20 bill. What should Kaley do?

_____

_____

_____

LEARNING ACTIVITY: MULTIPLE CHOICE

Circle the correct answer for each of the following questions.

1. _____ is calculated by dividing the total AR dollar amount by the average daily revenue of the practice.
   a. Accounts payable
   b. AR aging analysis
   c. Days in AR
   d. Remittance advice

2. The fee is determined by a physician or a practice's partners as a result of taking which of the following into consideration?
   a. Services involved
   b. Economic level of the community
   c. Prevailing fees in the community
   d. All of the above

3. It is _____ for a provider who is contracted with the patient's insurance provider to balance bill the patient.
   a. not allowed
   b. allowed
   c. required
   d. optional

4. Cycle billing requires approximately _____ percent of patient accounts to be billed each week.
   a. 10
   b. 15
   c. 20
   d. 25

5. PMS stands for
   a. practice management software.
   b. practice management system.
   c. practice maintenance system.
   d. practice maintenance software.

CRITICAL THINKING

Answer the following questions to the best of your ability. Use the textbook in considering the following questions.

1. Charles Burke, RMA, is working at the front desk of Pearson Family Medicine. His duties include checking in patients and collecting copayments. A sign posted near the desk states "Copayments are due at time of service." Frank Lewis arrives at the office in a visibly bad mood. He signs the patient sign-in sheet and sits in the overly crowded reception area. Charles realizes that Mr. Lewis has a $15 copayment that must be paid before he is seen by the physician. Mr. Lewis takes a call on his cell phone and begins arguing with the caller. How should Charles proceed in this situation and demonstrate professionalism with the patient?

   _____

   _____

   _____

   _____

   _____

2. Ada Stewart's patient account has a balance of $215.45, which has been past due for over 90 days. There is a notation in her financial record stating that Ms. Stewart had called the office 2 months earlier, when she received her monthly statement, and explained that she had lost her job but would be paying off her balance soon. DeShawn Heath, RMA, is making phone calls to all patients whose accounts are overdue. His next phone call will be to Ms. Stewart. How should DeShawn handle the phone call while being sensitive to the patient's situation?

   _____

   _____

   _____

   _____

   _____

RESEARCH ACTIVITY

Use Internet search engines to research the following topic and write a brief description of what you find. It is important to use reputable websites.

1. Research three collection agencies in your area that offer services for collecting overdue payments. List the advantages and disadvantages of using each of these three companies.

   _____

   _____

   _____

   _____

   _____

CHAPTER 18
Banking and Practice Finances

STUDENT STUDY GUIDE

Use the following guide to assist in your learning of the concepts from the chapter.

I. Financial Functions

1. Bookkeeping

    A. Most offices use _____ _____ for bookkeeping.

    B. List five types of transactions.

        i. _____ (resources)

        ii. _____ (debts)

        iii. _____ (revenue)

        iv. _____ (purchases)

        v. _____ (earnings)

    C. Fill in the basic accounting equation.

        _____ − _____ = _____

2. Accounting

    A. Accounting is the system of reporting the _____ _____ of a business.

    B. Monthly financial statements help physicians evaluate the _____ _____ of the practice and identify _____ that might be desirable.

3. _____ _____ is money owed to the practice for services provided.

4. Accounts Payable

    A. Accounts payable is money the medical practice _____ for services rendered.

    B. List eight examples of AP expenditures.

        i. _____

        ii. _____

        iii. _____

        iv. _____

v. _____

vi. _____

vii. _____

viii. _____

5. Banking

   A. Banking functions include _____ funds, writing _____,

   _____ funds between bank accounts, withdrawing _____,

   and _____ statements.

   B. List three types of bank accounts.

     i. _____

     ii. _____

     iii. _____

6. Computerized Accounting Systems

   A. Computerized accounting systems _____ cost and greatly reduce the risk of

   _____.

   B. _____ reports can be generated easily.

   C. Each user of a computerized accounting system should have a unique login consisting of a(n)

   _____ and _____.

7. Online Banking

   A. List five online banking functions.

     i. _____

     ii. _____

     iii. _____

     iv. _____

     v. _____

   B. A medical practice should _____ _____ to online accounts

   to only a few individuals and should change the logins frequently.

8. The Role of Medical Assistants in Practice Finances

   A. Roles vary by _____.

   B. MAs should be knowledgeable about _____ _____ and

   procedures and able to follow them exactly as _____.

   C. Legal and _____ behavior is essential.

9. Preventing Financial Fraud

   A. _____ is the unauthorized taking of funds.

   B. _____ rely heavily on one or two individuals to handle financial matters.

C. _____ _____ are a system of checks and balances to prevent embezzlement from occurring.

D. Two examples of internal controls are _____ _____ and _____.

II. Checks

1. Features of a Check

   A. _____ instrument

   B. Written and signed by a(n) _____ _____ of the check

   C. States a(n) _____ of money to be paid

   D. Payable on _____ or at a fixed date in the future

   E. Payable to the _____ of the check

2. Information on Checks (List 11 items.)

   A. _____

   B. _____

   C. _____

   D. _____

   E. _____

   F. _____

   G. _____

   H. _____

   I. _____

   J. _____

   K. _____

3. The ABA number identifies the area where the bank issuing the check is located and identifies the _____ _____.

4. Magnetic Ink Character Recognition

   A. The first series of numbers is the _____ _____ _____, which identifies the bank and its location.

   B. The second series of numbers identifies the _____ _____.

   C. The third series of numbers is the _____ _____.

5. Check Security

   A. Blank _____ and _____ stamps must be stored in a securely locked location to which only one or two people have access.

6. Advantages of Checks (List eight advantages.)

   A. _____

   B. _____

C. _____

D. _____

E. _____

F. _____

G. _____

H. _____

7. Special-Purpose Checks (List eight types of checks.)

A. _____

B. _____

C. _____

D. _____

E. _____

F. _____

G. _____

H. _____

8. Accepting Checks

A. When a check is received, it should be inspected for _____ and locked in a(n) _____ location.

B. A(n) _____ _____ is an individual who is authorized to sign the patient's check on her behalf.

C. A medical practice might consider the following types of checks too risky to accept.

   i. _____-party checks

   ii. Checks from _____-of-_____ banks

   iii. Cash _____

   iv. "_____ in Full"

9. Endorsement of Checks

A. Endorsement of a check is placed within the top _____ inches on the _____ side of the check as it is turned over.

B. An endorsement can consist of either a payee's _____ or _____ signature.

C. Checks are often endorsed as soon as they are _____.

10. Bank Hold on Accounts

A. _____ _____ _____ may be attached to the deposited funds that must "clear" before the bank knows the funds are present.

B. Funds cannot be used by the _____ until the check or funds have _____ and the hold is removed.

11. Returned Checks

    A. Checks may be returned if information is _____.

    B. More serious reasons for returned checks include _____ funds and stop-_____ orders.

III. Deposits

  1. Procedures Commonly Followed When Making Deposits

    A. Prepare and make deposits _____.

    B. Maintain all records of _____ _____ in a safe location.

    C. Compare the total on the _____ _____ against the total on the _____ _____ for checks and cash.

    D. Keep a duplicate copy of _____ on file in the office.

    E. Keep _____ _____ for deposits on file in the office.

    F. Immediately record deposits in the _____.

  2. Completing the Deposit Slip

    A. Deposit slips include the total dollar amounts of _____ and _____ being deposited.

    B. Entries should be printed in _____ _____.

    C. Check for _____ if the deposit slip total doesn't match the total on the day sheets.

    D. _____-_____ deposit slips are generated by accounting software based on payments entered into the computer since the last deposit.

  3. Deposits to Savings Accounts

    A. Cash and checks can be deposited or transferred into a savings account to earn _____ _____ than in a checking account.

    B. _____ _____ should specify the conditions in which deposits should to be made into a savings account.

  4. Making a Deposit

    A. Deposits can be made in person, by _____, by night _____, or by being picked up by a bank _____.

    B. _____ should never be sent in the mail.

    C. Online banking might allow you to deposit checks electronically by scanning the _____ and _____ (with _____) of each check.

  5. Accepting and Depositing Cash

    A. Currency should be checked with a(n) _____-detection device.

B. Bank statements should be reconciled as soon as they are _____, and errors should be corrected _____.

C. _____ accounts are easier to reconcile because there are fewer transactions.

D. With computerized reconciliation, the computer performs all the _____.

VI. Payroll

1. Preparing payroll requires calculating _____ _____, wages, and _____ for the entire staff; printing and _____ checks; and sending monies _____ to the appropriate places.

2. Payroll checks are generally issued _____, bi-weekly, or _____.

3. Fair Labor Standards Act

A. The FLSA is a federal law that classifies employees as _____ or _____ from earning overtime pay for hours worked in excess of _____ hours per week.

B. _____ employees must be paid for overtime hours.

C. The overtime pay rate is _____ times the normal pay rate.

D. Paid time off is not required by _____.

E. _____ employees receive a predetermined amount of money every pay period that is not dependent on the number of _____ worked.

4. Methods for Managing Payroll (List three methods.)

A. _____

B. _____

C. _____

5. Deductions

A. A(n) _____ _____ check is calculated by subtracting deductions from the gross wage.

B. Deductions are money withheld from the employee's paycheck for _____, health and life insurance _____, and other benefits.

C. Required withholdings

i. List the three types of taxes the federal government mandates that employers withhold and report.

a. _____

b. _____

c. _____

ii. Individual states may also have payroll withholding requirements for income tax, workers' _____, _____ tax, and short-term _____ insurance.

6. Completing Check Stubs

   A. A check stub provides a permanent record of the _____, _____, _____, and _____ of the check.

   B. Accounting software prints the check stub at the same time as the _____.

   C. A(n) _____ _____ is a full page and contains two or three detachable sections for transaction information.

7. Errors in Check Writing

   A. If a check has an error, it should be marked _____.

   B. Keep voided checks for when the bank statement is _____.

8. Mailing Checks

   A. Checks printed from computer software are often used with a window _____.

   B. _____ envelopes can be used for mailing checks.

   C. Do not _____ a check to an invoice because it could tear and become unacceptable for deposit.

9. Petty Cash

   A. Petty cash is kept for _____ purchases.

   B. It is kept _____ from cash received from patients.

   C. Expenses paid for from petty cash must be recorded in a daily _____ log or _____ pad.

V. Bank Statements

   1. Information Included on Bank Statements (List 10 examples.)

      A. _____

      B. _____

      C. _____

      D. _____

      E. _____

      F. _____

      G. _____

      H. _____

      I. _____

      J. _____

   2. Reconciliation

      A. Reconciliation is the process of comparing the data on _____ _____ with the _____ maintained in the medical office.

B. Bank statements should be reconciled as soon as they are _____, and errors should be corrected _____.

C. _____ accounts are easier to reconcile because there are fewer transactions.

D. With computerized reconciliation, the computer performs all the _____.

VI. Payroll

1. Preparing payroll requires calculating _____ _____, wages, and _____ for the entire staff, printing and _____ checks, and sending monies _____ to the appropriate places.

2. Payroll checks are generally issued _____, bi-weekly, or _____.

3. Fair Labor Standards Act

A. The FLSA is a federal law that classifies employees as _____ or _____ from earning overtime pay for hours worked in excess of _____ hours per week.

B. _____ employees must be paid for overtime hours.

C. The overtime pay rate is _____ times the normal pay rate.

D. Paid time off is not required by _____.

E. _____ employees receive a predetermined amount of money every pay period that is not dependent on the number of _____ worked.

4. Methods for Managing Payroll (List three methods.)

A. _____

B. _____

C. _____

5. Deductions

A. A(n) _____ _____ check is calculated by subtracting deductions from the gross wage.

B. Deductions are money withheld from the employee's paycheck for _____, health and life insurance _____, and other benefits.

C. Required withholdings

   i. List the three types of taxes the federal government mandates that employers withhold and report.

      a. _____

      b. _____

      c. _____

   ii. Individual states may also have payroll withholding requirements for income tax, workers' _____, _____ tax, and short-term _____ insurance.

D. _____ _____ often include premiums for health, life, and disability insurances; pension plan contributions; and union dues.

6. Deposit Requirements

A. The _____ _____ _____ imposes a severe penalty for failure to deposit federal tax money withheld from employee _____.

B. Quarterly report filings are due _____ 30, July 31, _____ 31, and January 31.

C. Federal unemployment tax is the sole responsibility of the _____ and is based on the employee's _____ _____ but must not be deducted from the employee's _____.

D. Few states require both employee and employer to make payments toward the _____ _____ _____ _____.

7. Year-End Reporting

A. W-2 forms report the following.

   i. The employee's _____ gross income

   ii. Federal, state, and local _____ withheld

   iii. Taxable _____ benefits

   iv. The employee's _____ _____ for the year

B. W-2 forms must be delivered by January _____ for the preceding calendar year.

C. The employer provides _____ copies of the W-2 form to each employee

KEY TERMINOLOGY REVIEW

Match each of the following terms with the correct definition.

a. accounts payable (AP)

b. assets

c. remittance slip

d. fidelity bond

e. embezzlement

1. _____ Also known as resources.

2. _____ The unauthorized taking of funds.

3. _____ Employee dishonesty coverage.

4. _____ Tear-off stub of an invoice being paid.

5. _____ Money that is owed to vendors, suppliers, utility companies, and others for services rendered.

APPLIED PRACTICE

Read the scenario and answer the questions that follow.

Scenario
Daniel Evans, CMA (AAMA), works as the administrative medical assistant for Happy Valley Medical Center. As part of his work responsibilities, Daniel must handle payroll, accounts payable, and banking procedures. It is Thursday, and Daniel must perform these duties.

1. Daniel must calculate the gross earnings for the two clinical medical assistants who work in the back office. The office pays its employees every week, for the previous week's work. For every hour over 40 hours worked, employees get paid time and a half. Last week, Shelby Coleman worked 43.5 hours. She earns $13.00 per hour. Chantal Jefferson worked 45 hours last week. Chantal earns $13.75 per hour.

   a. What are Shelby's gross earnings?

   _____

   b. What are Chantal's gross earnings?

   _____

2. Daniel Smith has received an invoice from a vendor that supplied the physician with new business cards. The invoice reads as follows:

SELECT STATIONERY UNLIMITED

Bill to: Happy Valley Medical Clinic
1129 Felicity Road
Springfield, PA 00010
Account #: 288901HVMC

Remit Payment to: Select Stationery Unlimited
PO Box 588
New York, NY 11110

Item Number	Description	Price	Total
0123	250 Business Cards	32.99	32.99
		Tax (5%)	1.65
		Shipping and Handling	4.95
		Total	$ 39.59

---

a. Complete the check according to how Daniel should pay this bill.

Happy Valley Medical Clinic	**13003**
1129 Felicity Road	_____ **20**___
Springfield, PA 00010	
Pay to the order of: _____	
_____ **dollars**	
MEMO:_____	_____

LEARNING ACTIVITY: MULTIPLE CHOICE

Circle the correct answer to each of the following questions.

1. Which of the following would be considered a deduction for the purposes of employee payroll?
   a. Federal tax withholding
   b. Vacation pay
   c. Overtime pay
   d. All of the above

2. Petty cash is available for incidentals such as
   a. small purchases.
   b. reimbursements.
   c. miscellaneous expenses.
   d. all of the above.

3. Which of the following is *not* an example of an AP expenditure?
   a. Rent
   b. Copayments
   c. Utilities
   d. Office supplies

4. A bill from the shipper that documents the total amount due is a(n)
   a. invoice.
   b. packing slip.
   c. purchase order.
   d. remittance slip.

5. The American Bankers Association (ABA) number is always located
   a. in the phone book.
   b. in the upper-right corner of a printed check.
   c. in the lower-left corner of a printed check.
   d. None of the above

6. Check stubs are used
   a. as permanent records of the date, amount, payee, and purpose of the check.
   b. as bookmarks.
   c. as examples of the correct way to write a check.
   d. for quarterly reporting forms.

7. How much is typically paid to employees as overtime wages?
   a. Twice the employee's normal rate of pay
   b. One and a half times the employee's normal rate of pay
   c. Three times the employee's normal rate of pay
   d. None of the above

8. The _____ IRS form is used to calculate the correct amount of withholdings from the employee's paycheck.
   a. Circular E
   b. W-2
   c. W-4
   d. None of the above

9. A money market account
   a. is an interest-bearing account.
   b. is used more as an investment tool.
   c. typically requires a minimum balance of $500.
   d. all of the above.

10. A payroll system that has 24 pay periods a year is
   a. weekly.
   b. bi-weekly.
   c. semi-monthly.
   d. monthly.

CRITICAL THINKING

Answer the following questions to the best of your ability. Use the textbook and other resources such as the Internet in considering the following questions.

1. Francie Weston, RMA, has been newly hired to work in a busy family practice clinic. When Francie looks at her first paycheck, she notices that a tax has been taken out for something called FICA. She asks her office manager to explain what this tax is. How might the office manager explain this tax to Francie?

   _____

   _____

   _____

   _____

   _____

2. Peyton has just been hired as an office manager for a brand new family medicine practice. The physicians of the practice would like her to establish a policy for paying bills for the practice. What types of things should Peyton consider when establishing a policy for paying bills?

   _____

   _____

   _____

   _____

   _____

RESEARCH ACTIVITY

Use Internet search engines to research the following topic and write a brief description of what you find. It is important to use reputable websites.

1. Look up three different software programs that can perform payroll functions. Create a list of the advantages and disadvantages of these three programs. Cite the websites used for your research.

   _____

   _____

   _____

   _____

   _____

CHAPTER 19
Medical Office Management

STUDENT STUDY GUIDE

Use the following guide to assist in your learning of the concepts from the chapter.

I. Systems Approach to Office Management

1. Management philosophy recommends a(n) _____ _____ when managing a medical office.

2. Personnel Management Responsibilities (List six responsibilities.)

   A. _____

   B. _____

   C. _____

   D. _____

   E. _____

   F. _____

3. Employee Records

   A. List the employee information that federal law requires an employer to maintain.

   i. _____

   ii. _____

   iii. _____

   iv. _____

4. Financial Management

   A. Duties include banking, _____, collections, and _____ collections.

5. Scheduling

   A. Ineffective scheduling affects employee _____ and sparks discontent among physicians and _____.

   B. _____ in the schedule is necessary to accommodate unexpected occurrences.

6. Facility and Equipment Management (List four duties in this category.)

   A. Facility _____ and planning

   B. Inventory _____

C. Maintenance of _____ and OSHA standards

D. Equipment _____

7. Clinical Office Management Duties

A. _____ clinical personnel

B. Keeping track of medical _____

C. _____ supplies

D. Meeting the _____ requests

E. Ensuring that proper _____ are followed

8. Communication

A. Important communication skills include _____ communication; oral
_____, including _____ and nonverbal; and patient
_____.

9. Legal Concepts

A. Though lawyers are often used, it is important to understand legal requirements with which
the _____ _____ must comply.

II. Role of the Office Manager

1. The office manager coordinates all _____ _____ conducted in the
medical office.

2. To be efficient, the office manager must have effective _____ and
_____ skills.

3. A good office manager strives to establish and implement a(n) _____
_____ to management.

4. Time Management

A. Time management requires the ability to _____ and _____
important tasks to complete them on schedule.

B. A(n) _____ list prioritizes tasks based on priority levels 1, 2, and 3.

C. Priority 1 tasks are done _____, and Priority 3 tasks are done
_____.

D. Always _____ _____ complete instructions rather than trust
them to memory.

5. Monthly Planning

A. List five items commonly included on a monthly office schedule.

i. _____

ii. _____

iii. _____

      iv. _____

      v. _____

B. List four items typically listed on a physician's calendar.

      i. _____

      ii. _____

      iii. _____

      iv. _____

C. Periodically compare the _____'s calendar with the master office calendar and make updates as necessary.

6. Staff Meetings

A. Staff meetings should be held on a(n) _____ basis to promote _____ and the flow of important information.

B. Meetings should be scheduled at times when all staff can be present, such as _____ or _____ office hours.

C. The office manager prepares the _____, frequently with input from the physician and other staff.

D. An agenda identifies items for _____ and limits the _____ allotted.

7. Motivating Employees

A. List 13 leadership qualities that employees expect of management.

      i. _____

      ii. _____

      iii. _____

      iv. _____

      v. _____

      vi. _____

      vii. _____

      viii. _____

      ix. _____

      x. _____

      xi. _____

      xii. _____

      xiii. _____

8. Leadership Styles
   A. Leadership style refers to the predominant way a manager _____
      _____ and _____ to those around him.
   B. Briefly describe each of the following types of leadership styles.
      i. Authoritarian—_____
      ii. Democratic—_____
      iii. Permissive—_____
      iv. Bureaucratic—_____
9. Types of Authority
   A. Reward-based power incorporates rewards in exchange for better _____
      _____ and teamwork.
   B. Legitimate authority and responsibility are given to people based on their
      _____.
   C. _____ authority is given to those who have a great deal of knowledge.
   D. Referent power is given out of high _____ and respect.
   E. Informative power is wielded by those with information that others _____ or
      _____.
   F. _____ _____ is the idea that if you know the right people, you
      can get what you need.
III. Creating a Team Atmosphere
   1. The office manager must realize that she is the team _____.
   2. Managers also must show that they are a(n) _____ part of the team.
   3. Team Size
      A. The size of a group can greatly affect the _____ of how it functions.
      B. A smaller group may have a more _____ atmosphere, and a larger group may
         have a more rigid _____.
   4. Team Personalities and Traits
      A. A team atmosphere can begin with staff members helping with the _____
         process.
      B. Staff members may be able to provide some insight into the _____ of a job
         candidate.
      C. A manager should look for staff members who complement each other's
         _____ and _____.
   5. Team Accountability
      A. If something goes wrong, the team must come together to _____ and
         _____ the problem.

6. Team Purpose and Goals

   A. Successful teams work with the same _____ in mind and approach a problem or task using _____ _____.

   B. Switching places or shadowing others helps team members experience the _____ and _____ of the office as a whole.

IV. Hiring Effective Staff Members

   1. Advertising a position is often done by placing ads in newspapers and _____ _____, with professional _____, on the Internet, at formal _____ programs, and at _____ agencies.

   2. Conducting Interviews

      A. Interviewing often begins with a short _____ interview.

      B. Interview questions

         i. The Equal Opportunity Employment Act of 1972 prohibits discriminating against applicants based on race, _____, religion, sex, or _____ _____ both during an interview and on a(n) _____.

         ii. Employers generally cannot ask _____-related questions or require medical _____ until after an applicant has been given a conditional job offer.

         iii. Employers can ask if the applicant will need a(n) _____ to perform a specific job duty.

      C. Assessing a good fit

         i. Ask applicants about past office _____ and what types of _____ they have worked with before.

         ii. Ask off-the-cuff questions to see how the applicant _____.

         iii. Sometimes it is better to hire someone with a little less _____ but who is a good _____ fit for the office.

      D. Checking _____ is done after conducting the interview.

   3. Hiring the Applicant

      A. After an applicant has accepted the position, all _____ _____ should be notified that the position has been filled.

      B. New employees should receive a job _____ and written confirmation of the job offer that includes the _____ and _____ offered.

      C. Examples of screenings required by some offices include the following.

         i. _____ screening

         ii. Acceptable _____ report

         iii. Acceptable _____ background check

iv. Pre-_____ physical

v. Body _____ testing and training

D. The new employee probationary period is usually _____ days.

E. List 13 subjects covered during new hire orientation.

i. _____

ii. _____

iii. _____

iv. _____

v. _____

vi. _____

vii. _____

viii. _____

ix. _____

x. _____

xi. _____

xii. _____

xiii. _____

F. At-will employment means that there is not an explicit _____ _____ between the employer and employee.

4. Performance Evaluations

A. Reviews provide employees feedback on how well they are performing in their _____ _____ and provide the opportunity for managers to introduce new _____ for staff.

B. List four types of evaluations.

i. _____

ii. _____

iii. _____

iv. _____

C. Conducting a performance evaluation

i. The manager must look at the employee's _____ as a whole.

ii. The manager should be open to understanding _____ the employee may be experiencing and reinforce what is _____.

iii. Objectively _____ the employee's performance and provide the employee _____ _____ that support your ratings.

iv. Evaluation should also include the employee's soft _____.

v. Provide employees with new _____ and also areas to _____ before the next evaluation.

vi. The formal _____ _____ should not be the first time the employee hears of any concerns.

vii. Employees may ask for a(n) _____ in _____.

viii. Document everything said during an evaluation in a(n) _____ manner.

5. Disciplinary Process

A. Discipline may range from a(n) _____ period to outright dismissal.

B. Sometimes _____ and _____ warnings are issued before corrective action is taken.

C. List four situations that may result in immediate discharge.

i. _____

ii. _____

iii. _____

iv. _____

D. All incidents should be carefully _____ in the _____'s file.

6. Human resources documentation should include licensure or _____, continuing _____ _____, training, and _____ and dues.

V. Policies

1. Personnel Policy Manual

A. This manual contains information about the employer–_____ relationship, the work _____, and the expectations of the facility.

B. General information includes policies relating to dress and _____ codes, punctuality, _____ safety, and the role of the employee in a(n) _____.

C. Grounds for _____ are also discussed.

D. A well-designed manual remains flexible and allows for _____.

2. Workplace Sexual Harassment

A. Harassment is unwelcome sexual _____, requests for sexual _____, and other verbal or _____ harassment of a sexual nature.

B. It is against the law to create a(n) _____ work environment in which employees must accept _____ advances or listen to inappropriate talk.

C. _____ _____ _____ means giving something for something else and is often referenced in terms of sexual harassment.

3. Workplace Bullying

   A. Workplace bullying is repeated abuse of employees that involves

      i. _____ abuse

      ii. Humiliation

      iii. _____

      iv. Threatening _____

      v. Interference with or _____ of work duties

4. Office Policies and Procedures Manual

   A. This manual describes how to carry out _____ within a particular medical practice.

   B. The manual provides detailed descriptions of standard _____ procedures and administrative and _____ tasks.

   C. A policy is a plan of _____, and a procedure describes the _____ to be performed to carry out the _____.

   D. The primary functions of the manual are to

      i. List the _____ to be performed within the office.

      ii. Standardize the _____ for each task.

      iii. Describe job _____ and titles.

   E. One person may be responsible for _____ of the manual, but input from a variety of personnel makes it better.

   F. The physician should provide the _____ _____ of all written policies and procedures.

VI. Travel and Speaking Arrangements

1. Travel arrangements can include making _____, _____, and car rental reservations, as well as preparing a printed _____ itinerary.

2. Determine the physician's preferences before making any plans.

3. Flight Information (List five examples.)

   A. _____

   B. _____

   C. _____

   D. _____

   E. _____

4. Hotel Information (List four examples.)

   A. _____

   B. _____

C. _____

D. _____

5. The physician may have you do _____ to help prepare for a speaking engagement.

6. When creating handouts, use impeccable _____ and _____.

VII. Medical Practice Marketing and Customer Service

1. Marketing promotes the _____ of a physician or group of physicians to a population of _____.

2. Patient Information Booklet

   A. This booklet contains information about

      i. _____ hours

      ii. Payment _____

      iii. Appointment and _____ policy

      iv. Telephone _____ service

      v. Information about the _____

      vi. After-hours _____

      vii. _____ to the facility

      viii. _____ information

   B. _____ _____ are helpful for those with special needs, and they teach methods of disease prevention.

3. Target Market

   A. _____ offered in a target market can affect the physician's office location.

   B. Types of services the practice could offer can be _____ and _____ to meet the expectations and needs of the target market.

   C. _____ must be put into place after determining services.

4. Marketing the Practice

   A. List three low-cost marketing tools.

      i. Free marketing through word of _____

      ii. Public relations activities such as local _____ and events

      iii. _____ for the practice

5. Customer Service

   A. Customer service delivered to patients can _____ patients in or _____ them away.

   B. Consider the following when evaluating customer service.

      i. What impression does the _____ have?

      ii. Are staff members helpful and _____?

iii. Are staff members _____ and considerate of the patient's

_____ and conditions?

C. Excellent customer service usually means increased _____ as a result of

increased patient _____.

KEY TERMINOLOGY REVIEW

Without using information from the textbook, write a sentence using each selected key term in the correct context.

1. *Colleagues*

   _____

   _____

2. *Discriminatory*

   _____

   _____

3. *Grievance*

   _____

   _____

4. *Itinerary*

   _____

   _____

5. *Probationary period*

   _____

   _____

APPLIED PRACTICE

Complete the following activities using your textbook and/or the Internet as reference.

1. Pretend that you are the office manager for a pediatric practice. You need to place an ad for a medical assistant position that has become available in your office. The position is part time and includes both administrative and clinical duties. Write the ad for the job description, including additional skills you think would be important for this position. Then indicate three resources you would use to place this ad.

   _____

   _____

   _____

   _____

   _____

2. Again, pretend that you are an office manager. Assign priority levels to the tasks listed on the following to-do list.

TO-DO LIST

Priority Level (1-3)	Task
	File monthly invoices.
	Create work schedule for the next 2 weeks.
	Discuss Dr. Turner's schedule changes.
	Return call to an upset patient.
	Create agenda for next month's staff meeting.
	Write ad for the part-time medical assistant position.
	Send a memo to staff about the pharmaceutical representative lunch next week.

LEARNING ACTIVITY: TRUE/FALSE

Indicate whether the following statements are true or false by placing a T or an F on the line that precedes each statement.

_____ 1. A new employee's probationary period is usually 21 days.

_____ 2. The clinical aspects of office management are separate from the administrative aspects.

_____ 3. At-will employment means that employers can terminate an employee without just cause.

_____ 4. Referent power is given to those with a great deal of knowledge.

_____ 5. A physician usually conducts staff meetings.

CRITICAL THINKING

Answer the following questions to the best of your ability. Use the textbook as a reference.

1. Teresa Clymer, CMA (AAMA), has just been promoted to office manager. In order to create a team atmosphere and ensure the building of a successful team, what factors should Teresa consider?

_____

_____

_____

_____

_____

2. Mavis Raschenko, RMA, has repeatedly received sexually explicit e-mails from her coworker Adam. He also has made unwanted advances toward Mavis, and she feels very uncomfortable going to work every day. How should Mavis handle the situation with Adam?

_____

_____

_____

_____

RESEARCH ACTIVITY

Use Internet search engines to research the following topic and write a brief description of what you find. It is important to use reputable websites.

1. Research the importance of conducting performance evaluations and explore the tools that are available to help perform this task in the medical office setting. Write an essay explaining what you have learned through your research. Cite your sources at the end of the essay.

_____

_____

_____

_____

CHAPTER 20
Body Structure and Function

STUDENT STUDY GUIDE

Use the following guide to assist in your learning of the concepts from the chapter.

I. Organization of the Human Body

   1. Complete the diagram of the organization of body. (Refer to Figure 20-1 in your textbook.)

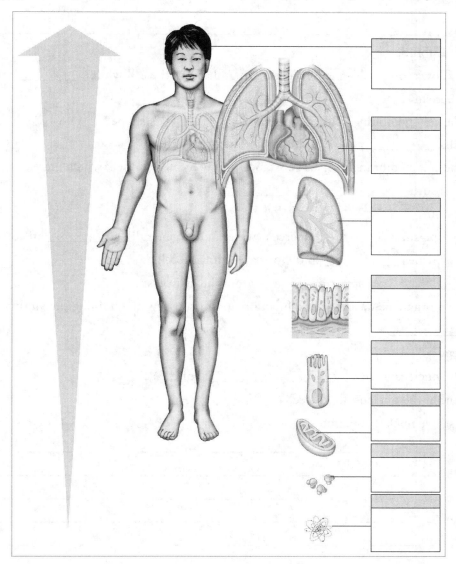

2. Atoms

    A. _____ and _____ constitute the majority of the anatomic mass and reside within the nucleus.

    B. _____, _____, and _____ combine to create elements.

3. Molecules

    A. A molecule is a chemical combination of _____ or more atoms.

    B. Molecules can take the form of _____, _____, or _____.

4. Cells

    A. The cell is the _____ block of the human body.

    B. List the three components that are common to all cells.

        i. _____

        ii. _____

        iii. _____

5. Cell Membrane

    A. It allows some substances to pass into and out of the cell while _____ the passage of other substances.

    B. The cell membrane helps maintain the _____'s shape.

    C. Cilia _____ the overall surface area of a cell.

    D. The cell membrane propels substances along a cell's surface, which increases the cell's ability to absorb _____ and _____.

6. Cytoplasm

    A. Cytoplasm is _____ percent water and is generally _____ in color.

    B. It provides _____ and work areas for the cell.

    C. _____ are structures found within the cytoplasm.

    D. Each organelle has a specific function and purpose in maintaining the vitality of the _____.

7. Nucleus

    A. The nucleus is the _____ _____ of the cell.

    B. Within the nucleus are the cell's _____.

    C. List five nucleic functions.

        i. _____

        ii. _____

        iii. _____

        iv. _____

        v. _____

8. Cell Division: Mitosis and Cytokinesis

   A. List the five phases of mitosis.

      i. _____

      ii. _____

      iii. _____

      iv. _____

      v. _____

   B. Cytokinesis divides the _____, _____, and cell membrane, completing the division of the original cell into two new _____ cells.

9. Meiosis

   A. Meiosis is the cellular division of _____ cells.

   B. A female gamete is a(n) _____, and a male gamete is a(n) _____ cell.

10. Tissues

   A. Specialized cells that have the same _____ and _____ form tissue.

   B. List four types of tissue found within the human body.

      i. _____

      ii. _____

      iii. _____

      iv. _____

   C. List three types of muscle tissue.

      i. _____

      ii. _____

      iii. _____

II. Body Organs and Systems

   1. A group of _____ with similar function come together to form organs.

   2. Body systems are groups of _____ that work together toward the same purpose: to sustain _____ within the _____ body.

III. Chemistry

   1. Passive and Active Transport

     A. Passive transport involves a number of processes, including _____, _____, and _____.

     B. Through active transport, _____ are able to obtain what they need through _____ fluid by two methods: phagocytosis and _____.

   2. Electrolytes

     A. Electrolytes break down into ions that are either _____ or _____ charged.

     B. Electrolytes carry _____ impulses to other cells.

C. Electrolytes that are lost must be _____ to keep their concentrations in the body fluids constant.

3. Metabolism

   A. Metabolism is the chemical processes in the body that maintain life, including the _____ and _____ of energy.

   B. _____ is a chemical process that builds things up.

   C. _____ is a chemical process that breaks down larger units into smaller ones.

IV. Genetics and Heredity

   1. Genetics is the study of the _____ makeup of animals or plants.

   2. Genetic Engineering

      A. Genetic engineering is generally considered to be the use of _____ by scientists intentionally to make _____ to the genetic makeup.

      B. Controversy surrounds whether genetic engineering is _____ or _____.

   3. Genetic Fingerprinting

      A. The _____ and _____ of a person's unique genetic makeup is known as genetic fingerprinting.

      B. DNA samples are obtained from hair, _____, _____ fluid, blood, or saliva, but any part of a(n) _____ can be used.

      C. Isolating a strand of DNA is done by using chemicals, such as _____, and _____ to separate the different parts of the DNA.

   4. Genetics, Heredity, and Disease

      A. Heredity is the _____ of genes from parent to child.

      B. Individuals carry _____ genes for each trait: one from the _____ _____ and one from the _____ _____.

   5. Genetic Disorders

      A. Mutations are changes in the _____ sequence of a(n) _____.

      B. Genetic mutations can occur at any time during _____.

      C. Albinism

         i. Albinism is a common _____ disorder.

         ii. It is a congenital but _____ disorder.

         iii. A mutation in a recessive gene causes a hereditary lack of pigment in the _____, _____, and eyes.

         iv. The patient is prone to _____ and may complain of _____ because protective melanin is not present.

      D. ADHD

         i. ADHD stands for _____-_____/_____ _____.

ii. It is characterized by a person having difficulty _____ attention and _____ and completing tasks.

iii. ADHD is _____ times more prevalent in _____ than in _____.

E. Cleft palate

i. Cleft palate is a(n) _____ defect in the roof of the mouth that occurs when the _____ bones of the skull do not close properly.

ii. The cleft causes a(n) _____ between the mouth and the nasal cavities.

iii. Cleft palate affects _____ more often than _____.

F. Color deficiency

i. This disorder was previously called _____ _____.

ii. It often entails difficulty distinguishing between _____ and _____.

iii. This condition is a(n) _____, sex-linked disorder, usually passed from mother to _____.

iv. With total color deficiency, a person is unable to perceive any color at all because of a defect in or absence of _____ in the _____.

G. Cystic fibrosis

i. Cystic fibrosis is usually diagnosed in _____.

ii. This disease causes mucus to become _____, dry, and _____.

iii. Mucus builds up and clogs passages, primarily in the lungs and the _____.

H. Down syndrome

i. Down syndrome occurs when a person has a(n) _____ chromosome at the _____ pair.

ii. A mother who gives birth after age _____ has an increased risk of delivering an infant with Down syndrome.

iii. _____ is generally used as a tool for diagnosing this disorder.

I. Fragile X syndrome

i. Fragile X syndrome also is known as _____-Bell syndrome, _____ _____ syndrome, and _____ syndrome.

ii. This condition is the most common form of inherited _____ _____.

iii. Generally, _____ are affected with moderate mental retardation and _____ with mild mental retardation.

J. Hemochromatosis

i. Hemochromatosis is characterized by an extreme accumulation of _____.

ii. It is common in the _____ population, affecting approximately _____ in _____ individuals of _____ ancestry.

iii. _____ deposits in the skin eventually cause _____ of the skin.

K. Hemophilia

    i. Hemophilia is a(n) _____, sex-linked disorder in which blood _____ time is greatly increased.

    ii. It is caused by a(n) _____ gene mutation in the _____ chromosome.

    iii. Females carry the _____ gene and transmit the disorder to their _____ offspring.

L. Klinefelter's syndrome

    i. Klinefelter's syndrome is a congenital _____ disorder.

    ii. Symptoms go unnoticed until _____.

    iii. This disorder also can lead to shyness, _____ difficulties, and _____ disorders.

M. Muscular dystrophy

    i. Muscular dystrophy is characterized by progressive _____ and weakening of muscles.

    ii. Muscular dystrophy occurs most frequently in _____.

    iii. The most common type is _____ muscular dystrophy, which accounts for _____ percent of all cases.

    iv. Death often occurs within _____ to _____ years after the onset of symptoms.

N. PKU

    i. PKU stands for _____.

    ii. PKU is caused by a recessive gene _____.

    iii. If the condition is not treated early, _____ _____ occurs because of brain damage.

O. Sickle cell anemia

    i. This chronic form of anemia is caused by a(n) _____ gene mutation.

    ii. It is also known as _____ SS disease.

    iii. It is most common in people of _____ or _____ descent.

P. Spina bifida

    i. Spina bifida is a congenital _____ tube defect.

    ii. Sometimes the _____ _____ and its membranes may _____ outside the body and be evident at birth.

    iii. Most often the abnormality occurs in the _____ region.

Q. Talipes

    i. Talipes is an inherited disorder of the _____.

    ii. It is referred to as _____.

    iii. Orthopedic shoes and _____ the foot may be treatment options.

R. Tay-Sachs disease

    i. Tay-Sachs disease is caused by a genetic mutation that targets the _____

        _____.

    ii. TSD tends to affect people of _____ and _____ European Jewish or French-Canadian ancestry.

    iii. This disease afflicts babies often around the age of _____ month(s).

S. Turner's syndrome

    i. Turner's syndrome is caused by all or part of one of the _____ chromosomes becoming lost before or immediately after _____.

    ii. _____ may be impaired.

    iii. The patient is usually _____ in stature.

APPLIED PRACTICE

1. Label the parts of the cell found in this image. (Refer to Figure 20-2 in your textbook.)

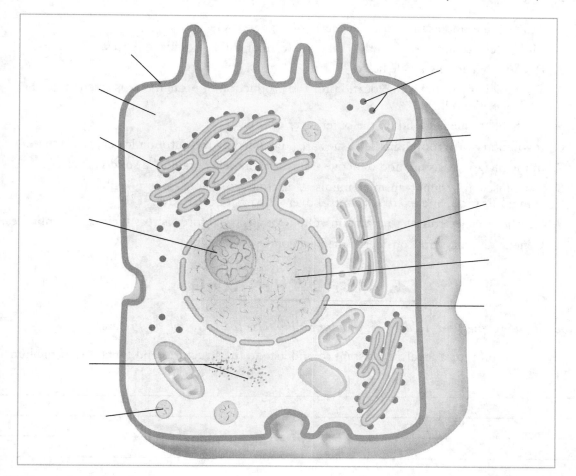

2. Label the stages of mitosis. (Refer to Figure 20-4 in your textbook.)

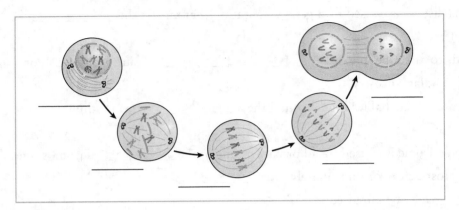

LEARNING ACTIVITY: TRUE/FALSE

Indicate whether the following statements are true or false by placing a T or an F on the line that precedes each statement.

_____ 1. Atoms are found at the most basic level of organization.

_____ 2. Molecules cannot move and thus take the form of solids, liquids, or gases.

_____ 3. DNA is shaped in a single helix.

_____ 4. The Golgi apparatus is the location for the production of protein that is essential to the vitality of the cell.

_____ 5. Epithelial tissue is found on the outer layer of skin.

_____ 6. Involuntary or smooth muscle tissues are controlled by the autonomic nervous system.

_____ 7. In the phagocytosis method of active transport, the cell "engulfs" a solid particle.

_____ 8. The muscular system transmits impulses, responds to change, is responsible for communication, and exercises control over all parts of the body.

_____ 9. Cells utilize electrolytes to maintain voltage or electrical force across their cell membranes.

_____ 10. Genetic disorders are considered medical conditions.

CRITICAL THINKING

Answer the following questions to the best of your ability. Use the textbook as a reference.

1. Why is it important for a medical assistant to understand the structures and functions of the human body?

_____

_____

_____

_____

_____

2. Arlene is taking a medical law and ethics class as a part of her training to become a medical assistant. She has been assigned to write one paragraph explaining why genetic engineering is considered an ethical issue. What information might Arlene include in her assignment?

_____

_____

_____

_____

_____

RESEARCH ACTIVITY

Use Internet search engines to research the following topic and write a brief description of what you find. It is important to use reputable websites.

1. Conduct further research on genetic engineering. Discover more about this fascinating topic and write a brief essay that explains what you learned through your research. Be sure to cite your sources.

_____

_____

_____

_____

_____

CHAPTER 21
The Integumentary System

STUDENT STUDY GUIDE

Use the following guide to assist in your learning of the concepts from the chapter.

I. Functions of the Integumentary System

   1. The skin works in multiple ways to provide _____ for the body.

   2. Functions of the Skin

     A. Protection

       i. The skin prevents _____ _____ from entering the body.

       ii. Protective pigmentation called _____ protects against the sun's UV rays.

     B. Regulation

       i. When body temperature rises and requires _____, the blood vessels in the skin _____.

       ii. When heat conservation is needed, the blood vessels in the skin _____.

     C. Sensory reception

       i. The integumentary system and the _____ system work together for the function of sensation.

       ii. Sensory reactions include responses to pressure, _____, _____, cold, _____, and more.

     D. Absorption

       i. _____ (through-the-skin) medications take advantage of the ability of the skin to absorb substances.

     E. Secretion

       i. _____ glands secrete perspiration, or _____.

       ii. _____ glands secrete oil for _____.

II. Structures of the Skin

   1. Three Layers of Skin

     A. The epidermis is divided into _____ layers.

     B. The dermis, or _____ _____, is made of _____ tissue.

     C. The subcutaneous tissue is the _____ layer.

2. Epidermis

   A. Stratum corneum

      i. The stratum corneum is the _____ layer of skin, which consists of dead cells filled with a protein called _____.

      ii. The stratum corneum forms a protective _____ for the body.

      iii. The _____ of the layer depends on the part of the body.

   B. Stratum lucidum

      i. The stratum lucidum is the _____ layer directly beneath the _____ _____.

      ii. Cells in this layer are either _____ or _____.

   C. Stratum granulosum

      i. The stratum granulosum consists of several layers of _____ cells that become part of the _____ lucidum and stratum _____.

      ii. Cells actively become _____, or hardened, after they lose their _____.

   D. Stratum germinativum

      i. The stratum germinativum is made of several layers of living cells that are still capable of _____, or cell division.

      ii. The stratum germinativum is most responsible for the _____ of the epidermis.

      iii. This layer contains _____.

3. Dermis

   A. The dermis is the _____ layer of the skin.

   B. It is composed of _____ tissue containing nerves and nerve endings, blood vessels, sebaceous and _____ glands, hair follicles, and _____ vessels.

   C. It is divided into two layers: the _____ layer and the _____ layer.

4. Subcutaneous Layer

   A. This layer is composed of _____ _____ tissue.

   B. Tissue helps support, nourish, insulate, and _____ the skin.

III. Accessory Structures of the Skin

   1. Hair

      A. The visible portion of hair is the _____.

      B. The _____ is found at the base of each hair follicle.

      C. With the exception of the _____ of the hands and the _____ of the feet, the entire body is covered by a very thin layer of hair.

2. Nails

  A. Fingernails and toenails are composed of hard _____.

  B. The nail bed is also called the _____.

  C. The light-colored, half-moon area at the base is the _____.

  D. Average nail growth is about _____ mm per week.

  E. Nail _____ may be adversely affected by disease.

3. Sebaceous Glands

  A. Sebaceous glands secrete _____.

  B. The function of sebum is to _____ and _____ hair and skin.

  C. In hair-covered areas, these glands are contained in hair _____.

  D. At hairless areas, sebum rises to the surface through _____.

4. Sudoriferous Glands

  A. Sudoriferous glands, or _____ glands, occur in nearly all regions of the skin.

  B. Sweat glands secrete _____, which helps cool the body through _____.

IV. Common Pathology of the Integumentary System*

1. Skin Cancer

  A. Skin cancer is the most _____ of all cancers.

  B. It affects more than _____ people each year in the United States.

  C. It occurs when normal skin cells undergo a change during which they _____ and _____ without the normal controls.

  D. As the cells multiply, they form a mass called a(n) _____.

2. Basal Cell Carcinoma

  A. Basal cell carcinoma is the most _____ form of skin cancer.

  B. It often appears as a change in the skin, such as a(n) _____, an irritation, or a(n) _____ that does not heal, or a change in a(n) _____ or mole.

  C. Although the _____ is the most common site, it may affect the head, neck, back, chest, or shoulders.

  D. Exposure to _____ is the most common cause of this cancer.

  E. Signs and symptoms of basal cell carcinoma

    i. Firm, _____ _____, including tiny blood vessels with a spiderlike appearance

    ii. Red, tender, _____ _____ that bleeds easily

    iii. Small fleshy bump with a smooth, pearly appearance, often with a(n) _____ center

---

*Pathological conditions discussed in the textbook but not listed in the student study guide will be covered in other workbook activities.

iv. Smooth, shiny bump that may look like a(n) _____ or _____

v. _____-like patch of skin, especially on the face, that is firm to the touch

vi. Bump that itches, bleeds, _____ _____, and then repeats the cycle and has not healed in _____ _____

vii. Change in the _____, _____, or _____ of a wart or mole

F. Treatment options for basal cell carcinoma

i. The most common treatment is _____ to destroy or remove the entire skin growth.

ii. Microscopically controlled surgery to remove skin cancer is very effective, with cure rates higher than _____ percent.

3. Squamous Cell Carcinoma

A. Squamous cell carcinoma is a malignant tumor that affects the _____ layer of the skin.

B. Risk factors for squamous cell carcinoma

i. _____ predisposition

ii. _____ pollution

iii. _____ to X-rays or other forms of radiation

iv. Exposure to _____

C. Signs and symptoms of squamous cell carcinoma

i. A(n) _____ _____, growth, or bump that is small, firm, reddened, nodular, coned, or flat

ii. A lesion with a(n) _____ or crusted surface or growth that is located on the face, _____, neck, hands, or arms

iii. Occasionally on the _____, _____, _____, or _____

D. Treatment options for squamous cell carcinoma

i. _____ removal of the tumor, including removal of the skin _____ the tumor

ii. _____ shaving to remove small tumors

iii. _____ _____ if broad areas of skin are removed

iv. _____ treatment

4. Malignant Melanoma

A. Malignant melanoma originates in the _____ of the skin.

B. Abnormal cellular growth often occurs in the melanocytes of a preexisting _____.

C. Malignant melanoma can be identified using the _____ rule.

    i. _____

    ii. _____ irregularity

    iii. _____ variegation

    iv. _____ greater than 6 mm

    v. _____ above the surrounding tissue

D. Treatment

    i. Early _____ is key to successful treatment.

    ii. The outlook is poor for those with _____ lesions.

5. Acne Vulgaris

A. Acne vulgaris occurs when oil and _____ _____ cells clog the skin's pores.

B. It most often affects _____, with more than 85 percent of them developing at least a mild form.

C. Signs and symptoms of acne vulgaris

    i. Skin blemishes are often _____ and _____.

    ii. With a mild case of acne, only _____ and _____ may be present.

    iii. Severe acne can mean hundreds of _____ or _____ that can cover the face, neck, chest, and back.

    iv. _____ _____ are pimples that are large, deep, and can leave scars on the skin.

D. Treatment options for acne vulgaris

    i. The _____ of the acne will determine the most useful and beneficial treatment.

    ii. Treatment may include _____ and gels applied to the skin as well as oral antibiotics.

6. Alopecia

A. Alopecia is _____ or _____ of hair.

B. The most common form is _____-_____ _____, also known as androgenic alopecia.

C. Alopecia areata causes _____ of baldness that come and go.

D. Signs and symptoms of alopecia

    i. Alopecia areata: Patches of baldness about the size of a(n) _____ _____

    ii. Androgenic alopecia: A set pattern of hair loss that starts with a(n) _____ hairline, followed by thinning of the hair on the _____ and temples

     iii. Women's hair gradually thins with _____, but women tend to lose hair only from the _____ of the head.

  E. Treatment options for alopecia

     i. Drugs and _____ can be rubbed on the scalp.

     ii. Shampoos and formulas are available for _____ _____ to the scalp.

     iii. Hair transplants help with the _____ of hair loss.

7. Cellulitis

  A. Cellulitis is a(n) _____ infection below the surface of the skin.

  B. Risk factors include diabetes and a(n) _____ immune system.

  C. Signs and symptoms of cellulitis

     i. Erythema, _____, swelling, and _____

     ii. Fever and _____ accompanying an infection

  D. Treatment options for cellulitis

     i. _____ and oral antibiotics are administered.

     ii. Severe cases may require _____ antibiotics.

8. Contact Dermatitis

  A. Contact dermatitis is a(n) _____ _____ of the skin caused by irritating substances.

  B. Signs and symptoms of contact dermatitis

     i. _____ and _____ skin

     ii. Vesicles (_____ _____) and rash

     iii. _____ and _____

     iv. _____ in the case of serious allergic reactions

  C. Treatments options for contact dermatitis

     i. _____ (anti-allergy medicines)

     ii. _____ _____ (creams to reduce inflammation)

     iii. _____ _____ (oral medications)

9. Calluses and Corns

  A. Calluses and corns are excessive growths of the _____ _____ layer of the epidermis that often occur on the hands and feet.

  B. They can be caused by physical _____ _____ or by other factors, such as ill-fitting shoes and hands being unprotected during manual labor.

  C. Signs and symptoms of a callus

     i. A callus is an area of _____ _____ that does not have an identifiable border.

ii. It may appear _____-_____, _____, or even
_____.

iii. It may be painless or may feel _____, throb, or burn.

D. Signs and symptoms of a corn

   i. A corn has a(n) _____ _____ and various textures.

   ii. Corns appear most commonly on the _____.

   iii. They may be hard or soft and are generally _____.

E. Treatment options for calluses and corns

   i. Treatment is necessary only if calluses and corns become _____ or
burdensome.

   ii. Placing bandages to reduce _____ and applying lotions or _____
to soften corns or calluses can be helpful.

10. Decubitus Ulcers

A. A decubitus ulcer is also called a(n) _____ _____ or a(n)
_____.

B. A decubitus ulcer typically occurs when _____ _____ is maintained
on a specific area of the skin.

C. Common locations include the coccyx, _____, heels, _____,
shoulders, _____, and back of the head.

D. Signs and symptoms: Four stages of a decubitus ulcer

   i. Stage I: _____ area on the skin that does not blanch (turn white) when
pressed.

   ii. Stage II: The skin has a(n) _____ or a(n) _____
_____. The area around the site may be red and irritated.

   iii. Stage III: The skin looks like a(n) _____ with damage to the tissue below
the skin.

   iv. Stage IV: The wound becomes so deep that there is damage to the tissue beneath the
_____ _____, including damage to _____ and muscle.

E. Treatment options for decubitus ulcers

   i. Treatment begins by relieving pressure through the use of _____ surfaces
and _____.

   ii. Decubitus ulcers are typically _____, which means cleaned of all toxins, and
then medicated and covered with special dressings to help in healing.

11. Eczema

A. Eczema is also called _____ _____.

B. It is a chronic skin condition caused by a(n) _____ _____ on the skin.

C. _____ tends to play a role.

D. Signs and symptoms of eczema

   i. Red and _____ skin caused by scaling, _____, and rashes

E. Treatment options for eczema

   i. Weeping lesions are treated with _____ _____ and dressings.

   ii. Severe cases and dry, scaly lesions may be treated with mild anti-itch _____ or low-potency topical _____.

   iii. Very severe cases may require _____ _____ and _____ _____ (TIMs).

12. Folliculitis

A. Folliculitis is an infection or inflammation of the _____ _____.

B. It most often appears in areas that become irritated by _____ or by the rubbing of clothes, or where follicles and pores are blocked by _____ and _____.

C. Common sites include the _____, the _____, under the arms, and on the legs.

D. Signs and symptoms of folliculitis

   i. A(n) _____ rash

   ii. Raised, red, often _____-filled lesions around hair follicles

   iii. _____ that occur in areas with a high concentration of hair follicles

   iv. _____ at the site of the rash and pimples

E. Treatment options for folliculitis

   i. Taking steps to minimize _____ to the hair follicles by avoiding clothes that rub against the skin

   ii. Shaving with a(n) _____ _____ instead of a razor blade

   iii. Keeping the skin clean using soap and water and _____ _____

   iv. Application of _____ _____

13. Hirsutism

A. Hirsutism is a condition of thick abnormal _____ _____ that affects men and women; _____ are more commonly affected.

B. Signs and symptoms of hirsutism

   i. Thick and _____ hair growth

   ii. Often linked to _____ disorders, such as problems with the ovaries or _____ glands

C. Treatment options for hirsutism

   i. Removing unwanted hair by shaving, _____, waxing, or using depilatory _____

ii. _____ and laser hair removal for more permanent hair removal

iii. _____-blocking medications

14. Keloids

A. Keloids typically appear following _____ or a(n) _____ but may also appear spontaneously after inflammation.

B. Signs and symptoms of keloids

i. Skin blemishes can appear _____ and raised and red or _____ in color.

ii. They often have a(n) _____-like appearance.

iii. Keloids also tend to be _____, bothersome, and _____ to the touch.

C. Treatment options for keloids

i. Common treatment includes _____ injections, surgery, and laser removal.

ii. Additional forms of treatment include _____, _____ injections, and application of _____ sheets.

15. Pediculosis

A. Pediculosis is a(n) _____ by eggs, larvae, or adult lice.

B. Forms of pediculosis include *Pediculus humanus capitis* (_____ _____), *Pediculus humanus corporis* (_____ _____), and *Phthirus pubis* (_____ _____).

C. Signs and symptoms of pediculosis

i. The most common symptom with all types of lice is _____.

ii. Head lice tend to cause itching on the back of the _____ or around the _____.

iii. Itching around the _____ is an indication of pubic lice.

iv. Body lice tend to travel to the body to feed on _____ and then return to _____.

D. Treatment options for pediculosis

i. Prescription and nonprescription medications are available, such as medicated shampoos and _____ rinses.

ii. Special combs are available to help remove _____ (lice eggs) from hair.

16. Psoriasis

A. Psoriasis affects an estimated _____ million Americans.

B. The condition has _____ and _____ characteristics.

C. It is thought to be caused by a buildup of _____ _____ cells that, rather than shed off, pile up and form _____ patches.

D. Signs and symptoms of psoriasis

    i. Psoriasis episodes may include redness, itching, and _____, dry silvery _____ on the skin.

    ii. _____ can be gradual or abrupt.

    iii. _____ have been attributed to infection, obesity, and lack of sunlight, as well as sunburn, stress, poor health, and cold climate.

    iv. When the case is severe and widespread, large quantities of _____ can be lost, causing _____ and severe secondary infections that can be serious.

E. Treatment options for psoriasis

    i. Common treatments include analgesics, sedation, _____ _____, retinoids, and antibiotics.

    ii. Mild cases are treated at home with _____ medications.

    iii. Severe lesions may require _____ for proper treatment.

17. Rosacea

A. Rosacea is a disorder primarily of the _____ _____.

B. It is often characterized by _____ and _____.

C. Signs and symptoms of rosacea

    i. _____ on the cheeks, nose, chin, or forehead

    ii. Small visible _____ _____ on the face, _____ on the face, and watery or irritated eyes

    iii. Over time, _____ that becomes ruddier and more persistent.

D. Treatment options for rosacea

    i. Therapies and medications are available to treat the symptoms, such as _____ antibiotic or cortisone-based _____.

    ii. Avoiding extreme _____ and temperature changes, reducing _____ intake, and use of _____ can help prevent or mitigate rosacea outbreaks.

18. Scabies

A. Scabies is a highly _____ disorder of the skin caused by the scabies mite or human _____ _____.

B. It is spread by _____ _____, such as shaking hands, sleeping together, or close contact with infected articles such as clothing, bedding, or towels.

C. Signs and symptoms of scabies

    i. A very small _____ blister

    ii. Intense _____ and a red _____ that occurs around the area

D. Treatment options for scabies

    i. Application of a lotion or cream with a 6–10 percent concentration of

        _____

    ii. _____ and _____ to relieve itching

19. Seborrheic Dermatitis

    A. Seborrheic dermatitis is a(n) _____ condition of the sebaceous or oil glands caused by an increase in _____.

    B. It is most common in infants and children and is frequently known as _____ _____.

    C. Signs and symptoms of seborrheic dermatitis

        i. Yellow or white scales that attach to the _____ _____

        ii. Thick or patchy crusts on the _____

        iii. Itching or soreness, as well as _____

    D. Treatment options for seborrheic dermatitis

        i. Application of low-strength _____

        ii. Shampooing the scalp daily with _____ _____

20. Tinea

    A. Tinea is a(n) _____ infection of the skin.

    B. It can appear _____ on the body.

    C. If the fungus is on the head, it is called _____ _____.

    D. Fungus on the feet is known as _____ _____, or athlete's foot.

    E. Fungus in the genital area is referred to as _____ _____, or, more commonly, _____ _____.

    F. Signs and symptoms of tinea

        i. A ring, often with _____, red, scaly _____

    G. Treatment options for tinea

        i. Tinea is treated with antifungal _____ or oral antifungal agents.

21. Urticaria

    A. Urticaria is better known as _____.

    B. It is caused by acute _____ to medications, food, or environmental stimuli.

    C. A major concern is that it can obstruct the _____ _____ in a severe reaction known as _____.

    D. Signs and symptoms of urticaria

        i. It occurs as _____ areas of pink, itchy, swollen patches of skin.

        ii. _____ and _____ sensations are common.

iii. Hives may vary in size from the diameter of a(n) _____ _____ to the diameter of a cereal bowl.

iv. Many times, the hives may _____, forming an even larger area of irritation and swelling.

E. Treatment options for urticaria

    i. Removal of the _____ _____

    ii. Treatment with _____ and _____

22. Vitiligo

A. Vitiligo is also known as _____.

B. It is a disorder that causes white patches and large areas of decreased _____ to form on the skin.

C. Patches form because of the destruction of _____.

D. Signs and symptoms of vitiligo

    i. It is marked by the early or premature _____ or whitening of body hair or by the depigmentation of skin or _____ membranes.

    ii. It begins to appear on the neck, _____, elbows, genitals, _____, or knees.

E. Treatment options for vitiligo

    i. Treatment is often aimed at _____ out skin tone and color.

    ii. _____ and _____ lotions may be used to even out the skin tone.

    iii. Medical treatments may include the use of _____ _____ therapy as well as topical ultraviolet therapy.

    iv. _____ _____, as well as a form of tattooing called _____, may also be successful.

23. Verrucae (Warts)

A. Verrucae is an infection caused by viruses in the _____ _____ (HPV) family.

B. Warts can grow on all parts of the body, including the _____, the inside of the mouth, the genitals, and the _____ _____.

C. A common wart is the _____ wart, which occurs on the soles of the feet.

D. Signs and symptoms of warts

    i. The _____ and _____ of a wart will vary with its location.

    ii. Warts may appear _____ or _____ and may vary in color from flesh-toned to red, pink, or white.

    iii. Warts may also appear as raised or _____ _____ _____.

E. Treatment options for warts

    i. Over-the-counter topical medications that contain _____ _____

    ii. _____, which means freezing the wart

    iii. Various _____ _____

    iv. In severe cases, _____ _____

V. Skin Care Treatments

  1. Botox

    A. This popular procedure is indicated for reducing _____.

    B. A very small, diluted amount of the toxin _____ _____ is injected into the wrinkle lines.

    C. The procedure is usually repeated every _____ to _____ months.

    D. Temporary side effects include headaches, bruising, and _____ _____.

  2. Chemical Peels

    A. Light chemical peel

      i. The purpose of this treatment is to reduce the size of _____, make the skin appear _____, and produce more _____ in the skin.

      ii. During a light chemical peel, only the _____ layer of the skin is stripped.

      iii. The procedure is completed in about an hour and leaves the skin _____ _____ for a short time.

    B. Medium chemical peel

      i. The purpose of this treatment is to _____ _____, resulting in much smoother skin than is achieved with a light chemical peel.

      ii. This treatment strips the _____ _____ and some underlying cells, causing collagen and elastin to be stimulated.

      iii. Recovery from a medium chemical peel can take up to _____ days because of the peeling, swelling, and redness that occur after treatment.

    C. Deep chemical peel

      i. This aggressive treatment can affect the layers of skin down to the _____ layer.

      ii. It is aimed at reducing all _____ of _____ in the face, with the exception of certain areas.

      iii. The healing process includes _____ pain.

      iv. _____ medications are required.

  3. Laser Resurfacing

    A. Short, pulsated _____ _____ are used to vaporize damaged or troublesome areas of the skin.

B. Full-face laser resurfacing takes approximately _____ to _____ hours.

C. Partial-face resurfacing takes _____ to _____ minutes.

D. Resurfacing results in the stimulation and production of new _____ and skin cells.

E. _____ ointment and sterile _____ are applied to reduce the incidence of infection.

4. Microdermabrasion

A. Microdermabrasion involves removing the top layer of _____ _____ cells.

B. Tiny _____ are used with abrasion and suction devices to produce healthier-looking skin.

C. This non-_____ and non-_____ approach is appealing to many patients who do not wish to pursue more aggressive skin-freshening treatments.

APPLIED PRACTICE

1. Using information found in the textbook, fill out the following table regarding integumentary disorders.

Disease	Symptoms	Treatment
Furuncles/carbuncles		
Herpes simplex		

(continued)

Disease	Symptoms	Treatment
Herpes zoster (shingles)		
Impetigo		

2. Label the structures of the skin.

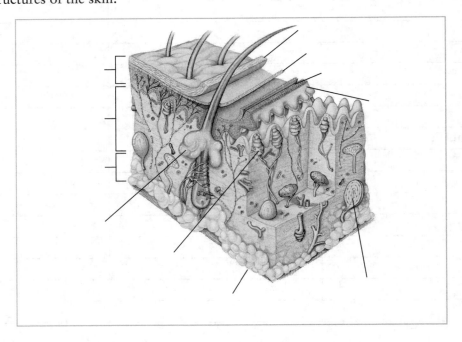

LEARNING ACTIVITY: TRUE/FALSE

Indicate whether the following statements are true or false by placing a T or an F on the line that precedes each statement.

1. _____ Keratin is a protective pigment used to guard the skin against ultraviolet rays.
2. _____ Sudoriferous glands secret sweat.
3. _____ The epidermis is divided into four layers.
4. _____ The reticular layer is the third layer of the epidermis.
5. _____ The body loses about 0.5 liters of fluid a day through perspiration.
6. _____ An abnormal mole is known as a malignant lesion.
7. _____ There are four stages of decubitus ulcers.
8. _____ Alopecia areata is another term for male-pattern baldness and is hereditary.
9. _____ Scabies is a form of tinea.
10. _____ Urticaria is another word for hives.

CRITICAL THINKING

Answer the following questions to the best of your ability. Use the textbook as a reference.

1. As you are helping a geriatric patient get into a gown for an examination, you notice that she has a dime-sized mole with an irregular border on her back. You realize that the patient likely cannot see it and may be unaware of it. Would you mention it to the patient or only to the physician? State the reason for your answer.

_____

_____

_____

_____

_____

2. Utilize Internet search engines to locate a reputable site that provides pictures of various skin conditions, including lice. Draw a picture of head lice and state how this condition is treated.

_____

_____

_____

_____

3. What possible advice could you give to a patient who has had a skin cancer removed today and works daily as a lifeguard in the sun?

_____

_____

_____

_____

_____

RESEARCH ACTIVITY

Use Internet search engines to research the following topic and write a brief description of what you find. It is important to use reputable websites.

1. Visit the Skin Cancer Foundation website, at www.skincancer.org. After reviewing the website, answer the following questions.

   a. What prevention information do you find most interesting. Why?
   b. Read the section Skin Cancer Facts. Which of the facts listed do you find most surprising?
   c. What can you do to further reduce your risk of developing skin cancer?

   _____
   _____
   _____
   _____
   _____

CHAPTER 22
The Skeletal System

STUDENT STUDY GUIDE

Use the following guide to assist in your learning of the concepts from the chapter.

I. Bones and Their Classification

1. Bone Classification (List six classifications of bones.)

    A. _____

    B. _____

    C. _____

    D. _____

    E. _____

    F. _____

2. Functions of Bones

    A. Bones provide _____, _____, and the framework of the body.

    B. They provide _____ for the body's internal organs.

    C. They serve as a storage place for _____ _____, _____, and _____.

    D. They play an important role in the formation of blood cells as _____ takes place in the _____ _____.

    E. They provide an area for the attachment of _____ muscle.

    F. They help make movement possible through _____.

3. Structures of Long Bones (List the term that matches each definition.)

    A. _____—the ends of a developing bone

    B. _____—the shaft of the long bone

    C. _____—the membrane that forms the covering of bones, except at their articular surfaces

    D. _____ _____—the dense, hard layer of bone tissue

    E. _____ _____—the narrow space or cavity throughout the length of the diaphysis

F. _____—the tough connective tissue membrane lining the medullary canal that contains the bone marrow

G. _____ (spongy) _____—the reticular tissue that makes up most of the volume of bone.

4. Bone Markings (List eight markings from Table 22-2.)

A. _____

B. _____

C. _____

D. _____

E. _____

F. _____

G. _____

H. _____

II. Joints and Movement

1. A(n) _____, also called a joint, is the point where two bones connect.

2. Joints are always classified according to the _____ of _____ they permit.

3. Types of Joints (List three types.)

A. _____

B. _____

C. _____

III. The Axial Skeleton

1. The axial skeleton consists of the skull, _____, _____, vertebrae, sacrum, and _____.

2. Five Vertebral Regions (List the regions.)

A. _____, consisting of the first 7 vertebrae

B. _____, the 12 middle vertebrae

C. _____ _____, the lowest 5 vertebrae

D. _____

E. _____, or tailbone

3. The ribs form a protective _____ that houses the _____, _____, and other vital components of the human body.

A. The rib cage consists of _____ pairs of ribs, which are divided into three categories: _____, _____, and _____ ribs.

IV. The Appendicular Skeleton

1. The appendicular skeleton is responsible for _____.

2. It consists of the upper and lower _____ as well as the clavicles, the _____, and the _____ girdle.

3. Upper Extremity Bones (List six bones.)

A. _____

B. _____

C. _____

D. _____

E. _____

F. _____

4. Lower Extremity Bones (List seven bones.)

A. _____

B. _____

C. _____

D. _____

E. _____

F. _____

G. _____

5. Bones of the Pelvic Girdle (List five bones.)

A. _____

B. _____

C. _____

D. _____

E. _____

V. Common Pathology Associated with the Skeletal System*

1. Scoliosis

A. Scoliosis is an abnormal _____ curvature of the spine.

B. It is often diagnosed in toddlers, _____, and adolescents.

C. Signs and symptoms of scoliosis

i. A scoliotic spine appears to have a(n) _____ or _____ shape.

ii. Those afflicted with scoliosis may often appear as if either their _____ or their _____ are uneven.

---

*Pathological conditions discussed in the textbook but not listed in the student study guide will be covered in other workbook activities.

D. Treatment options for scoliosis

    i. _____ braces

    ii. Physical _____

    iii. _____

2. Lordosis

  A. Lordosis is an exaggerated _____ curvature of the _____ spine.

  B. Signs and symptoms of lordosis

    i. It is commonly diagnosed in adults who are _____ and carry excess weight in their abdomen, as well as _____ women.

    ii. The most glaring sign is a severe inward curvature of the _____ _____.

  C. Treatment options for lordosis

    i. Treatment depends on the patient's overall _____ and age, as well as the severity of the condition.

    ii. The goal of treatment is to stop the _____ of the curvature and prevent spinal deformity.

    iii. A patient can slow the progression by losing excess _____ _____ and doing physical therapy to help maintain and _____ the core of the body.

3. Kyphosis

  A. Kyphosis is an exaggeration of the _____ _____ of the spine.

  B. Signs and symptoms of kyphosis

    i. Rounded appearance of the _____ back

    ii. Fatigue, _____ back pain, and either a tender or _____ feeling within the spine

    iii. In severe cases, _____ of _____

  C. Treatment options for kyphosis

    i. Physical therapy focusing on the _____ and _____ of the spine is common.

4. Bursitis

  A. Bursitis is inflammation of the bursa, which are small sacs of _____ around the _____.

  B. Bursitis generally results from overuse and _____ to joints.

  C. It occurs most frequently in the elbow, _____, _____, and hip.

  D. Signs and symptoms of bursitis

    i. Joint pain and _____ mobility

    ii. Swelling and _____ surrounding the joint

E. Treatment options for bursitis

    i. Treatments include rest, _____ medication, steroid _____, aspiration of excess _____ from the bursa, and antibiotics.

    ii. _____ _____ may also increase and promote and restore range of motion and movement of the joint.

5. Carpal Tunnel Syndrome

  A. Carpal tunnel syndrome occurs when pressure is placed on the _____ _____.

  B. _____ movements involving the wrist may contribute to the condition.

  C. Certain conditions increase the risk of carpal tunnel syndrome, including _____, diabetes, and _____ arthritis.

  D. Signs and symptoms of carpal tunnel syndrome

    i. Pain, _____, and _____ weakness

    ii. Hands and fingers feeling tingly, _____, and swollen

    iii. Pain and _____ radiating up the _____

  E. Treatment options for carpal tunnel syndrome

    i. Application of _____ _____ at night for several weeks

    ii. Hot and cold _____

    iii. Resting the _____ and _____ and avoiding the activities that trigger pain

    iv. Proper _____

    v. NSAIDs to relieve pain and reduce _____

    vi. _____ (sometimes called "water pills")

    vii. Injections of _____

    viii. A surgical procedure to decrease pressure on the _____ _____

6. Dislocations

  A. A dislocation occurs when a bone _____ out, or _____ from, the joint.

  B. _____ _____ on a joint may cause one of the bones that meet at that joint to become dislocated.

  C. Usually the joint _____ and ligaments tear when a dislocation occurs, and often the _____ are injured.

  D. Signs and symptoms of dislocations

    i. Bones appearing to be out of place or _____

    ii. _____ skin around the joint

    iii. Limited _____

        iv. Joint appearing bruised or _____

        v. Intense _____

  E. Treatment options for dislocations

        i. A procedure known as _____ is used to align and reposition the joint.

        ii. Pain relievers and _____ medications are often prescribed.

        iii. _____ _____ may be given for reduction procedures that are difficult and must be performed in an operating room.

7. Osteoporosis

  A. Osteoporosis is characterized by progressive loss of _____ _____ and thinning of bone _____.

  B. It affects more than _____ million Americans, mostly _____.

  C. Those with osteoporosis are subject to increased _____ potential, especially in the hips, _____, and wrists.

  D. Signs and symptoms of osteoporosis

        i. Common signs of osteoporosis are decreased _____ and a stooped _____.

        ii. _____ can be an indicator.

        iii. Additional signs and symptoms include back pain and _____ _____ throughout the body.

  E. Treatment options for osteoporosis

        i. Treatment is aimed at preventing more _____ loss, but the disease itself cannot be _____.

  F. Prevention methods for osteoporosis

        i. _____ _____ that are rich in vitamins and minerals

        ii. Weight-bearing _____ to strengthen weakened bones

        iii. _____ and _____ supplements added to the diet

        iv. Medications to help preserve _____ and decrease bone _____

8. Hallux Valgus

  A. Hallux valgus is the enlargement of the _____ _____ of the joint at the base of the big toe.

  B. It is most commonly known as a(n) _____.

  C. Signs and symptoms of hallux valgus

        i. _____ skin surrounds the _____ joint of the big toe.

        ii. The joint may be filled with _____ and feel _____ to the touch.

  D. Treatment options for hallux valgus

        i. Properly _____ _____ should be worn.

    ii. Proper _____ and _____ of the joint should be considered.

    iii. Pain medications and _____ medications may be used.

    iv. Foot _____ may be required for severe cases.

9. Hammertoe

  A. Hammertoe is a condition in which the toe bends into a hammer shape or claw shape because of the _____ _____ of the proximal interphalangeal joint.

  B. It may also be hereditary or result from a(n) _____ _____ to the foot.

  C. Signs and symptoms of hammertoe

    i. Pain and visible joint _____

  D. Treatment options for hammertoe

    i. Analgesics, _____, and specially designed _____

    ii. In severe cases, _____ _____ of the toe

10. Rickets

  A. Rickets is an early childhood disease caused by deficiencies of _____, vitamin _____, and _____.

  B. Signs and symptoms of rickets

    i. _____ and _____ of the bones

    ii. Increased likelihood of bone _____

    iii. Impaired _____ associated with decreased height and muscle _____

    iv. Decreased _____ _____ and weakness

  C. Treatment options for rickets

    i. Correcting vitamin deficiency by increasing _____ and _____ intake

    ii. Comfort measures, including _____ and application of_____ and _____

11. Osteomalacia

  A. Osteomalacia is adult onset of _____.

  B. Causes include _____, liver disease, _____ _____, and side effects associated with _____ medications.

  C. Signs and symptoms of osteomalacia

    i. Bone _____

    ii. _____ legs

    iii. Frequent _____

  D. Treatment options for osteomalacia

    i. Increasing _____ and _____ intake

    ii. Comfort measures to relieve _____

APPLIED PRACTICE

1. Using information found in the textbook, fill in the following table. Compare similarities and differences between the different types of arthritis.

Type of Arthritis	Symptoms	Treatment
Arthritis		
Osteoarthritis		
Rheumatoid arthritis		
Gouty arthritis		

2. Refer to the textbook and label the following features of the skeletal system.

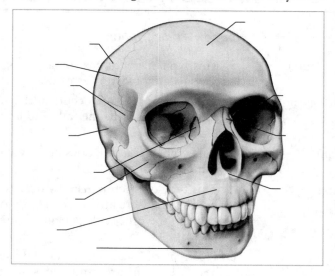

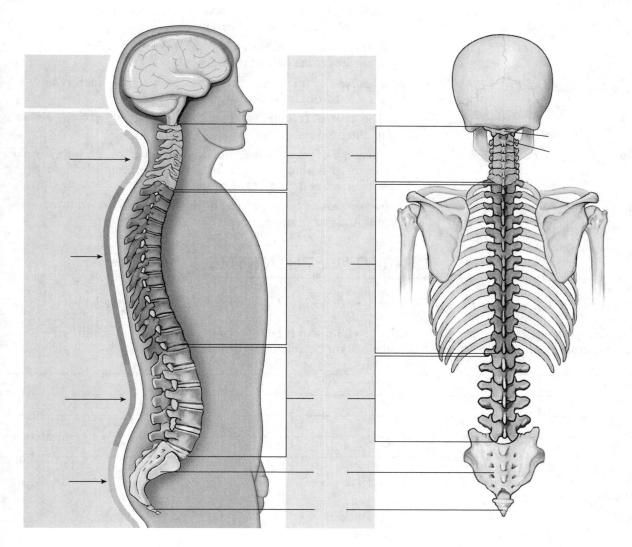

LEARNING ACTIVITY: MATCHING

Match the name of each fracture with the correct description.

1. _____ Closed (simple)

2. _____ Open (compound)

3. _____ Comminuted

4. _____ Transverse

5. _____ Greenstick

6. _____ Spiral

7. _____ Colles

8. _____ Pott

9. _____ Compression

10. _____ Epiphyseal

a. This type of fracture is spread along the length of a bone and is produced by twisting stresses.

b. This type of fracture occurs in the vertebrae after severe stress, such as when someone falls and lands with a significant amount of force.

c. This type of fracture does not involve a break in the skin. It is completely internal.

d. This type of fracture usually occurs in young children, whose bones are still relatively soft. Only one side of the shaft is broken; the other side is bent, similar to breaking a green plant stick.

e. This type of fracture is commonly seen in children in areas of bone where the growth plate is undergoing calcification (a hardening process of the calcium in the bones) and the chondrocytes (cartilage-forming cells) are dying.

f. This type of fracture occurs in the ankle and affects both bones of the lower leg (the tibia and fibula).

g. This type of fracture is dangerous because the fracture has broken through the skin.

h. This type of fracture is a break in the shaft of the bone across its longitudinal axis.

i. This type of fracture is frequently the result of reaching forward to stop or cushion a fall. This fracture is exemplified by a break in the distal portion of the radius.

j. In this type of fracture, part of the bone is shattered into a multitude of bony fragments.

CRITICAL THINKING

Answer the following questions to the best of your ability. Use the textbook as a reference.

1. If a patient has an injury to the skeletal system and is being seen in the medical office for an appointment, how might the medical assistant be able to assist this patient?

   _____

   _____

   _____

   _____

2. List the risk factors associated with osteoporosis and write a profile that depicts a patient who has the disease.

_____

_____

_____

_____

_____

RESEARCH ACTIVITY

Use Internet search engines to research the following topic and write a brief description of what you find. It is important to use reputable websites.

1. Conduct further research on two conditions/diseases of the skeletal system. These conditions can be ones that are found in the textbook or others that you may be interested in learning more about. Write an essay about what you learned, including how the disease presents itself, the possible cause of the condition, the treatment, and technology that may be available in the future to address the condition/disease. Be sure to cite your sources.

_____

_____

_____

_____

_____

CHAPTER 23
The Muscular System

STUDENT STUDY GUIDE

Use the following guide to assist in your learning of the concepts from the chapter.

I. Functions of Muscle (List five functions.)

1. _____

2. _____

3. _____

4. _____

5. _____

II. Types of Muscle Tissue

1. Muscle tissue has the ability to _____, which produces the movement of _____ and _____ body parts.

2. Muscles are composed of 75 percent _____; 20 percent _____; and 5 percent _____, lipids, inorganic _____, and nonprotein _____ compounds.

3. Skeletal Muscle

   A. Skeletal muscle is called _____ or striated (which means _____ in appearance).

   B. Skeletal muscle helps us perform skeletal movement because it is _____ to the _____ of the body.

   C. Skeletal muscle is responsible for _____ movements, meaning that it is under _____ _____.

4. Smooth Muscle

   A. Smooth muscle is _____ muscle.

   B. It is found in the body's _____ (organs).

   C. It is not _____ controlled, meaning it is not controlled by _____ thought.

5. Cardiac Muscle
   A. Cardiac muscle is found in the _____.
   B. Cardiac muscle cells are both _____ and involuntary.
   C. Cardiac muscle tissues are supplied with _____ _____ that
      carry messages to and from the _____ _____ system.

III. Energy Production for Muscle
   1. Muscles use energy in the form of _____ _____, a type of chemical
      _____ created within the body's cells.
   2. This type of energy is needed for _____ or repeated muscular
      _____.
   3. There are two types of ATP: _____ and _____.
   4. Oxygen Debt and Muscle Fatigue
      A. Oxygen debt may occur when the skeletal muscles are used _____ for more
         than 1 or 2 _____.
      B. When oxygen is lacking, the body is unable to produce energy through _____
         means, and the _____ method of creating energy is activated.
      C. The body can use anaerobic energy for only about _____ _____.
      D. _____ _____ usually develops as a result of an accumulation of
         lactic acid.
      E. Accumulation of _____ _____ decreases the muscle's ability to
         contract.
         i. This causes the muscle to become incredibly _____, and muscles may
            _____.

IV. Structures of Skeletal Muscles
   1. Structures of Skeletal Muscles (List five structures; see Table 23-1.)
      A. _____
      B. _____
      C. _____
      D. _____
      E. _____
   2. Attachments to Skeletal Muscles
      A. The _____ is a muscle's attachment point to a bone that is primarily
         _____ or still.
      B. The _____ is the attachment point of the other end of that muscle to a bone
         that _____.

C. Muscles perform in groups according to three categories: _____ _____ or _____, _____, and _____.

V. Major Skeletal Groups

1. Muscles are often identified according to their _____ size, _____, shape, or number of _____ to the muscle.

2. Muscle Groups (List six groups of muscles, not specific muscles.)

   A. _____

   B. _____

   C. _____

   D. _____

   E. _____

   F. _____

VI. The Pathology of the Muscular System*

1. Atrophy

   A. Atrophy is loss of muscle _____ and _____ that occurs when muscles aren't used over a long period of time.

   B. It results from bed _____ and _____, and it can also be caused by malnutrition and _____.

   C. Signs and symptoms of atrophy

      i. _____ _____ of a muscle group

      ii. Extreme _____ and _____ associated with atrophic muscle groups

   D. Treatment options for atrophy

      i. Exercise, particularly _____ exercise of the immobilized muscle

      ii. Active exercise of _____ _____ to prevent atrophy

2. Fibromyalgia

   A. Fibromyalgia is characterized by musculoskeletal _____ and _____.

   B. It occurs more often in _____ than _____.

   C. Signs and symptoms of fibromyalgia

      i. _____ to _____ muscle pain and fatigue

      ii. _____ disorders

      iii. _____ bowel syndrome

---

*Pathological conditions discussed in the textbook but not listed in the student study guide will be covered in other workbook activities.

iv. Depression

v. Chronic _____

D. Treatment options for fibromyalgia

   i. There is _____ _____.

   ii. Emphasis is often placed on improving the patient's _____.

   iii. Medications prescribed include muscle _____, pain

   _____, antiinflammatory drugs, _____, and

   _____ drugs.

   iv. Other treatments frequently employed include _____, acupuncture,

   acupressure, _____ techniques, and massage.

3. Ganglion Cyst

   A. A ganglion cyst is a(n) _____ saclike _____ or fluid-filled cyst.

   B. Typically the cysts develop over a(n) _____ or _____.

   C. Signs and symptoms of ganglion cysts

      i. Often _____

      ii. Very _____ if its location causes it to press on a(n) _____

      iii. Possible _____

   D. Treatment options for ganglion cysts

      i. Treatment is not necessary if a cyst is _____ and painless.

      ii. _____ drugs can be used to reduce swelling and _____.

      iii. Often _____ is performed.

4. Lyme Disease

   A. Lyme disease is caused by the _____ _____ bacterium.

   B. The bacterium is transmitted through the _____ of an infected

   _____.

   C. Signs and symptoms of Lyme disease

      i. Round _____ rash

      ii. Headache, _____, neck stiffness, and _____

   D. Treatment options for Lyme disease

      i. If detected early, _____ _____ is possible.

      ii. Antibiotics prescribed include erythromycin, _____, or

      _____.

      iii. If not detected early, Lyme disease can result in _____,

      _____, _____, and nervous system disorders.

5. Muscular Dystrophy
    A. MD progressively _____ and causes degeneration of the body's
        _____ muscles, thereby reducing control of _____.
    B. Types of MD (List nine types.)
        i. _____
        ii. _____
        iii. _____
        iv. _____
        v. _____
        vi. _____
        vii. _____
        viii. _____
        ix. _____
    C. Signs and symptoms of MD
        i. General signs and symptoms that are common in all forms and are specific to muscle
            groups include muscle _____, loss of _____, and
            immobility.
        ii. More varied signs and symptoms include difficulty _____ and frequent
            _____, delayed development of _____
            _____, and mental _____.
    D. Treatment options for MD
        i. There is no _____ for any form of MD.
        ii. _____ _____ is implemented to sustain and build muscle
            strength and overall _____.
        iii. _____ devices provide support.
        iv. _____ _____ is especially important for those whose
            respiratory muscles and overall respiratory system is affected by the disease.
        v. Medications often prescribed include _____, _____, and
            _____.

6. Myasthenia Gravis (MG)
    A. MG is a chronic _____ neuromuscular disease.
    B. Its Latin origin means "_____ _____ weakness."
    C. It most commonly occurs in _____ _____ women and older
        _____ but can occur at any age.

D. Signs and symptoms of myasthenia gravis

    i. The primary symptom is _____ _____.

    ii. Muscle weakness increases during periods of _____ and improves after periods of _____.

E. Treatment options for myasthenia gravis

    i. There is no _____ for MG.

    ii. Medications may be given to decrease the production of _____.

    iii. Medications to improve _____ _____ as well as neuromuscular _____ are also prescribed.

7. Tendonitis

A. Tendonitis is often caused by excessive and _____ _____.

B. Inflammation occurs when the _____ _____ of the tendon begin to tear.

C. List the areas commonly associated with tendonitis.

    i. _____

    ii. _____

    iii. _____

    iv. _____

D. Signs and symptoms of tendonitis

    i. _____ and _____ commonly surround the affected area.

    ii. Burning sensations surround the _____ and inflamed _____.

E. Treatment options for tendonitis

    i. Tendonitis should lessen with _____ over time.

    ii. Support and protect the tendons by _____ any areas of the tendon that are being _____ during use.

    iii. It is important to _____ up the tendon, reduce the _____, and minimize any _____.

    iv. _____ _____, including exercises to increase range of motion, has proven to be very beneficial.

8. Tetanus

A. Tetanus is an infectious disease caused by the bacterium _____ _____.

B. It usually enters the body through a(n) _____, a cut, or a(n) _____ wound.

C. This bacterium is commonly found in _____, _____, and manure.

D. Signs and symptoms of tetanus

    i. Profoundly painful _____ _____ all over the body

    ii. A(n) _____ _____ that results in the mouth being unable to open (lockjaw)

    iii. Difficulty _____ because of neck _____

    iv. Stiffness of the _____, _____, and back muscles

    v. _____

E. Treatment options for tetanus

    i. Prevention is best, through _____.

    ii. For an unvaccinated person, treatment includes the administration of _____, administration of _____, and vaccination.

APPLIED PRACTICE

1. Using the textbook, fill in the sections of the table below.

Disease/Injury	Symptoms	Treatment
Rotator cuff tears		
Shin splints		

Disease/Injury	Symptoms	Treatment
Sprains		
Strains		

2. Label the major muscles shown in the diagram below.

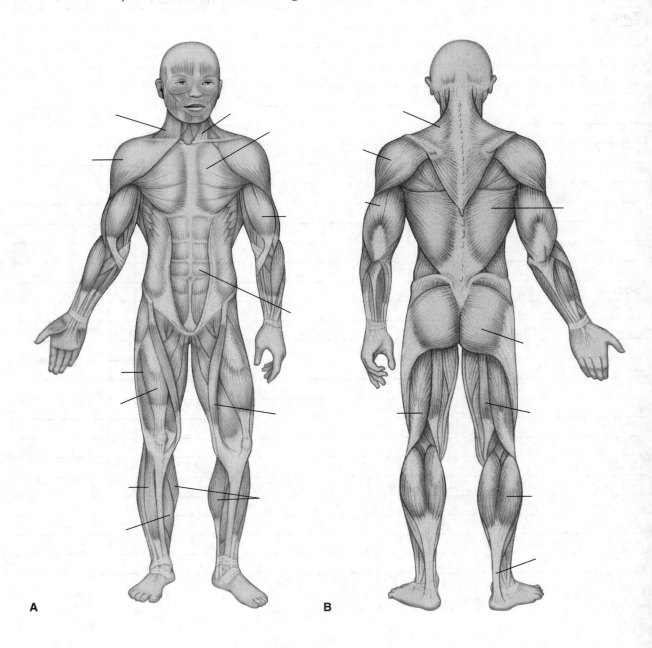

A

B

LEARNING ACTIVITY: FILL IN THE BLANK

Use the following list of words to fill in the blanks within the paragraph below. Use your textbook as reference.

circulatory   glycogen   nutrition
fascia   lengths   oxygen
fibers   muscles   shapes

The muscular system is composed of all the _____ within the body. Muscle fibers are made

of different _____ and _____ and vary in color from white to deep red. The

muscle _____ are held together by connective tissue. The connective tissue is held together

by a fibrous sheath called _____. Each fiber within a muscle also has its own nervous

system connection with a stored supply of energy in the form of _____. Muscle must be

supplied with proper _____ and _____ to perform properly. The muscular

system is well permeated by vessels from both the _____ system and the lymphatic system.

CRITICAL THINKING

Answer the following questions to the best of your ability. Use the textbook as a reference.

1. With children, why are injections usually given in the vastus lateralis muscle? When should the gluteus maximus muscle be used when giving an injection to an adult?

   _____

   _____

   _____

   _____

2. How does regular exercise help older adults stay healthy?

   _____

   _____

   _____

3. Christopher was working on his father's farm, planting crops and spreading manure as fertilizer. He didn't realize that he had an open cut on his hand while he was working. A few days later, he developed body spasms, and his jaw became locked. What is the likely diagnosis Christopher may be given by a physician? Could it have been prevented? Explain your answer.

   _____

   _____

   _____

   _____

RESEARCH ACTIVITY

Use Internet search engines to research the following topic and write a brief description of what you find. It is important to use reputable websites.

1. Conduct research on one of the various forms of muscular dystrophy. What are signs, symptoms, and treatments that are specific to the form of MD you have chosen? Include additional information about the disease that you find to be interesting. Be sure to cite your resources.

   _____

   _____

   _____

   _____

   _____

CHAPTER 24

The Nervous System

STUDENT STUDY GUIDE

Use the following guide to assist in your learning of the concepts from the chapter.

I. Sections and Functions of the Nervous System

    1. The central nervous system (CNS) includes the _____ and the _____ cord.

    2. The _____ _____ system is made up of nerves that connect the CNS to the other parts of the _____.

    3. Subsections of the peripheral nervous system (PNS) include the _____ nervous system and the _____ nervous system.

    4. Functions of the Nervous System

        A. It detects and interprets _____ _____.

        B. It uses that information to _____ _____ about how it is being received.

        C. It carries out _____ _____ based on the decisions made.

II. Structural Units of the Nervous System

    1. Nervous system tissue is made up of specialized _____ _____ called neurons and supporting tissue structures known as _____.

    2. Types of Neurons (List three types.)

        A. _____

        B. _____

        C. _____

    3. Nerve Fibers

        A. A nerve fiber is a single _____ process.

        B. The nerve fibers in the peripheral nervous system are wrapped in protective membranes called _____.

        C. Myelinated sheaths have both an inner sheath of myelin and an outer sheath, or neurilemma, composed of _____ _____.

        D. Schwann cells are needed for the process of _____ a damaged nerve fiber.

E. Nerve fibers of the _____ _____ system do not contain Schwann cells.

F. Damage to nerve fibers of the CNS is _____, whereas damage to a peripheral nerve can be _____.

4. Nerves

A. A nerve is a(n) _____ _____ of nerve fibers found outside the CNS.

B. Nerves are often categorized as _____ (conducting impulses to the CNS) or _____ (conducting impulses from the CNS to muscles, organs, and glands).

5. Tracts

A. A tract is a group of _____ _____ within the CNS.

B. Nerve fibers that are housed within the nerve tract must have the same _____, _____, and _____.

6. Nerve Impulses and Synapses

A. A nerve impulse begins with _____, which occurs at the receptor.

B. When the _____ is stimulated, it reacts by initiating a chemical change or _____.

C. When a receptor reacts to a stimulus, the resulting impulse is transmitted from the _____ _____ to other _____.

III. Central Nervous System

1. This portion of the nervous system receives impulses from the _____ _____, processes the _____, and responds with appropriate _____.

2. The brain and the spinal cord are divided into _____ matter and _____ matter.

A. Gray matter consists of _____ cell bodies and true _____.

B. White matter consists of the _____ nerve fibers.

3. The Brain

A. The brain is the _____ mass of nervous tissue in the body.

B. List the three membranes of the brain (innermost to outermost).

   i. _____

   ii. _____

   iii. _____

4. The Cerebrum

A. The cerebrum is the _____ portion of the mature brain.

B. It is divided into two mirror-image portions called _____

_____.

C. The outer covering of the cerebrum is called the _____ cortex.

D. List the lobes of the cerebral cortex.

    i. _____ lobe—deals with reasoning, personality and emotions, problem solving, planning, parts of speech, and movement.

    ii. _____ lobe—perceives stimuli related to touch, pain, temperature, and pressure; recognizes and differentiates size, shape, and color.

    iii. _____ lobe—perceives and recognizes auditory stimuli (hearing) and memory; interprets organizing and sequencing of items and events.

    iv. _____ lobe—primarily concerned with the aspects of vision; perceives and recognizes printed words.

5. Diencephalon

A. The _____ and _____ make up the diencephalon.

B. This portion of the brain serves as a(n) _____ _____ for all sensory impulses except for _____.

6. Brain Stem

A. The brain stem contains the midbrain, the _____, and the _____ oblongata.

B. These structures relay important information to the cerebrum, including _____, _____, and other _____ data.

7. Cerebellum

A. The cerebellum is the second-_____ portion of the brain.

B. It is located in the back of the skull, just above the _____ and below the _____.

C. It plays an important part in the coordination of _____ _____.

D. It is responsible for adjusting _____ _____ to automatically maintain _____.

8. Spinal Cord

A. The spinal cord extends from the base of the _____ _____ to the junction between the first and second _____ vertebrae.

B. It conducts _____ _____ from the rest of the body to the brain and sends _____ _____ from the brain to the rest of the body.

9. Cerebrospinal Fluid (CSF)

A. CSF is often considered to be the _____ of the nervous system.

B. Functions

    i. CSF serves as a(n) _____ to protect the brain and spinal cord.

    ii. It nourishes the brain and spinal cord with _____ and

    _____.

    iii. It acts as a vesicle to carry _____.

IV. Peripheral Nervous System

  1. The nerves of the PNS connect the CNS to sensory organs and to other organs of the body,

    _____, _____ vessels, and _____.

  2. Cranial and Spinal Nerves

    A. Cranial nerves originate in the _____ and are identified by

    _____ numerals.

    B. They are arranged in _____ pairs to each side of the brain and are named for the

    _____ or area of the body they serve.

    C. There are _____ pairs of spinal nerves that are connected to the spinal cord, and each pair

    is named for the region of the _____ _____ where it exists.

  3. Somatic Nervous System

    A. This division of the PNS is made up of nerves that connect to the _____

    muscles, the _____ organs, and the _____.

    B. It is called the "voluntary" nervous system because it connects to muscles and other

    structures that are under _____ _____ of the body.

    C. It is responsible for processing _____ information received from the

    _____, ears, _____, and touch.

  4. Autonomic Nervous System

    A. This division controls _____ bodily functions.

    B. Some functions under its control include _____ rate, the control of

    _____ _____ tissue, _____ secretion, sweating,

    and _____ blood pressure.

    C. It is divided into two counteracting systems that work together to maintain

    _____.

    D. Sympathetic division of the ANS

      i. The sympathetic division of the ANS is found in the spinal nerves of the

      _____ and _____ spine.

      ii. It is responsible for the "_____-or-flight" response, during which a

      person experiences increased _____ in conjunction with increases in

      _____ rate and other bodily _____.

E. Parasympathetic division of the ANS

    i. The first stages of the parasympathetic nervous system response are formed by _____ nerves and _____ nerves.

    ii. The response of the parasympathetic division has a(n) _____ and _____ effect.

    iii. The phrase used with this subsystem is "_____ and _____."

V. Common Pathology of the Nervous System*

  1. Alzheimer's Disease

    A. Alzheimer's disease is a progressive, _____ disease that attacks the brain and its cognitive function.

    B. More than _____ _____ people are affected with the disease.

    C. Signs and symptoms of Alzheimer's disease

       i. Inability to remember _____ events

       ii. Inability to _____ thoughts

       iii. _____ that becomes difficult to understand and follow

       iv. Decline in skills related to _____ and writing

       v. _____ changes

    D. Treatment options for Alzheimer's disease

       i. Medications may _____ the progression of the disease in the early stages.

       ii. Patients must continue to take medication throughout their _____ to avoid regression.

       iii. Older adults who maintain _____ _____ and engage in _____ stimulating activities may be less prone to develop Alzheimer's disease.

  2. Amyotrophic Lateral Sclerosis

    A. ALS is of unknown _____; heredity and _____ factors could be associated with the disease.

    B. It breaks down _____ neurons.

    C. Signs and symptoms of ALS

       i. Loss of control of _____ muscle movement, including that of the arms, legs, and trunk, is common.

       ii. Slurred _____; muscle _____; and difficulty _____, specifically chewing and swallowing, are common initial symptoms.

*Pathological conditions discussed in the textbook but not listed in the student study guide will be covered in other workbook activities.

      iii. Depending on the form of ALS, the loss of _____ _____

         (dementia) or sensory symptoms may occur.

  D. Treatment options for ALS

      i. There is no known _____.

      ii. Medications as well as _____, physical, and _____

        therapy can help to slow the _____ of symptoms.

3. Bell's Palsy

  A. Bell's palsy is weakness or _____ of the muscles that control

      _____ on one side of the face.

  B. It often has a(n) _____ onset.

  C. It is caused by damage to a(n) _____ _____, one of which runs

    beneath each ear to the muscles on the same side of the face.

  D. Signs and symptoms of Bell's palsy

      i. _____ paralysis of the face

      ii. Facial _____ and lack of expression on the afflicted side

      iii. Headaches, changes in _____, and excessive _____ or

         _____

  E. Treatment options for Bell's palsy

      i. _____ at the onset can reduce swelling and inflammation.

      ii. _____, ointments, and eye _____ may be prescribed to

        treat and protect the eye.

      iii. Without treatment, it may resolve on its own in a few _____ or

        _____.

4. Disk Disorders

  A. Disk disorders occur when the intervertebral _____ between the spinal

    vertebrae _____, creating pain and _____ of stature.

  B. Signs and symptoms of disk disorders

      i. Pain can be very _____ and sometimes _____.

      ii. Decreased _____ of the affected region is also common due to the severe

        pain.

      iii. Leg _____ and other _____ weakness may occur.

      iv. _____ is also associated with disk disorders.

  C. Treatment options for disk disorders

      i. _____ rest

      ii. _____ or _____ therapy

      iii. Muscle _____

iv. _____

v. _____ therapy for ruptured or slipped disks

vi. _____ therapy, acupuncture, and _____

5. Encephalitis

   A. Encephalitis is often caused by a(n) _____ infection.

   B. It primarily affects _____ and _____ people.

   C. Signs and symptoms of encephalitis

      i. Headache, sudden _____, vomiting, sensitivity to _____, stiff _____ and back, confusion, _____, clumsiness, and _____ are common.

      ii. Emergency treatment is required if there is loss of _____ or decreased _____, seizures, muscle _____, or impaired _____.

   D. Treatment options for encephalitis

      i. _____

      ii. _____ medications

      iii. _____

      iv. _____ to decrease inflammation

      v. _____ to control irritability and agitation

6. Epilepsy and Seizures

   A. _____ are disorders associated with misfiring or interference of electrical impulses within the brain.

   B. _____ is a disorder characterized by recurring seizures.

   C. The cause of epilepsy is often _____.

   D. Signs and symptoms of epilepsy and seizures

      i. Seizures temporarily interfere with _____ control, movement, _____, vision, or _____ of one's surroundings.

   E. Treatment options for epilepsy and seizures

      i. Medication is often used to reduce the _____ and the _____ of seizures.

      ii. In very severe cases of epilepsy, _____ may be required.

      iii. It is important to minimize exposure to or circumstances that _____ seizure activity.

7. Huntington's Chorea

   A. Huntington's chorea is a progressive degenerative disorder of the cerebral and _____ _____.

B. It is also referred to as _____ _____.

C. Signs and symptoms of Huntington's chorea

    i. Uncontrolled movements of the _____, _____, and _____ of the body

    ii. Increased irritability, _____ swings, _____, and anger

    iii. _____ movement

    iv. Rigidity

    v. Problems with _____ and coordination, difficulty _____, and slurred _____

D. Treatment options for Huntington's chorea

    i. Antidepressants, mood _____, and _____ drugs are often used.

    ii. The medication _____ is specifically approved and used to reduce jerking and movements.

    iii. There is currently _____ _____ for the disorder.

    iv. Most patients die within _____ year(s) of being diagnosed.

8. Hydrocephalus

A. Hydrocephalus commonly occurs in _____.

B. It is characterized by an excessive number of CSF _____ in the brain, causing the brain to _____ against the skull.

C. Without proper treatment, this condition can result in _____ _____.

D. Signs and symptoms of hydrocephalus

    i. Enlarged _____

    ii. Among infants, _____, sleepiness, _____, and seizures

    iii. Among older children and adults, _____, coordination and gait _____, nausea and _____, _____ disturbance, drowsiness, and _____ changes

E. Treatment options for hydrocephalus

    i. A surgically inserted _____ creates an exit for the excessive _____ to drain off the brain, allowing it to be redistributed to the rest of the body.

9. Meningitis

A. Meningitis is an infection of the meninges that surround and protect the _____ and _____ cord.

B. It may be caused by a virus or _____.

C. Bacterial meningitis, if left untreated, has a high _____ _____.

D. Signs and symptoms of meningitis

    i. _____ stiffness, headache, vomiting, _____ fever, and chills

    ii. _____ (sensitivity to light)

    iii. Increased _____

    iv. Decreased desire to _____ or _____

    v. Difficulty _____

E. Treatment options for meningitis

    i. Immediate _____ _____ is necessary for a positive outcome.

    ii. _____ are used to treat the bacterial infection.

    iii. _____ medications can reduce brain swelling.

    iv. General _____ and anticonvulsants may be used.

    v. To prevent the spread of this disease, _____ may be required.

    vi. _____ types of vaccinations are available to guard against contracting meningitis.

10. Multiple Sclerosis

A. MS is an autoimmune disease in which the body attacks and destroys its own _____ that surrounds the nerves of the brain and _____ _____.

B. As the myelin is damaged, scarlike tissue begins to develop and becomes very _____ and _____; this is known as sclerosis.

C. The sclerotic tissue impedes the transmission of _____ _____, resulting in difficulty with movement, _____, or sensation.

D. Signs and symptoms of MS

    i. _____ vision

    ii. Dizziness

    iii. Paralysis

    iv. Loss of _____

    v. Problems with speech and _____

    vi. Depression and _____ changes

    vii. Pins-and-needles _____

    viii. _____ incontinence

    ix. Numbness

       x. _____ stiffness

      xi. Uncontrollable _____

  E. Treatment options for MS

      i. Treatment depends on the type and _____ of the disease.

      ii. Drug therapy is used to minimize the _____ and symptoms, delay the _____ of the disease, and improve the overall _____ of life.

11. Neuralgia

  A. Neuralgia is a general term for _____ _____.

  B. The causes of neuralgia are _____.

  C. Signs and symptoms of neuralgia

      i. Neuralgia involves brief but possibly _____ pain.

      ii. It is often described as _____ pain along the course of the affected nerve.

      iii. Patients who have long suffered with _____ may also suffer from neuralgia.

  D. Treatment options for neuralgia

      i. Treatment varies depending on the cause, _____, and severity of the pain and other factors.

      ii. Rest, _____, and _____ are used to aid in pain relief.

      iii. Mild over-the-counter _____ may be used.

      iv. Other treatments may include the use of _____, narcotic _____, nerve blocks, and anesthetic agents that are administered via local _____ or _____ procedures to decrease the sensitivity of the nerve.

12. Parkinson's Disease

  A. Parkinson's disease is a(n) _____ disorder.

  B. It is caused by the _____ of nerve cells in the parts of the brain that control _____.

  C. Parkinson's disease is attributed to a combination of _____ factors, aging, and environmental _____.

  D. Signs and symptoms of Parkinson's disease

      i. Tremor of a(n) _____, especially when the _____ is at rest

      ii. Slow _____ or a(n) _____ to move

      iii. _____ limbs

      iv. A shuffling _____ and a stooped _____

      v. Reduced _____ expression and a soft _____

vi. The disease may also cause _____, personality change, dementia, _____ disturbances, speech _____, and _____ difficulties.

vii. Parkinson's tends to _____ over time.

E. Treatment options for Parkinson's disease

    i. _____ is commonly used to treat the symptoms of Parkinson's but must eventually be _____.

    ii. _____ intervention can help minimize the effects of involuntary _____ caused by this disease; however, few patients are _____ for surgical treatment.

13. Sciatica

A. Sciatica is pain that runs along the sciatic _____.

B. It is often caused by _____ related to a pinched root or excessive _____ on the sciatic nerve.

C. Signs and symptoms of sciatica

    i. Sharp pain runs from the lower _____ down the back of the _____.

    ii. Pain may be worse during periods of _____, at night, and with _____ changes.

    iii. _____ and _____ sensations may also be present with sciatica.

D. Treatment options for sciatica

    i. Analgesics, _____, and _____ are medications commonly used to treat the symptoms of sciatica.

    ii. Cold or _____ _____ may be beneficial.

    iii. Rest and restriction of _____ that cause pain and discomfort often help.

    iv. Gentle _____ _____ are helpful in increasing tolerable movements.

    v. In extreme cases, _____ intervention may be necessary.

14. Spinal Cord Injuries

A. Damage, _____, or a break in the _____ _____ can result in paralysis.

B. _____ refers to paralysis from approximately the shoulders down.

C. _____ refers to paralysis from approximately the waist down.

D. _____ occurs when paralysis affects one side of the body.

E. Signs and symptoms of spinal cord injuries

    i. Complete _____ from the point of injury and _____ is the most common sign of paralysis.

    ii. _____ and feeling are lost in conjunction with the loss of movement.

F. Treatment options for spinal cord injuries

    i. Treatment is aimed at reducing _____ associated with paralysis through effective and careful _____ of the patient.

    ii. _____ therapy may also be helpful.

15. Stroke

A. Stroke is the _____-leading cause of death in the United States.

B. The _____ _____ dies when the blood supply to the brain is impaired by _____ or _____.

C. Brain cells can die when the _____ supply is interrupted for more than a few minutes.

D. Signs and symptoms of stroke

    i. _____ or weakness on one side of the body

    ii. Confusion or trouble _____

    iii. _____ disturbances in one or both _____

    iv. _____

    v. Loss of _____ or coordination

    vi. Severe _____ with no known cause

E. Treatment options for stroke

    i. _____ intervention is vital.

    ii. Physicians will attempt to stabilize the patient by either _____ blood clots or stopping the _____.

    iii. _____ may be necessary.

    iv. Medications will be administered to control _____ of the brain and _____ _____.

    v. Medications and treatments are given after the incident to _____ the chance of _____.

16. Transient Ischemic Attacks

A. Transient ischemic attacks are commonly known as _____.

B. They generally resolve on their own without _____, though they are frequently precursors of a true _____.

C. Signs and symptoms of transient ischemic attacks

    i. Temporary sudden weakness, _____, and change of _____

D. Treatment options for transient ischemic attacks

    i. Patients must seek _____ _____ if they have suffered a TIA.

    ii. _____ and aspirin therapy are often used to reduce the risk of blood clot formation.

E. Steps to reduce risk of TIA or stroke

    i. Cease _____

    ii. Stop _____ and maintain a healthy _____

    iii. Decrease _____ consumption

    iv. Lower blood _____

    v. Control _____

17. Traumatic Brain Injuries

A. Epidural and _____ hematomas can develop when the head receives a blow.

B. Traumatic brain injuries can result in _____ or _____.

C. Signs and symptoms of traumatic brain injuries

    i. Signs and symptoms vary depending on the _____ that causes the trauma.

    ii. Common symptoms include loss of _____, headache, _____, dizziness, _____ and vomiting, _____ vision, and ringing in the _____.

    iii. Behavioral, _____, and sleep pattern changes may also be indicative of a more _____ trauma to the brain.

D. Treatment options for traumatic brain injuries

    i. Treatment depends on the _____ of trauma.

    ii. Medications or procedures to reduce _____ and pressure on the brain are initiated if swelling is present.

    iii. _____ _____ are often indicated, but special caution must be used as some can cause more bleeding.

    iv. _____ exercises are usually needed.

    v. Medications to suppress _____ are frequently prescribed following brain trauma.

APPLIED PRACTICE

1. Using the textbook, fill in the sections of the table below.

Type of Headache	Symptoms	Treatment
Migraine headaches		
Tension headaches		
Cluster headaches		
Post-traumatic headaches		

2. Using your textbook, label the image below of the different parts of the brain.

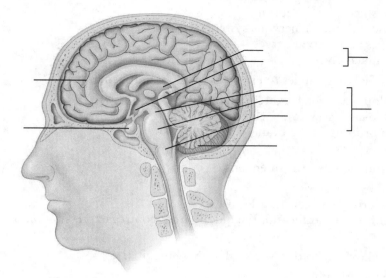

LEARNING ACTIVITY: MULTIPLE CHOICE

Circle the correct answer to each of the following questions.

1. Which of the following applies to a cerebrovascular accident?
   a. It is the third-leading cause of death in the United States.
   b. It is caused by a virus.
   c. Muscle tissue dies when the blood supply to a part of the brain is decreased.
   d. All of the above

2. Which of the following are signs and symptoms of encephalitis?
   a. Headache
   b. Stiff neck and back
   c. Drowsiness
   d. All of the above

3. Sciatica
   a. usually causes mild to moderate pain.
   b. is caused by inflammation due to a pinched nerve root.
   c. usually occurs on both sides of the body.
   d. All of the above

4. Which of the following diseases has an unknown etiology?
   a. ALS
   b. TIA
   c. Parkinson's disease
   d. Multiple sclerosis

5. The corpus callosum
   a. controls most of the body's functions.
   b. is divided into gray and white matter.
   c. joins the right and left hemispheres of the brain.
   d. All of the above

6. Which of the following makes up the central nervous system?

   a. Nerve tracts and motor neurons
   b. Somatic and autonomic nervous systems
   c. Spinal nerves and cranial nerves
   d. Brain and spinal cord

7. Which of the following applies to epidural and subdural hematomas?

   a. They develop when the head receives a blow.
   b. They are typically seen in the elderly.
   c. They are a bruising of the brain.
   d. None of the above

8. Which of the following is true of epilepsy?

   a. It is caused by a bacterium.
   b. It is characterized by recurring seizures.
   c. It is a weakness or paralysis of the muscles that control expression on one side of the face.
   d. All of the above

9. Which of the following is *not* associated with meningitis?

   a. It is similar to encephalitis.
   b. It may be caused by a virus or bacteria.
   c. It has a high death rate if untreated.
   d. It is an autoimmune disease.

10. Motor neurons are

    a. greatly affected in ALS.
    b. considered afferent nerves.
    c. housed within the nerve tract.
    d. structurally like a stem.

CRITICAL THINKING

Answer the following questions to the best of your ability. Use the textbook as a reference.

1. A patient, a 57-year-old female named Katie Gilpatrick, has come into the office and is exhibiting signs of high stress. How can the medical assistant help reduce Ms. Gilpatrick's stress level during the appointment?

   _____

   _____

   _____

   _____

   _____

2. Allison is a 23-year-old female who is epileptic and has had a severe seizure within the past 2 days. She is concerned about transportation to and from her college classes. She asks you, the medical assistant working with her physician, for advice. Why is it important to be aware of the laws in your state regarding driving and neurological disorders?

   _____

   _____

   _____

   _____

   _____

3. Loretta Nydriski is a 60-year-old patient who is being seen for observable right-side facial drooping, specifically near the mouth. The patient states that she "woke up this way," and she "can't feel anything on the entire right side of my face." What would you suspect the diagnosis might be on the basis of her symptoms, and what is the treatment for this condition? *(Medical assistants never make a diagnosis; this is a question about your knowledge of the signs and symptoms of various conditions that are presented in the textbook.)*

_____

_____

_____

_____

RESEARCH ACTIVITY

Use Internet search engines to research the following topic and write a brief description of what you find. It is important to use reputable websites.

1. Visit the Parkinson's Disease Foundation website, at www.pdf.org. Type "Science News" in the Search box at the top of the page. Choose an article of interest and provide a summary of the information discussed in the article. Discuss what interested you most about the article that you selected.

_____

_____

_____

_____

CHAPTER 25

The Special Senses

STUDENT STUDY GUIDE

Use the following guide to assist in your learning of the concepts from the chapter.

I. The Eye and the Sense of Vision

    1. The eye is a(n) _____, _____-filled organ composed of specialized structures that work together to facilitate vision.

    2. Nerves in the eye are essential in the _____ of _____.

    3. Nerves of the Eye

        A. The nerves of the eye control the amount of _____ entering the eye through the _____.

        B. They focus light on the _____ by using the _____.

        C. They transmit the resulting images from the _____ to the _____.

    4. Structures of the Eyeball

        A. Outer Layer of the Eyeball (List the structures only.)

            i. _____

            ii. _____

            iii. _____

        B. Middle Layer of the Eyeball (List the structures only.)

            i. _____

            ii. _____

            iii. _____

            iv. _____

        C. Inner Layer of the Eyeball

            i. The innermost layer of the eye is the _____.

            ii. Photosensitive cells in the retina called _____ and _____ translate light rays into nerve impulses that are transmitted to the _____.

            iii. Rods react to _____ light and are used in _____ vision; cones are sensitive to _____ light and are used to see color.

iv. The optic nerve enters at the _____ _____ and carries incoming information from the eye to the brain.

D. The External Structures of the Eye

i. The eyelids, or _____, close over the eyeballs, protecting them from intense light, foreign matter, and impacts.

ii. Light enters through the _____ _____, the opening between the superior and inferior eyelids.

iii. _____ in the margins of the eyelids further protect the eye from foreign matter.

iv. The superior and inferior palpebrae meet at the _____ at each _____ of the eye.

v. The _____ is a mucous _____ that lines the underside of the eyelids and the anterior part of the eyeball.

vi. Tears are produced, stored, and removed by the structures that make up the _____ _____.

vii. The _____ _____ secretes tears through ducts on the surface of the conjunctiva of the upper lid.

viii. The _____ _____ collect and drain the tears into the _____ _____, which empties into the _____ _____, which empties into the nasal cavity.

II. Common Refractive Disorders

1. _____ problems occur because light rays change direction when they pass through the eye.

2. Myopia (Refer to Table 25-1 in the textbook.)

A. Myopia is also called _____.

B. Objects that are _____ away tend to be blurry and difficult to see.

C. It is easier to see objects that are _____ to the eye.

3. Hyperopia (Refer to Table 25-1 in the textbook.)

A. Hyperopia is also called _____.

B. Objects that are _____ to the eye are harder to decipher and blurred.

C. It is easier to see things that are _____ away.

4. Presbyopia (Refer to Table 25-1 in the textbook.)

A. As with _____, with presbyopia there is difficulty focusing and seeing objects that are close.

B. This specific disorder is directly related to the _____ _____.

5. Astigmatism

A. Astigmatism is a condition caused by an irregularity in the curvature of the

_____ and _____.

B. This irregular shape causes light not to focus on the _____ but rather to

spread out over a(n) _____.

C. Signs and symptoms of astigmatism

i. _____ near or distant vision

ii. Possibly _____ and _____

D. Treatment options for astigmatism

i. _____ lenses

ii. Surgery to reshape the _____

6. Strabismus

A. Strabismus is also called _____ eyes or wall eyes.

B. The eyes are _____ and do not focus on the same image.

C. It is caused by abnormal _____ control and weakness in the

_____ ocular muscles of the eye.

D. Signs and symptoms of strabismus

i. Poor _____ perception

ii. _____ vision

E. Treatment options for strabismus

i. Eyeglasses

ii. Eye _____

iii. Wearing a patch over the _____ eye to force the

_____ eye to become stronger

iv. _____ to realign the eyes

III. Pathology and Disorders Related to the Eye

1. Blepharitis

A. Blepharitis is _____ of the eyelids, particularly near the

_____ hair follicles.

B. Signs and symptoms of blepharitis

i. Redness, _____, and _____ of the eyelids

ii. _____ sensations

iii. Development of _____ that covers the eye

C. Treatment options for blepharitis

i. Warm _____ _____

ii. Ophthalmic _____ therapy

2. Conjunctivitis

    A. Conjunctivitis is commonly known as _____.

    B. This highly _____ condition is _____ of the conjunctiva

    C. Signs and symptoms of conjunctivitis

        i. An early symptom is the feeling of a(n) _____ _____ in the eye.

        ii. Other common symptoms include _____ in the sclera, increased _____ production, a thick yellow _____ that crusts over the _____, itchy eyes, _____ eyes, _____ vision, and greater sensitivity to _____.

    D. Treatment options for conjunctivitis

        i. _____ the eyes and applying _____ compresses is an effective home remedy.

        ii. Over-the-counter _____ _____ are used to keep eyes lubricated.

        iii. _____ eyedrops may be required.

        iv. Isolation during the first _____ _____ of antibiotic therapy is recommended.

3. Hordeolums

    A. Hordeolums are also known as _____.

    B. They are very common and frequently _____.

    C. They are often caused by the _____ bacterium.

    D. Signs and symptoms of hordeolums

        i. Redness and _____ are followed by itching, _____, and discomfort in the upper or lower _____.

        ii. A hordeolum develops as a(n) _____-filled _____ at the base of an eyelash.

    E. Treatment options for hordeolums

        i. They often resolve on _____ _____.

        ii. A(n) _____, _____ compress applied to the area may help relieve the pain.

        iii. Patients should avoid _____ the affected eye and never _____ a hordeolum.

        iv. _____ creams or _____ may be applied to accelerate healing.

v. A physician may need to _____ and _____ a hordeolum to assist in the healing process; particularly if _____ is affected.

4. Cataracts

   A. A cataract is a(n) _____ or opacity of the _____ that prevents light from entering the eye.

   B. Signs and symptoms of cataracts

      i. As cloudiness begins to develop, _____ begins to decrease.

      ii. Vision may be fuzzy, _____, or filmy.

      iii. Sufferers may also experience a lack of _____ _____ and see halos around lights.

      iv. _____ vision suffers.

      v. The patient may also experience _____ vision or problems with bright _____.

   C. Treatment options for cataracts

      i. Eyeglasses, _____ lenses, and stronger _____ may be sufficient for early cataracts.

      ii. _____ is eventually the only effective treatment.

5. Retinal Detachment

   A. Retinal detachment occurs when a retina has separated from the underlying _____ _____.

   B. Damage may start as small _____ or _____ and later, if left untreated, develop into full _____.

   C. When such a separation occurs, vision is _____.

   D. If the detachment is detected _____, it can be repaired and the vision _____.

   E. Signs and symptoms of retinal detachment

      i. An increase in _____ or flashes of _____ in the field of vision

      ii. Feeling as if a(n) _____ has obscured part of the vision

   F. Treatment options for retinal detachment

      i. Treatment for small holes or tears is usually _____ surgery or cryotherapy.

      ii. For retinal detachment, more _____ surgery requiring a hospital stay is generally recommended.

6. Macular Degeneration

   A. Macular degeneration is the _____ of the _____.

B. It is a(n) _____ disease and one of the leading causes of
_____ among people over the age of 55.

C. The two types of macular degeneration are _____ and
_____.

D. Signs and symptoms of macular degeneration

   i. Dry macular degeneration: a decline in _____ vision, increasing
_____ of overall vision, and a need for _____
illumination for reading and close work

   ii. Wet macular degeneration: visual _____ and a blurry spot in the
_____ vision

E. Treatment options for macular degeneration

   i. There is no known _____ or _____ for dry
macular degeneration.

   ii. If performed early, _____ _____ may halt the
progression of wet macular degeneration.

7. Amblyopia

A. Amblyopia is also known as _____ _____ and is a
disorder often seen in _____.

B. It is caused by improper development of the nerve pathway from the
_____ to the _____, which causes the affected eye to
send _____ _____ to the brain.

C. Signs and symptoms of amblyopia

   i. Eyes that appear to turn _____ or _____

   ii. Decreased _____

   iii. Faulty depth _____

D. Treatment options for amblyopia

   i. Treatment for underlying conditions, such as _____ or
_____ disorders, must first be completed.

   ii. A(n) _____ may be worn over the strong eye to force the brain to
interpret the images from the afflicted eye to foster development of the nerve pathway
from that eye.

8. Corneal Abrasion

A. A corneal abrasion is a(n) _____ or _____ on the
cornea.

B. Most corneal abrasions result from _____ or _____.

C. Other causes include improperly fitting _____ _____

    and _____ _____ becoming stuck in the eyelid.

D. Signs and symptoms of corneal abrasion

    i. A corneal abrasion can be very _____ and irritating.

    ii. Other symptoms include _____ vision, excessive tearing,

        _____ feeling on the cornea, and possibly _____.

    iii. The patient will be very _____ to light and will have difficulty

        _____ the affected eye.

E. Treatment options for corneal abrasion

    i. Mild _____ and resting the eyes

    ii. If the abrasion becomes _____, antibiotic eyedrops or

    _____

9. Glaucoma

    A. Glaucoma affects people of all _____ and all _____.

    B. It is characterized by increased _____ in the eye.

    C. Left untreated, the pressure can lead to damage of the _____

    _____ and eventual _____.

    D. There are two basic types of glaucoma: _____ and

    _____.

    E. Signs and symptoms of open-angle glaucoma

      i. This chronic condition is sometimes referred to as _____ glaucoma.

      ii. It is _____ and is often referred to as the "silent thief" of

      _____.

      iii. Once symptoms begin to occur, damage is _____

      _____.

    F. Signs and symptoms of closed-angle glaucoma

      i. Sharp eye _____

      ii. Decreased _____ vision

      iii. Red _____ eyes

    G. Treatment options for glaucoma

      i. Medications such as _____ _____ to reduce

      intraocular pressure

      ii. Laser and _____ surgery

10. Nystagmus

    A. Nystagmus is characterized by involuntary, repetitive, rhythmic _____

    _____.

B. Signs and symptoms of nystagmus

    i. _____ eye movements, which may be lateral,

    _____, or even circular

C. Treatment options for of nystagmus

    i. It is important to address the underlying cause, which might be a(n)

    _____, a(n) _____, alcohol abuse, or retinal

    maldevelopment.

11. Retinopathy

A. Retinopathy is a disease of the retina that is caused by either recurring or

    _____ damage.

B. Diabetic patients are prone to _____ _____.

C. Nerve damage can result from _____ _____ and can

    lead to permanent _____.

D. _____ _____ disease, trauma, and other disorders can

    cause _____ retinopathy.

E. Symptoms vary based on the type of _____ that is diagnosed.

F. Treatment lies in treating the _____ _____ causing

    the disorder.

IV. The Ear and the Sense of Hearing

1. Anatomy of the Ear

A. The Outer Ear

    i. _____, or auricle

    ii. Auditory canal, or _____ _____

    iii. _____ _____ or eardrum

    iv. _____

B. The Middle Ear

    i. The middle ear contains three small bones, or _____: the

    _____ (_____), _____ (_____), and

    _____ (_____).

    ii. The function of the middle ear is to transmit sound _____,

    _____ the air pressure on both sides of the

    _____ membrane, and protect the ear from potentially damaging

    _____ noise.

    iii. The _____ _____, or auditory tube, extends 3 to

    4 cm from the middle ear to the nasopharynx.

C. The Inner Ear

    i. The inner ear is a maze of canals within a bony labyrinth in the

       _____ bone.

    ii. The _____, _____, and three

       _____ canals make up the labyrinth.

    iii. The cochlea, which is the organ of hearing, is a bony spiral structure that resembles

       a(n) _____ _____.

    iv. The vestibule is the fundus of the internal auditory _____ and

       controls the sense of _____.

V. Hearing Loss

  1. The study of _____ disorders, including hearing _____, is audiology.

  2. Two Types of Hearing Loss

    A. Conductive hearing loss

      i. Conductive hearing loss is a(n) _____ condition.

      ii. It could be caused by _____ ear infections, _____

       ear, fluid accumulation within the _____ ear, impacted

       _____, and allergies.

      iii. It can be _____ corrected by treating the underlying cause or can be

       _____ corrected.

    B. Sensorineural hearing loss

      i. Sensorineural hearing loss is _____ hearing loss caused by damage

       to the _____ or to nerve pathways from the

       _____ ear to the _____.

      ii. It can be caused by malformation of the auditory _____, head

       _____, aging, and exposure to _____

       _____.

      iii. _____ _____ can be helpful to those who have

       only partial hearing loss.

      iv. New advances in medicine, specifically _____ _____,

       are helping to change the outlook for those with this condition.

VI. Pathology Related to the Ear

  1. Impacted Cerumen

    A. This condition is _____ that has accumulated and

      _____ to the point that it obstructs the auditory canal.

    B. It generally affects _____ adults.

C. It is often caused by the patient trying to _____ earwax at home by placing external _____ into the ear in an attempt to _____ it.

D. Signs and symptoms of impacted cerumen

    i. Blocked or muffled _____

    ii. A(n) _____ feeling in the ear

    iii. _____

E. Treatment options for impacted cerumen

    i. It may be possible to _____ the wax and remove it by _____ the ear with an ear syringe.

    ii. In the medical office this procedure is termed _____.

2. Ruptured Tympanic Membrane

  A. Injuries can occur when objects entering the ear _____ the membrane or when unequal _____ _____ on both sides of the membrane causes a rupture.

  B. Signs and symptoms of ruptured tympanic membrane

    i. Sharp, _____ _____ in the affected ear may be followed by drainage of fluid.

    ii. Tinnitus, _____ loss, and _____ (dizziness) are also common symptoms.

    iii. _____ and _____ may accompany vertigo.

  C. Treatment options for ruptured tympanic membrane

    i. A ruptured membrane is able to heal _____ any treatment.

    ii. Treatment that is usually provided includes _____ medications to prevent infection and analgesics to reduce _____.

3. Otitis Media

  A. Otitis media is inflammation of the _____ ear.

  B. It can be caused by _____ or _____ infections, often secondary to sore throats and colds.

  C. It occurs in _____ more frequently than in _____.

  D. Signs and symptoms of otitis media

    i. Infants and _____ may tug at the affected ear.

    ii. The child may also be unusually irritable or _____, have a(n) _____, and have difficulty _____.

    iii. _____ may drain from the ear.

  E. Treatment options for otitis media

    i. The main goal is to eliminate the cause of _____.

ii. _____ _____ help to kill bacteria and eliminate the source of the infection.

iii. _____ help reduce swelling by shrinking the blood vessels in the Eustachian tubes.

iv. Tubal _____ may be necessary every 1 to 2 days.

v. Recurrent ear infections may be treated with _____.

4. Otosclerosis

A. Otosclerosis is a condition characterized by abnormal bone _____ _____ around the stapes.

B. Signs and symptoms of otosclerosis

i. The overgrowth causes gradual _____ _____ in one or both ears.

ii. Some people may also experience _____ and dizziness.

C. Treatment options for otosclerosis

i. Mild cases may be treated with a(n) _____ _____.

ii. More severe cases may require _____.

5. Tinnitus

A. Tinnitus is _____ in the ears.

B. It is a common condition that afflicts approximately _____ _____ Americans.

C. It may be caused by hearing _____, loud noise, certain _____, and other health problems such as _____ and tumors.

D. Signs and symptoms of tinnitus

i. Ringing, _____, or roaring in one or _____ ears

E. Treatment options for tinnitus

i. Maskers may be worn like a hearing aid to help mask or drown out the tinnitus through the production of _____ _____.

ii. _____ _____ have also proven to be helpful by enhancing sounds that need to be heard while lessening the effects of tinnitus.

iii. Alternative therapies include _____ techniques, _____, and _____.

6. Ménière's Disease

A. Ménière's disease is named after a(n) _____ physician who first described the syndrome.

B. This disease affects a person's _____ and _____.

C. Signs and symptoms of Ménière's disease

   i. Four main symptoms are loss of _____, _____ in the ear, _____, and _____.

   ii. Other symptoms include nausea, _____, _____, and headaches.

   iii. Symptoms often occur suddenly, without _____, and they may occur _____ or infrequently.

D. Treatment options for Ménière's disease

   i. Treatment is aimed at controlling _____ through lifestyle modifications.

   ii. Low-sodium diets and _____ drugs to reduce fluid _____ are often implemented.

   iii. Avoiding excessive _____ and alcohol is also beneficial.

   iv. Medications that control _____ and improve blood _____ in the inner ear may be beneficial.

   v. Eliminating _____ use and reducing _____ levels may also reduce the severity of symptoms.

7. Presbycusis

A. Presbycusis is a type of hearing loss involving the gradual _____ of the sensory receptors in the _____.

B. Factors that lead to presbycusis include changes due to _____ of the ear, prolonged exposure to _____ _____, infection, _____, and side effects of certain _____.

C. Signs and symptoms of presbycusis

   i. Presbycusis generally occurs in _____ ears.

   ii. It causes problems with hearing both the _____ and the _____-pitched tones of conversation.

   iii. Hearing loss is generally _____.

D. Treatment options for presbycusis

   i. Treatment is generally achieved through the use of a hearing _____.

   ii. If hearing loss is severe enough, _____ _____ may be suggested by a physician.

VII. The Senses of Taste and Smell

1. The nose is the _____ _____ for the sense of smell.

2. Once a smell receptor is activated, it sends the information to the brain via the _____ nerves.

3. The sense of taste and the sense of smell function together to create a combined effect that is interpreted by the _____.

4. _____ _____ are microscopic bumps on the tongue, the roof of the mouth, and the walls of the throat.

5. Five types of taste cells are _____, _____, _____, _____, and _____.

VIII. The Sense of Touch

1. Touch is our oldest, most _____ sense.

2. The sense of touch is found over the _____ _____.

3. Nerve endings in the _____ transmit information to the spinal cord, which in turn sends messages to the _____, where the feeling is registered.

4. The more _____ _____ there are in a given area of the body, the more _____ it is.

APPLIED PRACTICE

1. Label the parts of the eyeball and its anatomical structures.

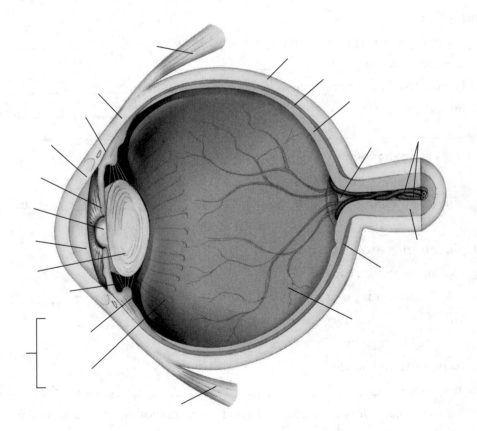

2. Label the parts of the ear and its anatomical structures.

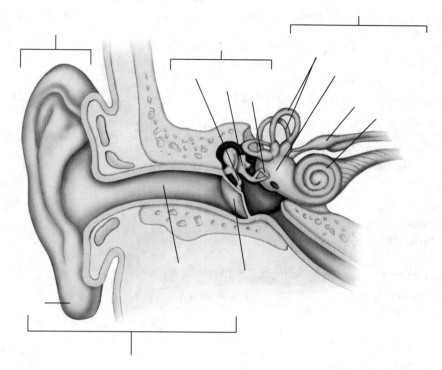

LEARNING ACTIVITY: MULTIPLE CHOICE

Circle the correct answer to each of the following questions.

1. Normal age-related hearing loss is termed

   a. tinnitus.
   b. presbycusis.
   c. diplopia.
   d. sensorineural hearing loss.

2. How can intraocular pressure be reduced?

   a. Eyedrops
   b. Laser surgery
   c. Conventional surgery
   d. All of the above

3. Swimmer's ear is also known as

   a. otosclerosis.
   b. otitis media.
   c. otitis externa.
   d. presbycusis.

4. Which of the following is *not* a part of the inner ear?

   a. Cochlea
   b. Eustachian tube
   c. Vestibule
   d. Labyrinth

5. Refraction problems
   a. involve the inability to focus correctly and occur because light rays change direction when they pass through the eye.
   b. are typically seen more in children than in the elderly.
   c. include conditions such as blepharoptosis.
   d. involve all of the above.

6. The use of an eye patch is recommended for
   a. glaucoma.
   b. nystagmus.
   c. strabismus.
   d. corneal abrasion.

7. Hypertensive retinopathy is caused by
   a. a variety of factors.
   b. high blood pressure.
   c. low blood pressure.
   d. diabetes.

8. Recurrent ear infections may be treated with
   a. myringotomy.
   b. keratotomy.
   c. osteotomy.
   d. none of the above.

9. Tastes and smells are most acute
   a. at birth.
   b. by the toddler stage.
   c. in young adults.
   d. in older adults.

10. A common disorder of the outer ear is
    a. otosclerosis.
    b. tinnitus.
    c. otitis media.
    d. impacted cerumen.

CRITICAL THINKING

Answer the following questions to the best of your ability. Use the textbook as a reference.

1. Wilma McAffee is a 78-year-old patient who has been having difficulty hearing. After an examination, it is determined that she has a buildup of ear wax in her ear. What is the term for the buildup of earwax? Might Wilma have contributed to her condition in any way? Since her hearing condition is temporary, which form of hearing loss would Ms. McAffee be suffering from?

_____

_____

_____

_____

_____

2. Stephanie Mulligan is being seen at Pearson Physicians Group because her lower eyelid has begun to droop outward. She states, "The dryness in my eye is driving me crazy." What condition might Ms. Mulligan be diagnosed with? What are the causes and treatments available for this condition? *(Medical assistants never make a diagnosis; this is a question about your knowledge of the signs and symptoms of various conditions that are presented in the textbook.)*

_____

_____

_____

_____

_____

RESEARCH ACTIVITY

Use Internet search engines to research the following topic and write a brief description of what you find. It is important to use reputable websites.

1. Visit different websites that deal with speech and hearing loss. What information can you find to help families with speech and hearing deficiencies? What websites did you find most useful? Could these websites be beneficial to staff members of an eye, ear, nose, and throat (EENT) practice? If so, why?

_____

_____

_____

_____

_____

CHAPTER 26
The Cardiovascular System

STUDENT STUDY GUIDE

Use the following guide to assist in your learning of the concepts from the chapter.

I. Structures of the Cardiovascular System

  1. The Heart

    A. The heart lies to the _____ of the chest's midline.

    B. The heart is similar in size and shape to a(n) _____.

    C. Describe the three layers of the heart.

      i. Pericardium—_____

      ii. Myocardium—_____

      iii. Endocardium—_____

    D. The _____ is a wall that separates the sides of the heart.

    E. The atria are the two _____ chambers of the heart.

    F. The ventricles are the two _____ chambers.

  2. Blood Vessels

    A. Arteries are the vessels that carry the blood _____

    _____ from the heart.

      i. The largest artery is the _____.

      ii. Arteries divide into _____ and smaller _____ as they spread out to all parts of the body.

      iii. _____ are the smallest and connect to the tiny capillaries that make direct contact with individual body _____.

    B. _____ transport blood from all parts of the body back to the heart.

      i. The smallest veins, called _____, branch off from the tiny capillaries and then join to form the full-sized veins.

      ii. Veins are _____ but thinner-walled than arteries and contain _____ that prevent blood from flowing backward.

    C. Capillaries are _____ blood vessels with walls that are just one _____ thick.

3. The Vascular System of the Heart

   A. The heart's dense musculature requires its own _____

   _____.

   B. Coronary arteries supply _____ blood to the heart.

   C. This is blood that directly _____ the heart muscle itself.

   D. Deoxygenated blood is drained into the coronary _____ by the coronary

   veins and then back into the right _____ for oxygenation.

II. How the Cardiovascular System Functions

   1. The heart is responsible for the movement of _____ through the

   cardiovascular system and throughout the entire body, providing _____ and

   _____ to cells and removing _____.

   2. Blood Flow Through the Heart

      A. The _____ vena cava brings blood from the head and upper

      _____.

      B. The _____ vena cava brings blood from below the

      _____.

      C. The _____ _____ receives all the blood from the

      superior and inferior vena cava.

      D. It pumps the blood through the _____ valve into the right ventricle.

      E. The right ventricle pumps the blood out through the pulmonary valve into the

      _____ _____, which carries the blood to the

      _____.

      F. The _____ vein carries the oxygenated blood from the lungs and empties

      it into the left _____ of the heart.

      G. The blood leaves the left atrium through the _____ valve, which is also

      called the _____ valve.

      H. Blood then enters the left _____.

      I. Blood leaves the left ventricle through the _____ valve and enters the

      _____.

      J. From the aorta the blood begins its journey through the various _____

      that branch off from the aorta to all the different _____ of the body.

   3. Conduction System of the Heart

      A. A(n) _____ conduction system is responsible for initiating the beats that

      send blood flowing through and from the heart.

B. The _____ _____ is considered the pacemaker of the heart and is located in the upper portion of the wall of the _____ _____.

   i. The SA node signals the right and left _____ to contract by discharging electrical signals.

C. The _____ _____ is located between the atria and ventricles in the _____ layer of the heart.

   i. The AV node _____ _____ the impulse for a moment to allow the atria time to finish contracting before the ventricles begin their contraction.

D. The _____ of _____ is also known as the atrioventricular (AV) bundle and is located in the septum of the heart.

E. As the impulse nears the end of the cardiac circuit, it travels from the bundle branches into the _____ fibers.

F. Purkinje fibers are responsible for relaying _____ _____ to the cells of the ventricles, prompting the ventricles to _____.

4. The Cardiac Cycle

A. The cardiac cycle consists of all the events that occur during one complete _____.

B. The heart beats about _____ times per minute.

C. List the four phases of the cardiac cycle.

   i. _____

   ii. _____

   iii. _____

   iv. _____

III. Pulmonary and Systemic Circulation

1. Pulmonary Circulation

A. Pulmonary circulation is the route blood takes from the _____ to the _____ via the pulmonary artery.

B. The function of pulmonary circulation is to carry _____ blood from the right side of the heart to the lungs and then to carry the _____ blood back to the left side of the heart.

2. Systemic Circulation

A. Systemic circulation is the route blood takes around the _____.

B. The function of systemic circulation is to deliver _____ blood and other nutrients to body cells and to carry _____ _____ and waste products away from the cells for elimination from the body.

IV. Blood Pressure

1. _____ _____ is defined as the force exerted by the blood against the inner walls of the arteries.

2. Blood pressure is usually measured in the _____ artery with a sphygmomanometer.

3. Systolic blood pressure measures _____ _____ when blood pressure is at its _____.

4. _____ blood pressure is the measurement obtained when the _____ relax and blood pressure is at its _____.

5. Pulse Pressure

   A. Pulse pressure is the _____ between the systolic and diastolic blood pressures.

   B. It indicates the tone of the _____ _____.

   C. It can be helpful when assessing a patient's risk profile for _____ _____.

V. Blood

1. Blood is a type of _____ tissue.

2. Blood _____ are the formed elements of the blood.

3. _____ is the fluid portion of the blood.

4. The amount of blood that circulates in a person's body is known as _____ _____.

5. Composition of Blood

   A. Red Blood Cells (RBCs)

      i. RBCs are produced in the red bone _____.

      ii. Mature red blood cells contain _____, which carries oxygen from the lungs to cells throughout the body.

   B. White Blood Cells (WBCs)

      i. WBCs help fight _____.

      ii. Five types of WBCs are neutrophils, _____, _____, monocytes, and _____.

   C. Blood Platelets

      i. Platelets are also known as _____.

    ii. Platelets control the loss of blood through the process of _____, or

       the formation of a(n) _____ at the point of

       _____.

  D. Blood Plasma

    i. Plasma is the _____ portion of the blood.

    ii. Plasma is 91 percent _____.

    iii. The other 9 percent is a mixture of proteins, _____, gases,

       electrolytes, _____, hormones, _____, and waste

       products.

    iv. Plasma constitutes about _____ percent of the total volume of

       whole blood.

6. Functions of Blood (List three functions.)

  A. _____

  B. _____

  C. _____

VI. Blood Types

  1. Blood type is based on whether the blood contains or lacks specific _____

    and _____.

  2. Blood type is determined by _____.

  3. Blood Types

    A. Type A—Type A _____ on the surface of the red blood cells and anti-B

       antibody in the _____. People with Type A blood can only be given Type

       _____ blood.

    B. Type B—Type _____ antigen on the surface of the red blood cells and anti-_____ antibody

       in their plasma; people with Type B blood can only be given Type B blood.

    C. Type AB—Type AB has both A and B _____ on the red blood cell

       surfaces and _____ anti-A nor anti-B antibodies. The majority of all

       people with type AB blood can receive all ABO blood types since their plasma lacks

       _____.

    D. Type O—Neither A nor B _____ are found on the red blood cells;

       however, _____ anti-A and anti-B antibodies are in the plasma. People

       with type O blood are considered _____ _____

       because their blood can be administered to most people regardless of the recipient's blood

       type.

  4. Rh Factor

    A. Rh factor is another _____ of a person's blood.

B. Rh positive means a person _____ the Rh antigen.

C. Rh negative means a person _____ _____ have the Rh antigen.

D. _____ can arise if an Rh-negative individual is given Rh-positive blood.

E. The Rh factor plays an important role during _____.

    i. When an Rh-positive fetus mixes with the mother's Rh-negative blood, the mother will develop _____ against the fetus's _____.

    ii. The first Rh-positive fetus generally _____ _____ suffer any effect.

    iii. If a second Rh-positive fetus is conceived, the fetus's _____ will be attacked by the mother's _____ almost immediately.

    iv. This can lead to a(n) _____ _____, erythroblastosis fetalis, in which the baby is born severely _____.

    v. This can be prevented by giving the drug _____ to the Rh-negative mother to inhibit the production of antibodies against the Rh antigen.

VII. Common Pathology Associated with the Cardiovascular System*

  1. Anemia

    A. Anemia is a condition in which the blood has an abnormally low number of _____ _____ cells.

    B. It can occur if the RBCs do not contain enough _____ or if the hemoglobin that is present is _____.

    C. Common causes of anemia

      i. Decreased production of healthy red cells by the _____ _____

      ii. Increased _____ (erythrocyte destruction)

      iii. Blood loss from heavy _____ _____, traumatic _____, or internal _____

    D. List five types of anemia.

      i. _____

      ii. _____

      iii. _____

      iv. _____

      v. _____

    E. Signs and symptoms of anemia

      i. The hallmark symptoms are increased _____ and _____.

*Pathological conditions discussed in the textbook but not listed in the student study guide will be covered in other workbook activities.

    ii. Other symptoms and signs include weakness, heart _____ and

        tachycardia, _____ of breath, dizziness, _____,

        _____ complexion, tinnitus, difficulty _____,

        and interrupted _____ patterns.

    iii. _____ is also common among anemic patients.

    iv. Sickle cell anemia is characterized by pain in the _____, joints, and

        _____. Infections and heart _____ may also

        occur with sickle cell anemia.

    v. Signs and symptoms of aplastic anemia can include bleeding in the

        _____ membranes, infections with _____ fevers,

        _____, and dyspnea.

F. Treatment options for anemia

    i. Treatment depends on the _____ and cause.

    ii. Injections of vitamin _____ may be necessary.

    iii. Oral dietary _____ including iron, _____

        _____, and vitamin B12 have also been effective.

    iv. Elimination of specific medications that suppress the body's _____

        _____ may be needed.

    v. Blood _____, analgesics, and _____ may also be

        required for more serious forms of the disorder.

2. Aneurysm

A. Aneurysm is caused by _____ walls of blood vessels that may become

   abnormally _____.

B. List common locations of aneurysms.

    i. _____ (aortic aneurysm)

    ii. _____ (cerebral aneurysm)

    iii. _____ (popliteal artery aneurysm)

    iv. _____ (splenic artery aneurysm)

    v. _____ (mesenteric artery aneurysm)

C. Signs and symptoms of aneurysm

    i. Symptoms vary depending on the aneurysm's _____.

    ii. An aneurysm near the body's surface may be distinguished by a(n)

        _____, throbbing mass.

    iii. Aneurysms within the body or brain often have _____ _____ and

        frequently go _____ until the aneurysm _____.

iv. A ruptured aneurysm leads to massive _____

_____ and is often _____.

D. Treatment options for aneurysm

   i. _____ intervention may be needed to repair and prevent

   _____ of the vessel.

   ii. A(n) _____ may be used to keep the vessel open and reinforce the

   wall.

   iii. A healthy diet and _____ may help prevent certain types of

   aneurysms.

   iv. Maintaining healthy blood _____ and _____

   levels is beneficial.

3. Arrhythmia

   A. Arrhythmia is a(n)_____ _____ caused by a

   disturbance of the _____ conductivity of the heart.

   B. List the two main categories of arrhythmia.

   i. _____—abnormally rapid rate of more than _____ beats per minute.

   ii. _____—abnormally slow rate of less than _____ beats per minute.

   C. Signs and symptoms of arrhythmia

   i. _____

   ii. _____

   iii. _____

   iv. _____

   v. _____

   vi. _____

   vii. _____

   D. Treatment options for arrhythmia

   i. Often arrhythmias are treated with _____.

   ii. Serious conditions may require _____ or implantation of a(n)

   _____.

4. Arteriosclerosis

   A. Arteriosclerosis is commonly known as _____ of the

   _____.

   B. It develops when the walls of the arteries become _____ and lose

   _____.

   C. Eventually _____ deposits in the artery walls develop areas that are hard

   and _____.

D. Signs and symptoms of arteriosclerosis

    i. It is not always recognized _____ or easily.

    ii. Precursor signs and symptoms include _____

        _____ pressure, recurrent _____ infections, and

        impaired _____.

E. Treatment options for arteriosclerosis

    i. Many _____ _____ are available.

    ii. The most effective treatments treat the _____

        _____.

5. Atherosclerosis

A. Atherosclerosis is hardening and _____ of the arteries from a buildup of

   _____ material and _____ within the vessel.

B. It often results from unhealthy lifestyle factors including smoking, high

   _____, excessive _____ consumption, and a poor

   _____.

C. Other conditions that often are related to atherosclerosis include _____

   and _____.

D. Atherosclerosis is the leading cause of _____ _____

   _____.

E. Signs and symptoms of atherosclerosis

    i. Angina may occur during _____ or other exertive

        _____.

    ii. _____ of breath and _____ may accompany

        angina.

    iii. If the blockage is large, angina can occur with _____ or no activity.

F. Treatment options for atherosclerosis

    i. Typically, angina decreases with _____ and

        _____.

    ii. _____ is a prescription medication that _____

        blood vessels and improves the flow of _____ blood to the heart.

    iii. Lifestyle changes include avoiding _____ foods, decreasing

        _____ consumption, stopping _____, and

        engaging in _____ _____.

    iv. Surgical intervention to _____ and remove the

        _____ clogs may be required.

6. Cardiac Tamponade

   A. Cardiac tamponade is pressure on the heart muscle caused by _____ or _____ collecting in the _____ sac that surrounds the heart.

   B. The pressure prevents the _____ from expanding, making it impossible for the heart to _____ enough blood for the body.

   C. Signs and symptoms of cardiac tamponade

      i. _____ of breath

      ii. Pale or _____ skin

      iii. Chest _____

      iv. _____

      v. _____

      vi. Anxiety and a feeling of _____ _____

   D. Treatment options for cardiac tamponade

      i. It requires an immediate procedure called _____.

      ii. _____ medications and _____ therapy may also be used to help reduce the workload of the heart.

7. Cardiogenic Shock

   A. Cardiogenic shock is a collapse of the _____ system.

   B. It is characterized by the inability of the _____ to pump enough blood to the body's _____.

   C. Signs and symptoms of cardiogenic shock

      i. Chest _____ and pressure

      ii. Change in _____

      iii. Rapid _____ and _____

      iv. Heavy _____

      v. _____

      vi. Decreased _____

   D. Treatment options for cardiogenic shock

      i. _____ medical treatment is necessary.

      ii. It is likely to include medications to restore _____ _____ and normal rhythm, _____ therapy, and _____ medications.

      iii. Heart _____ or the insertion of a(n) _____ may be required.

8. Endocarditis

   A. Endocarditis is inflammation of the _____ of the heart, including the

       _____ _____.

   B. It is most commonly caused by a(n) _____ _____.

   C. It frequently affects patients with existing abnormal conditions of the

       _____ _____.

   D. Signs and symptoms of endocarditis

      i. Weakness

      ii. _____

      iii. _____

      iv. Diaphoresis

      v. _____

      vi. Swelling in the _____ and legs

   E. Treatment options for endocarditis

      i. Antibiotics may be given _____ followed by

       _____ antibiotics over a 6-week period.

      ii. In serious cases, _____ _____ replacement might

       be necessary.

9. Myocarditis

   A. Myocarditis is _____ of the muscular layer of the heart.

   B. Signs and symptoms of myocarditis

      i. Symptoms generally resemble those of the _____, including fever,

       _____ _____, dyspnea, general _____

       and malaise, fainting, and decreased _____ _____.

      ii. The most frequent symptom of myocarditis is _____

       _____.

   C. Treatment options for myocarditis

      i. Reduction of the inflammation with _____ medications

      ii. _____ if necessary

      iii. Bed _____

      iv. A(n) _____-_____ diet

      v. _____ to remove excessive fluid from the body

10. Pericarditis

   A. Pericarditis is inflammation of the _____ that _____

    the heart.

B. It is most commonly caused by a(n) _____ _____ and may also accompany other diseases.

C. Signs and symptoms of pericarditis

    i. Sharp, _____ chest pain

    ii. _____

    iii. _____

    iv. Dyspnea, especially while _____ down, taking a _____ breath, or _____

D. Treatment options for pericarditis

    i. Analgesics

    ii. _____ to help reduce the amount of fluid around the heart

    iii. Antibiotics or _____ to treat the infection

    iv. _____ for chronic cases

11. Congestive Heart Failure

A. Congestive heart failure is a condition in which the heart is unable to pump _____ blood to the body's other organs.

B. Congestive heart failure results from several other conditions, including the following.

    i. _____

    ii. _____

    iii. _____

    iv. _____

    v. _____

    vi. _____

C. Signs and symptoms of congestive heart failure

    i. Shortness of _____ and general _____ and fatigue

    ii. Trouble simply _____ across a(n) _____ without becoming out of breath and _____

    iii. Swelling, usually in the _____ and _____ but sometimes in other parts of the body, including the _____

    iv. Shortness of breath that is pronounced when the person is lying _____

    v. Increased frequency of _____ during the night

    vi. Weight _____ that often occurs _____ because of the increased fluid and resulting edema

    vii. Cough, decreased _____, and irregular _____

D. Treatment options for congestive heart failure

    i. Rest, proper _____, and maintenance of a healthy

       _____

    ii. Revising daily _____ that may aggravate _____

    iii. Oxygen _____

    iv. Medications such as _____ inhibitors, _____

       blockers, _____, diuretics, and _____

12. Cor Pumonale

A. Cor pumonale is known as _____-sided heart disease.

B. It is a result of prolonged _____ of the pulmonary arteries and right

   _____ of the heart.

C. Signs and symptoms of cor pumonale

    i. Pain toward the _____ of the chest

    ii. Frequent _____ episodes during activity

    iii. Peripheral swelling of _____ and _____

    iv. _____ or wheezing

D. Treatment options for cor pumonale

    i. Medications that improve _____ _____ are

       usually prescribed.

    ii. Anticoagulants to _____ the blood or antihypertensive medications

       and diuretics to _____ _____ pressure may also

       be prescribed.

    iii. If medications fail, a(n) _____ or heart-lung transplant might be

       necessary.

13. Coronary Artery Disease

A. Coronary artery disease is also known as _____

   _____ _____.

B. It is the _____ of the coronary arteries that supply blood to the heart,

   which results from a buildup of _____ on the artery walls.

C. It is the most common form of _____ _____ and the

   leading cause of _____ in the United States.

D. Signs and symptoms of coronary artery disease

    i. _____ of breath

    ii. Fatigue with _____ and a(n) _____ sensation of

       the heart

iii. Edema in the _____

iv. A feeling of overall _____ and _____

E. Treatment options for coronary artery disease

i. _____ medications may be prescribed if hypertension is an underlying cause of CAD.

ii. _____ is administered during bouts of angina to help relieve chest pain.

iii. _____, taken in low doses on a daily basis, is also used to treat CAD.

iv. Medications can help lower _____ levels.

v. Patients are advised to make _____ changes that will assist in their progress.

14. Heart Attack/Myocardial Infarction/Cardiac Arrest

A. Cardiac arrest occurs when the blood supply to a part of the _____ has stopped, causing tissue damage or death from oxygen _____.

B. The main causes of myocardial infarctions include coronary artery disease, particularly _____, and _____.

C. Depending on the extent of the damage, a patient may suffer _____ or _____ from a heart attack.

D. _____ _____ is the total cessation of heartbeat and _____, and it may occur suddenly, with no prior _____ of a heart attack.

E. Signs and symptoms of cardiac arrest

i. The most common symptom is chest pain that is often described as _____ or squeezing, with a feeling of _____, heaviness, or _____ in the center of the chest.

ii. This pain may radiate down the _____ arm or into the neck or _____.

iii. A woman is more likely to feel pain in the _____, which may radiate across the _____ and up into the _____.

iv. _____, shortness of breath, nausea, _____ or dizziness, and an overall feeling of _____ _____ are also common symptoms experienced by women.

F. Treatment options for cardiac arrest

i. For a patient in cardiac arrest, cardiopulmonary _____ and _____ within the first few minutes increase the survival rate.

ii. _____ can stop some heart attacks in progress.

iii. _____, which is surgical vessel repair, is frequently performed to reopen blocked coronary arteries.

iv. _____ are used to hold the arteries open, allowing more blood flow.

v. In severe cases a(n) _____ artery _____ graft will be attempted to bypass the blocked artery using a(n) _____ from the leg or arm.

vi. Immediate _____ is key to survival.

15. Hemophilia

A. Hemophilia is a blood _____ disorder.

B. It is caused by a genetic defect of the _____.

C. Signs and symptoms of hemophilia

i. Excessive bleeding, or _____, is the primary sign of hemophilia.

ii. A hemophiliac may display signs including excessive _____ _____, heavy bleeding from a(n) _____ cut, and the _____ of bleeding after it has ceased for a short time.

iii. Signs of internal bleeding include easily _____ and blood appearing in _____ or _____.

D. Treatment options for hemophilia

i. Hemophilia is treated by _____ the deficient clotting factor in a process called _____ therapy.

16. Leukemia

A. Leukemia is a cancer of the _____ _____ and blood.

B. There are two types of leukemia.

i. Acute leukemia—A(n) _____ form of cancer. The increased number of abnormal cells crowd out the _____ _____ cells. This increases the body's risk of _____ and developing anemia. Another characteristic is a lack of _____, which means the patient may be at risk for extensive bleeding.

ii. Chronic leukemia—This form is _____ aggressive than acute leukemia because the abnormal cells accrue over a(n) _____ _____ of time.

C. Whether leukemia is lymphocytic or _____ depends on whether the cancer has struck _____ or myeloid cells, which are _____ _____ cells.

D. Signs and symptoms of leukemia

    i. _____

    ii. _____

    iii. _____

    iv. _____

    v. _____

    vi. _____

    vii. _____

    viii. _____

    ix. _____

    x. _____

    xi. _____

E. Treatment options for leukemia

    i. _____, radiation, and bone _____ transplantation

    ii. _____ drugs to kill leukemia cells

    iii. High-energy _____ to irradiate the cancer cells

17. Stroke

A. Stroke is sometimes called a(n) _____ _____.

B. It occurs when the _____ _____ to part of the brain is suddenly interrupted.

C. Signs and symptoms of stroke

    i. Numbness or _____ on one side of the body

    ii. _____ or trouble speaking

    iii. _____ problems

    iv. Severe _____

    v. Loss of _____ or coordination

    vi. Severe _____

D. Evaluate a patient for stroke by using the FAST acronym.

    i. _____—If a stroke is suspected, ask the individual to smile to determine whether one side of the face droops.

    ii. _____—To evaluate balance, ask the individual to hold out both arms. Does one arm drift downward?

    iii. _____—Ask the individual to repeat a simple phrase to assess the speech; look for signs of slurring or strange inflections.

    iv. _____—If a person demonstrates any of these signs, time is valuable, and treatment must be sought immediately by calling 911.

E. Treatment options for stroke

    i. Treatment is aimed at controlling factors that may place a patient

    _____ _____ for stroke or a(n)

    _____ of stroke.

    ii. Rehabilitation may be necessary to help the patient with _____ and

    _____, which are often affected.

    iii. Medications can prevent the formation of _____.

18. Thrombophlebitis

    A. Thrombophlebitis occurs when a(n) _____ _____

    causes inflammation in one or more veins, typically in the _____

    extremities.

    B. _____ thrombophlebitis occurs when the affected vein is near the surface

    of the skin.

    C. Signs and symptoms of thrombophlebitis

    i. Redness, _____, warmth, _____, and a dull ache

    or _____ may occur in the affected area.

    ii. Superficial veins visibly display as hard and red _____ of

    _____ vein just under the skin.

    iii. Deep veins in the leg may become swollen, _____, and

    _____, particularly when the person _____ or

    walks.

    D. Treatment options for thrombophlebitis

    i. Superficial vein thrombosis: Home remedies include limb _____,

    _____ application, and the use of _____.

    ii. Deep vein thrombosis: An injection of a(n) _____ medication often

    prevents the clot from growing.

    iii. Additional treatments may include the application of _____

    _____ to constrict the superficial veins and increase blood flow in

    the _____ _____.

    iv. A(n) _____ or bypass surgery may be required to remove an acute

    clot blocking a(n) _____ or abdominal vein.

19. Transfusion Incompatibility Reaction

    A. A severe transfusion reaction can occur if a patient is administered the

    _____ _____ of blood.

    B. Signs and symptoms of transfusion incompatibility reaction

    i. Signs and symptoms arise rapidly with collapse of the _____ system.

    ii. Symptoms of shock, such as _____, restlessness, and shortness of
        _____, are dramatic.

C. Treatment options for transfusion incompatibility reaction

    i. Transfusion of donor blood must be _____ immediately.

    ii. Normal _____ will be infused into the bloodstream intravenously.

    iii. If the reaction is more aggressive, administration of _____ may be
        needed.

20. Valvular Heart Disease

  A. Valvular heart disease is _____ to or a defect in one of the four valves of
    the heart.

  B. _____ _____ is one of the most common types of
    valvular heart disease.

    i. The mitral valve is unable to _____ _____

    ii. This deficiency prevents proper _____ _____
        and causes a buildup of blood in the left _____.

    iii. This can cause the _____ _____ to swell and
        may lead to other problems, including a backup of blood and body fluid in the lung
        tissue.

  C. Signs and symptoms of mitral stenosis

    i. A(n) _____ _____ may be audible with a
        stethoscope.

    ii. Generally mild signs and symptoms include increased fatigue,
        _____, and frequent _____ infections,
        discomfort with increased _____, edema of the
        _____ and _____, and heart palpitations.

  D. Treatment options for mitral stenosis

    i. Medication can strengthen _____ _____.

    ii. Short or long-term _____ may be required if bacterial
        _____ is involved.

    iii. Surgery to replace the damaged _____ may be required.

21. Varicose Veins

  A. Varicose veins are gnarled, _____ veins, usually superficial veins in the
    _____.

  B. They may be caused by prolonged periods of standing, _____,
    _____, or aging.

C. Signs and symptoms of varicose veins

    i. The limbs may feel heavy and _____.

    ii. When severe cases develop and are untreated the affected veins can

        _____, resulting in varicose _____ on the skin.

D. Treatment options for varicose veins

    i. Treatments aimed at symptom relief include such measures as moderate

        _____, avoiding long periods of _____,

        _____ the legs, and wearing support stockings.

    ii. _____ _____ may decrease the size and visibility

of the affected veins.

APPLIED PRACTICE

1. Using the textbook, fill in the table below.

Disease	Symptoms	Treatment
Hypertension		
Prehypertension		

Disease	Symptoms	Treatment
Hypotension		

2. Using the textbook, label the interior view of the heart chambers.

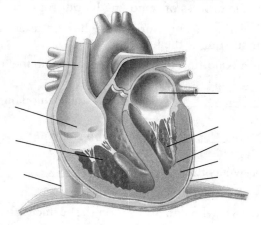

3. Using the textbook, label the conduction system of the heart.

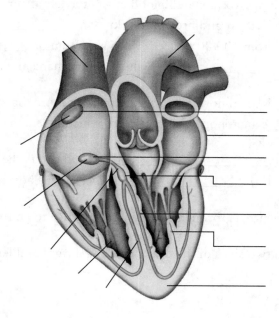

LEARNING ACTIVITY: FILL IN THE BLANK

Using words from the list below, fill in the blanks to complete the following statements.

agglutination
buffers
cardiac arrest
congestive heart failure
hypertension
myocardial infarction
pericardium
pulmonary artery
septum
tricuspid valve

aneurysm
Bundle of His
cardiac tamponade
defibrillation
hypotension
myocardium
prehypertension
pulmonary vein
tachycardia
venipuncture

1. The medical term for high blood pressure is _____.

2. The middle layer, or heart muscle, is called the _____.

3. _____ is the process of removing blood from the veins for examination.

4. _____ is defined as pressure on the heart muscle caused by blood or fluid collecting in the pericardial sac that surrounds the heart.

5. _____ is a condition in which the heart is unable to pump sufficient blood to the body's other organs.

6. Symptoms of a(n) _____ include a squeezing pain or heavy pressure in the middle of the chest.

7. Performing _____ on a patient who is having a heart attack but still has a pulse may be harmful.

8. The AV bundle is also known as the _____.

9. The _____ is the outer lining of the heart.

10. _____ occurs when an antigen on the surface of red blood cells binds to antibodies in the plasma.

11. On its return from the lungs, oxygenated blood enters the left atrium via the _____.

12. The total cessation of heartbeat and breathing is known as _____.

13. Blood pressure ranging from 120/80 to 139/89 is a symptom of _____.

14. The blood contains _____, which are mechanisms within the blood that balance the pH level.

15. _____ is an abnormally fast heartbeat of more than 100 beats per minute.

16. _____ is an abnormal condition in which a person's blood pressure is much lower than usual.

17. After going through the _____, the blood enters the right ventricle.

18. Common locations for a(n) _____ include the aorta, brain, leg, spleen and intestine.

19. Blood leaves the right ventricle through the pulmonary valve to go to the lungs, via the _____.

20. The wall that separates two sides of the heart, creating a right and left side, is called the _____.

CRITICAL THINKING

Answer the following questions to the best of your ability. Use the textbook as a reference.

1. You are working at the reception desk at Pearson Physicians Group. Mr. Donaldson has been waiting 5 minutes for his appointment. He is sitting in a chair with his left arm in front of his chest. His face appears as if he is in pain. He seems short of breath, and there appears to be some bluing of the skin near his lips. What is your first thought about this patient? How might you handle this situation? *(Medical assistants never make a diagnosis; this is a question about your knowledge of the signs and symptoms of various conditions that are presented in the textbook.)*

_____

_____

_____

_____

2. Monique La'Nosta has a history of hypertension and coronary artery disease. She was seen in the office 4 days ago for fatigue. Today, she has returned, with complaints of shortness of breath and being exhausted after brief activity. She has gained 10 pounds since her last office visit. What cardiovascular disease might Ms. La'Nosta be suffering from? What led you to make your decision? What would explain the patient's sudden weight gain? *(Medical assistants never make a diagnosis; this is a question about your knowledge of the signs and symptoms of various conditions that are presented in the textbook.)*

_____

_____

_____

_____

3. Adam Welch is a 32-year-old man who has had consistent blood pressure readings that average around 162/104. He has been diagnosed with hypertension. Based on his average readings, which stage of hypertension would Mr. Welch be assigned? What lifestyle changes might Mr. Welch want to consider in order to help decrease his blood pressure?

_____

_____

_____

_____

RESEARCH ACTIVITY

Use Internet search engines to research the following topic and write a brief description of what you find. It is important to use reputable websites.

1. Visit www.americanheart.org and navigate through the website. Pay particular attention to the section For Healthcare Professionals. Explain what information you think is most useful in this section and why.

   _____

   _____

   _____

   _____

   _____

CHAPTER 27
The Immune System

STUDENT STUDY GUIDE

Use the following guide to assist in your learning of the concepts from the chapter.

I. Function and Structures of the Immune System

  1. Functions of the Lymphatic System

    A. Maintaining _____ _____ by draining excess fluid from _____ and returning this fluid to the bloodstream

    B. Acting as a(n) _____ _____ system for wastes produced by cells

    C. Working in conjunction with the _____ system to absorb and transport fatty acids from the digestive tract to the _____

    D. Defending the body against _____ and other harmful agents

  2. Overview of the Lymphatic System

    A. The lymphatic system is a network of vessels, _____, and _____ that more or less parallel in function, but are separate from, the blood _____ of the circulatory system.

    B. _____ comes from blood plasma that has leaked out from capillaries.

    C. The lymphatic system collects the lymph and returns it to the _____.

  3. Lymphatic Pathways

    A. Fill in the image below to indicate the structures of lymphatic pathways from smallest to largest.

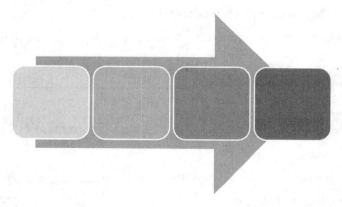

4. Lymph Nodes
   A. Lymph nodes come in many different sizes and _____, but most are bean shaped and about _____ _____ long.
   B. Lymph nodes have multiple _____ _____—vessels that bring lymph into the node.
   C. Lymph is circulated out of the node through _____ _____— vessels that carry it away from the node to the rest of the body.
   D. B lymphocytes are responsible for production of _____.
   E. When a(n) _____ enters the body, the B cells that produce antibodies against that particular antigen rapidly undergo _____ and divide in order to seek out and help to destroy the antigen.
   F. In addition to the part of the lymph node cortex that contains B lymphocytes, the rest of the lymph node cortex contains _____ _____.
   G. T lymphocytes promote _____ through a cell-mediated _____.
      i. Instead of producing _____ to attack the antigen as B lymphocytes do, T lymphocytes attack directly by _____ themselves to the _____ on the cells of the foreign substance.
   H. Some B and T lymphocytes become _____ _____, whose function is to "remember" the pathogen, which enables them to identify and _____ _____ if that same pathogen enters the body again.
5. Spleen
   A. The spleen is located in the upper-_____ _____ of the abdomen.
   B. It is the _____ lymphatic organ.
   C. The tissue of the spleen is either _____ or _____ pulp.
   D. Red pulp removes damaged _____ _____ cells and also acts as a storage site for _____.
   E. White pulp of the spleen is where the _____ _____ occurs.
   F. The white pulp is composed of both _____ and _____ lymphocytes.
6. Tonsils
   A. There are three sets of tonsils: _____, _____, and _____.
   B. They filter _____ and aid in the formation of _____ blood cells.
7. Bone Marrow and Thymus
   A. Bone marrow and the thymus are considered _____ lymphatic organs.
   B. The majority of the body's _____ are produced here.

C. Bone marrow contains _____ _____ that develop into all the cells of the _____.

D. The thymus gland is located behind the _____, in the _____ mediastinum.

   i. It is divided into an outer cortex and an internal _____.

   ii. The thymus manufactures _____-fighting _____ _____ and helps distinguish normal T cells from those that attack the body's own tissues.

II. The Immune Response and the Body's Defenses

1. The _____ _____ occurs when the cells, tissues, and organs that make up the immune system work together to _____ _____ and substances that invade body systems and cause illness and disease.

2. Antibodies work together to respond to a(n) _____ that has been detected in the body.

3. Once _____ have been created to attack a specific antigen, the person cannot get sick from the same _____ again.

4. This is the same reason _____ are given to protect against specific diseases.

5. Antibodies must work together with _____ _____, which will _____ antigens that have been tagged by antibodies.

6. Immunosuppressants and Immunity

A. Immunosuppressants are medications that _____ the immune system to keep it from working as _____ and _____ as it normally would.

B. Immunosuppressants are usually given after a(n) _____ _____ to prevent rejection of the organ.

C. There are three types of immunity.

   i. Innate immunity is passed down from _____ to _____.

   ii. Active immunity is not present at birth.

     a. Acquired active immunity develops after exposure to a live _____.

     b. Artificial acquired active immunity is induced by a(n) _____.

   iii. Passive immunity is not a(n) _____ form of immunity.

     a. _____ _____ _____ occurs when antibodies are passed to an infant through breast milk.

     b. _____ _____ _____ occurs when urgent treatment is needed for an already immune individual.

III. Common Pathology Associated with the Immune System

1. Autoimmune diseases occur when the body begins to attack its _____ healthy _____ and _____.

2. There are many autoimmune diseases.

   A. Rheumatoid arthritis is an autoimmune disease that attacks the _____ _____.

   B. Multiple sclerosis is an autoimmune disease that attacks the _____ _____.

   C. Crohn's disease is an autoimmune disease of the _____ _____.

   D. Glomerulonephritis is an autoimmune disease of the _____ _____.

3. Acquired Immunodeficiency Syndrome (AIDS)

   A. AIDS is a(n) _____ disease of the immune system

   B. It develops as the _____ _____ to HIV infection.

   C. Signs and symptoms of AIDS

      i. People with HIV can be _____ for up to 10 years after contracting the virus.

      ii. Progression to full-blown _____ is diagnosed when a T lymphocyte count is below _____.

      iii. Fever; _____ loss; diarrhea; swollen _____ glands; and ulcers of the _____, mouth, and _____ are common symptoms of AIDS.

      iv. Meningitis; _____; and yeast infections afflicting the _____, esophagus, and _____ are also common.

      v. _____ _____ is a skin cancer marked by red lesions and is seen in AIDS patients.

   D. Treatment options for AIDS

      i. There is currently _____ _____ for HIV and AIDS.

      ii. Treatment is aimed at improving the _____ and _____ of life through _____ treatment.

      iii. _____ drugs can suppress replication of the virus.

4. Allergies

   A. An allergy is an abnormal reaction, or _____, to a substance that doesn't normally cause a reaction in most people.

   B. Allergic reactions may be _____ or may be _____.

   C. _____ is an extreme, rapidly progressing, and often life-threatening allergic response.

   D. Signs and symptoms of allergies

      i. Local or systemic inflammatory reactions are characterized by redness, _____, and _____.

  ii. Respiratory symptoms include _____, sneezing, _____, and nasal _____.

  iii. Allergic conditions include _____ (skin inflammation), _____ _____ (irritation of the nasal passages), hay fever, _____ asthma, _____ (hives), and food allergies.

  iv. Anaphylaxis also involves swelling in the _____ and _____ that can cause breathing difficulties, _____, and death.

 E. Treatment options for allergies

  i. Treatment includes medications such as the antihistamine diphenhydramine (_____), allergy testing to determine the exact _____, and desensitization.

  ii. _____ counteracts the effects of an allergic reaction and is given to someone experiencing anaphylaxis.

5. Cancer

 A. Cancer cells are _____ in their form and function.

 B. They make use of the body's resources at the expense of _____ _____ through their uncontrolled growth and reproduction.

 C. Cancer cells join together to form _____ or masses.

 D. _____ occurs when cancer cells break away from a(n) _____ and travel to other areas of the body, where they keep growing and form new tumors.

 E. Signs and symptoms of cancer

  i. Cancer signs and symptoms are vast and depend on the _____ of the _____.

  ii. Generalized symptoms that often occur with most forms of cancer include extreme _____, decreased _____, unintentional and often _____ weight loss, and _____ and chills.

 F. Treatment options for cancer

  i. Cancer may be treated with _____, _____, _____, or a combination of all three.

  ii. The choice of treatment generally depends on the _____ of cancer and the _____ of the tumor.

  iii. The TNM system of staging tumors measures three criteria—_____, _____ _____ involvement, and _____.

6. Chronic Fatigue Syndrome (CFS)

 A. CFS is a continual sense of tiredness that is not helped by periods of _____ or _____.

B. Many physicians consider CFS to be a shared condition of many _____ and possibly _____ diseases.

C. Some believe that a(n) _____ immune system is the culprit.

D. Signs and symptoms of CFS

    i. Intense and continual fatigue lasting for at least _____ _____ that is not relieved with rest, lack of _____, depression and _____, and _____ disorders.

    ii. Flulike symptoms including _____ _____, low-grade _____, _____ lymph nodes, and _____ may also be associated with CFS.

E. Treatment options for CFS

    i. Treatment begins with a thorough evaluation of the patient's prior _____ _____.

    ii. Medications to treat _____ and _____ may be prescribed.

    iii. A healthy _____, incorporating _____ into daily life, and proper knowledge and implementation of _____ _____ techniques are helpful.

    iv. Rest, _____, and _____ mechanisms for dealing with stress are also important factors in treatment.

7. Infectious Mononucleosis

A. Infectious mononucleosis is caused by the _____-_____ virus.

B. Mononuclear _____ _____ cells multiply in number and increase.

C. This virus is commonly spread through _____ and is often called the _____ _____.

D. Signs and symptoms of infectious mononucleosis

    i. _____

    ii. _____

    iii. _____

    iv. _____

    v. _____

    vi. _____

    vii. _____

E. Treatment options for infectious mononucleosis

    i. _____ symptoms because the virus _____ be treated

    ii. Getting plenty of _____

    iii. Gargling with _____ _____

    iv. Taking analgesics and _____

    v. Taking _____ for severe swelling of the throat

8. Lymphedema

  A. Lymphedema derives from a damaged or dysfunctional lymphatic system that results in an accumulation of _____ _____, which causes _____.

  B. It is considered either primary or secondary. (Describe both.)

    i. Primary—_____

    ii. Secondary—_____

  C. Signs and symptoms of lymphedema

    i. Swelling at the _____ _____

    ii. Swelling limited to one _____ or one _____ as the lymphatic fluid pools in the affected extremity

  D. Treatment options for lymphedema

    i. _____ may be encouraged to help with movement and directing the accumulated fluid away from the extremity.

    ii. _____ _____ and bandages are also used to put pressure on the extremity.

    iii. A specialized massage, called _____ _____ _____, is available for some patients.

    iv. _____ _____ _____ is use of several treatments.

9. Rheumatoid Arthritis

  A. Rheumatoid arthritis occurs when the body's _____ _____ attack tissue in the joints, leading to pain and _____ of the articular cartilage.

  B. Patients often have a shorter _____ _____ than their healthy peers.

  C. Signs and symptoms of rheumatoid arthritis

    i. Pain, _____, and _____ in the joints of the wrists, _____, knees, _____, and ankles.

    ii. _____ joint stiffness is common.

     iii. Over time, joints will have decreased _____ of _____ and become _____.

     iv. Numbness, _____, and _____ sensations may also be felt near the affected joint.

     v. Fatigue, poor _____ _____, and _____ are also common.

  D. Treatment options for rheumatoid arthritis

     i. Drugs are used to treat and _____ the _____ and to help the patient have a better quality of life.

     ii. Antiinflammatory medications, _____, and _____ promote joint strengthening and mobility.

     iii. On initial diagnosis, _____-modifying _____ drugs are often prescribed.

10. Systemic Lupus Erythematosus (SLE)

  A. SLE is called a systemic disorder because its effects may appear in many _____ of the _____.

  B. Incidents that have been linked to triggering lupus include _____, illness due to _____, pregnancy, and even exposure to _____.

  C. Signs and symptoms of SLE

     i. Signs and symptoms of SLE mimic those of _____, making it difficult to _____ SLE.

     ii. Pain and swelling in the _____ are common.

     iii. General fatigue, _____, chills, _____ changes, and headache occur.

     iv. _____ loss, _____ sores, and sensitivity to _____ are also attributed to this disease.

     v. A butterfly rash covers the _____ of the nose and the _____, and it worsens in _____.

     vi. _____, raised _____ known as discoid lupus erythematosus appear.

     vii. Vasculitis, or _____ blood vessels, is common.

  D. Treatment options for SLE

     i. Treatment is usually aimed at reducing the _____ _____ and controlling _____ using corticosteroids.

     ii. _____ drugs may be prescribed to alleviate other symptoms.

APPLIED PRACTICE

1. Label the components of the lymphatic system.

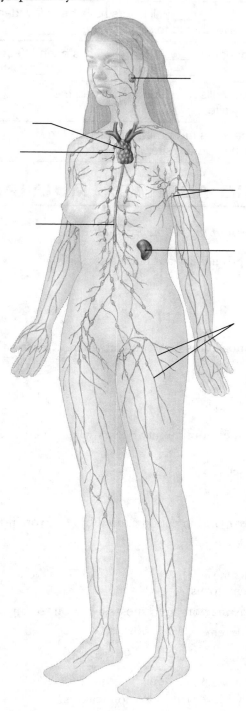

2. Fill in the blank spaces in the table below. Use your textbook for reference.

Stage 0	With early detection, _____ cancer cells are only a few layers deep. This is termed _____ in _____.
Stage I	_____ cell layers have been invaded by cancer cells, and some cells may have spread to surrounding _____.
Stage II	Surrounding _____ has been affected by cancer cells, but the cancer is _____ at the _____ site of cancer.
Stage III	Cancer cells have spread beyond the _____ _____ to nearby sites.
Stage IV	Cancer cells have metastasized to other _____ _____ other than the primary site.

LEARNING ACTIVITY: MULTIPLE CHOICE

Circle the correct answer to each of the following questions.

1. The cells responsible for production antibodies are

    a. T cells.
    b. B cells.
    c. A cells.
    d. M cells.

2. Which of the following substances may cause an allergic reaction?

    a. Dust
    b. Mold
    c. Pollen
    d. All of the above

3. Which of the following types of immunity occurs when a person is exposed to a live pathogen?

    a. Active
    b. Artificially acquired active
    c. Acquired active
    d. Natural

4. Which of the following is a viral infection caused by the Epstein-Barr virus?

    a. Infectious mononucleosis
    b. Lymphedema
    c. Chronic fatigue syndrome
    d. Systemic lupus erythematosus

5. Which of the following risk factors predisposes a person to cancer?

    a. Suppressed immune system
    b. Exposure to radiation
    c. Viruses
    d. All of the above

6. Which statement is *false* with regard to mononucleosis?

    a. It is caused by a herpes virus.
    b. It is common among toddler patients.
    c. It is characterized by an increase in white blood cells.
    d. It is often spread through saliva.

7. Which of the following allow the body to remember and recognize previous invading organisms?
   a. Lymphocytes
   b. Neutrophils
   c. Phagocytes
   d. Leukocytes

8. T lymphocytes attack directly by binding themselves to the antigens on the cells of the foreign substance. This process is known as
   a. active immunity.
   b. acquired active immunity.
   c. humoral immunity.
   d. cell-mediated response.

9. The thymus gland begins to decrease in size after
   a. birth.
   b. childhood.
   c. puberty.
   d. pregnancy.

10. Which of the following contains stem cells that create all the cells that make up the tissues and structures of the immune system?
    a. Bone marrow
    b. Liver
    c. Thymus gland
    d. Lymph nodes

CRITICAL THINKING

Answer the following questions to the best of your ability. Use the textbook as a reference.

1. Roman Antonelli is a 71-year-old patient at Pearson Physicians Group. Over the past 3 years, he has been experiencing an increased number of infections. He has been told he is more susceptible to developing autoimmune diseases. Explain why Mr. Antonelli is facing these new health challenges.

   _____

   _____

   _____

   _____

2. Brody Frenn is an 8-year-old boy who has recently been diagnosed with leukemia. His outlook is promising because his cancer has been diagnosed as stage I. Brody is scared and doesn't understand what cancer is. He asks you to explain how he got cancer and what stage I means. What will you say to Brody?

   _____

   _____

   _____

   _____

RESEARCH ACTIVITY

Use Internet search engines to research the following topic and write a brief description of what you find. It is important to use reputable websites.

1. Research an autoimmune disease that is of interest to you. Identify the signs and symptoms of the disease, how a diagnosis is made, and treatment options. Also, research support groups, societies, or foundations for that disease. Write an essay on your findings and be sure to cite the websites where you found your information.

   _____

   _____

   _____

   _____

   _____

CHAPTER 28
The Respiratory System

STUDENT STUDY GUIDE

Use the following guide to assist in your learning of the concepts from the chapter.

I. Overview of the Respiratory System

   1. Inhaled air passes from the _____ into blood in the capillaries, which carry the _____ to the body's _____.

   2. _____ _____ that has been picked up as a waste product of the cells is passed from the capillaries into the alveoli.

   3. The pathway for respiration through the respiratory tract is the mouth, _____, trachea, _____, bronchioles, and _____.

   4. Actions of inhalation and exhalation are achieved by the alternating _____ and _____ of the respiratory muscles.

II. Structures of the Respiratory Tract*

   1. Structures of the Upper Respiratory Tract (List four structures.)

      A. _____

      B. _____

      C. _____

      D. _____

   2. Structures of the Lower Respiratory Tract (List five structures.)

      A. _____

      B. _____

      C. _____

      D. _____

      E. _____

III. Mechanism of Breathing

   1. Two processes of ventilation are _____ and _____.

   2. Respiratory centers of the brain are located in the _____ _____ and the pons.

---

*The structures of the respiratory tract will be covered in more detail later, in other activities in this chapter.

3. Respiratory Muscles

    A. The diaphragm is a(n) _____-shaped muscle below the lungs that separates the _____ cavity from the _____ cavity.

    B. External intercostal muscles pull the ribs _____ and _____.

    C. Internal intercostal muscles pull the ribs _____ and _____.

4. Dyspnea is _____ breathing.

5. Apnea is the _____ of breathing for more than _____ seconds.

6. Orthopnea is trouble breathing unless a certain _____ is _____.

7. Inhalation

    A. The _____ system sends a(n) _____ to the diaphragm and external intercostal muscles.

    B. The diaphragm contracts and _____.

    C. At the same time, the external intercostal muscles contract to pull the _____ upward and outward, which increases the size of the _____.

    D. The increase in the size of the chest cavity _____ _____ within the chest so that _____ air, which is now under greater pressure, flows into the _____.

8. Exhalation

    A. The diaphragm and the intercostal muscles _____, and the thorax returns to its resting _____ and _____.

    B. This reduction in size of the thoracic cavity builds pressure _____ the chest cavity until it is greater than environmental air _____, which causes air to _____ _____ of the lungs.

    C. The elastic recoil of _____ _____ aids in quiet expiration.

    D. Forceful expiration involves the _____ intercostals and _____ muscles.

IV. Common Pathology Associated with the Respiratory System

1. Lack of oxygen in the body is termed _____.

2. _____ is also known as asphyxia.

3. Asthma

    A. Asthma is a chronic inflammatory disease of the _____.

    B. It typically occurs when _____ or other irritating substances cause swelling in the lining of the _____ and _____ tubes, aggravating sensitive tissues.

    C. Excessive _____ is created within the respiratory tract in an attempt to _____ the offending intruder.

D. The presence of excessive mucus can cause _____ or a sense of struggling to _____.

E. Signs and symptoms of asthma

    i. _____ and difficulty _____ are classic signs of asthma.

    ii. Congestion, _____, and _____ in the chest may occur, which can cause anxiety in the patient.

    iii. Symptoms may be worse in the _____ and at _____.

F. Treatment options for asthma

    i. _____ to open the bronchial passages

    ii. _____-acting beta 2 medications

    iii. Inhaled _____

4. Chronic Obstructive Pulmonary Disease (COPD)

A. COPD consists of two related diseases: chronic _____ and _____.

B. It is characterized by chronic obstruction of the _____ of air in and out of the _____.

C. It is generally _____ and progressively _____ over time.

D. Smoking is responsible for _____ to _____ percent of cases of COPD in the United States.

E. Signs and symptoms of COPD

    i. Shortness of _____ and difficulty breathing, particularly with _____

    ii. An increased number of respiratory _____

    iii. Wheezing, a persistent _____, regular production of _____, fatigue, tightness in the _____, and inability to catch one's _____

F. Treatment options for COPD

    i. There is no _____.

    ii. Treatment strategies include the following.

        a. Smoking _____

        b. _____ to open the airways and decrease airway inflammation

        c. Vaccination against _____ and _____

        d. Regular oxygen _____

        e. Pulmonary _____

        f. Proper _____ and minimal _____

5. Bronchitis

    A. Bronchitis is a respiratory disease marked by inflamed _____ _____ in the bronchial passages.

    B. There are two forms:

        i. Acute—Lasting less than _____ _____ and generally caused by _____ lung infections but can also be caused by _____ infections

        ii. Chronic—Recurring frequently for more than _____ _____ and may be caused by _____ attacks of acute bronchitis

    C. Signs and symptoms of acute bronchitis

        i. _____ cough

        ii. Yellow, _____, or _____ phlegm, which usually appears _____ to _____ hours after the cough begins

        iii. Coughing up _____ (hemoptysis)

        iv. Low-grade _____ and chills

        v. _____ and tightness in the chest

        vi. Pain below the _____ during deep breathing

        vii. Shortness of _____

    D. Signs and symptoms of chronic bronchitis

        i. Persistent _____ that produces yellow, white, or green _____ (for at least _____ months of the year and for more than _____ consecutive years)

        ii. Sometimes wheezing and _____

    E. Treatment options for acute bronchitis

        i. Getting plenty of _____

        ii. Drinking lots of _____

        iii. Avoiding _____ and fumes

        iv. Using an inhaled _____

        v. Taking cough _____

        vi. Taking antibiotics if there is a(n) _____ _____ present

    F. Treatment options for chronic bronchitis

        i. Routine use of _____ or oral steroids

        ii. _____ to thin mucus

        iii. With severe cases, supplemental _____

6. Emphysema

    A. Emphysema is a long-term, _____ disease of the lung and also a form of COPD.

B. Permanent holes develop in the _____ _____, making them unable to hold their shape properly on _____.

C. Signs and symptoms of emphysema

    i. Shortness of _____ is the most common symptom.

    ii. Severe breathing difficulties may cause the patient's complexion, _____, or _____ beds may turn bluish in appearance.

    iii. Coughing, sometimes caused by the production of _____, and _____ may also be symptoms.

    iv. Rapid _____, decreased _____, and intolerance for _____ are also common.

D. Treatment options for emphysema

    i. Most doctors require _____ _____.

    ii. _____ are usually the first medications prescribed.

    iii. Steroids and _____, if an infection is present, may be prescribed.

    iv. _____ therapy may be needed.

    v. _____ rehabilitation can help.

    vi. In severe cases, surgery to remove the _____ may be necessary.

7. Common Cold

A. A cold is a(n) _____ _____ of the upper respiratory tract.

B. The _____ is the most common culprit.

C. Cold viruses are transmitted through _____ which can travel _____ to _____ feet through the air.

D. Signs and symptoms of the common cold

    i. The cold usually appears _____ to _____ days after exposure to a cold virus.

    ii. Common symptoms are runny or _____ nose, _____ or sore throat, cough, _____, slight body _____, mild headache, sneezing, _____ eyes, low-grade fever of less than _____°F, and mild _____.

    iii. Nasal discharge may become _____ and turn _____ or green as the cold runs its course.

E. Treatment options for the common cold

    i. Medications can relieve some _____, though they can't shorten the _____ of the illness.

    ii. Mild _____ _____ may be helpful for fever, sore throat, and headache.

iii. _____ or decongestants may be useful for runny nose and nasal

   _____.

   iv. It is helpful to take _____ to help slow the spread of cold

   _____.

8. Hay Fever

   A. Hay fever is sometimes called seasonal allergic rhinitis or _____.

   B. It is a seasonal allergy in which the _____ _____ of the nose
   become inflamed.

   C. The most likely cause of hay fever is the _____ of trees, plants, and
   _____ carried by the wind and air.

   D. Signs and symptoms of hay fever

   i. Repeated and prolonged _____

   ii. Stuffy and _____ nose

   iii. Redness, _____, and _____ of the eyes

   iv. Itching of the nose, _____, mouth, and _____

   v. _____ problems

   vi. Impaired senses of _____ and _____

   vii. Difficulty breathing and increased coughing from postnasal drip at _____

   E. Treatment options for hay fever

   i. Avoid the _____ that causes the reaction.

   ii. Air filters can _____ air and remove _____ allergens.

   iii. _____ medication may be taken.

   iv. In more severe cases, _____ may be prescribed.

   v. Immunotherapy, or _____ _____, are also helpful in reducing
   symptoms.

9. Influenza

   A. Influenza is an illness caused by _____ that infect the respiratory tract.

   B. Influenza is more _____ than other viral infections.

   C. It has a rapid and quick _____ of symptoms.

   D. The three types of influenza are _____, _____, and _____.

   E. Type _____ is most problematic for humans.

   F. Signs and symptoms of influenza

   i. _____ usually 100°F to 103°F in _____ and often higher in

   _____

   ii. _____ cough

   iii. _____ throat

     iv. _____ or stuffy nose

     v. Headache

     vi. _____ aches

     vii. Chills

     viii. _____ fatigue

G. Treatment options for influenza

     i. _____ medications can shorten the course of influenza but must be taken within the first _____ day(s) after the onset of the first symptoms.

     ii. Medications including pain relievers (_____) and fever reducers (_____) may be prescribed.

     iii. The best defense against influenza is an annual influenza _____.

10. Legionnaires' disease

A. Legionnaires' disease is a lung _____ caused by breathing in a mist of _____ that has been contaminated with the _____ bacterium.

B. This bacterium tends to thrive in _____ water.

C. Signs and symptoms of Legionnaires' disease

     i. Symptoms start _____ to _____ days after exposure and infection.

     ii. Symptoms include high fever with _____, severe _____, shortness of _____, _____ cough, fatigue, and muscle _____ and pains.

     iii. Severe cases may lead to diarrhea, _____, _____ confusion, and kidney and _____ damage.

D. Treatment options for Legionnaires' disease

     i. _____ can fight the *Legionella* infection.

     ii. In severe cases, _____ _____ may be necessary to help with breathing difficulties.

     iii. _____ and _____ replacement might be indicated if the patient is dehydrated because of extreme illness.

11. Lung Cancer

A. Lung cancer is the leading cause of cancer deaths in both _____ and _____ in the United States and throughout the _____.

B. _____ is the most significant factor in the development of lung cancer.

C. _____ smoke is another cause for lung cancer; _____ nonsmokers die each year.

D. Two main types of cancer are _____ cell lung cancer and _____ cell lung cancer.

E. Signs and symptoms of lung cancer

    i. Early stages of lung cancer can be _____.

    ii. As symptoms progress, patients experience the following.

        a. Persistent _____

        b. Coughing up _____

        c. _____ of breath

        d. Wheezing and _____ pain

        e. Recurring _____ infections

        f. Excessive _____

        g. Decreased _____ and weight loss

    iii. With advanced stages of cancer, symptoms include _____ pain, _____ changes, and _____ skin or eyes.

F. Treatment options for lung cancer

    i. Treatment depends on the type of lung cancer and the _____ at which it is diagnosed.

    ii. The most widely used therapies for lung cancer are surgery, _____, and _____ therapy.

12. Pertussis

A. Pertussis is also called _____ _____.

B. It is characterized by _____ and _____ coughing spells.

C. It is caused by _____ _____, a highly contagious bacterium spread through _____ _____.

D. Vaccination is available and is first given when an infant is _____ month(s) old.

E. Signs and symptoms of pertussis

    i. Cough, _____ nose, and a(n) _____-grade fever are common symptoms.

    ii. _____ becomes difficult.

    iii. _____ coughing ends in a noise that sounds like a "_____."

    iv. Some patients may _____ or even lose _____ for a short period of time.

    v. Infants also tend to experience episodes of _____.

F. Treatment options for pertussis

    i. _____ can be effective if pertussis is diagnosed early.

    ii. Infants and children may be hospitalized and monitored due to decreased _____ and violent _____ spells.

iii. In the hospital, _____ therapy, oxygen _____ with high levels of humidity, IV _____, and _____ may be administered.

13. Pleurisy

A. Pleurisy is a(n) _____ of the pleura.

B. It can result from a number of diseases and disorders, including complications from _____ surgery.

C. Signs and symptoms of pleurisy

   i. The chief symptom is _____, intense shooting or stabbing _____ pain, and usually the pain is located directly _____ the area of inflammation.

   ii. Pain is most severe with _____.

   iii. Holding one's _____ often provides relief from the pain.

   iv. Talking, _____, and sneezing also produce intense _____.

   v. Pain may be referred to the _____, _____, or _____.

   vi. _____ is shallow.

   vii. _____ of the patient's lips or nail beds is common.

D. Treatment options for pleurisy

   i. Underlying disease or disorder must be _____.

   ii. _____ and antiinflammatory medicines help with chest pain associated with breathing.

   iii. _____-based cough syrups are prescribed to help ease the pain associated with a(n) _____ _____.

14. Pneumonia

A. Pneumonia is a(n) _____ of the lung or lungs.

B. It can be caused by bacteria, viruses, fungi, or chemical irritants.

C. Signs and symptoms of pneumonia

   i. Chest pain, especially when _____

   ii. Increased tiredness and _____

   iii. A cough that produces green _____ or pus-like sputum

   iv. _____ aches

   v. Fever, chills, and rapid and _____ breathing

D. Treatment options for pneumonia

   i. Fluids, rest, and _____ (if the pneumonia is caused by bacteria)

   ii. Nonprescription drugs for _____ relief

iii. Oxygen therapy and _____ treatments to thin out and remove secretions

iv. _____ in the case of severe pneumonia for careful monitoring and treatment

v. Pneumococcal _____ for prevention

15. Pulmonary Edema

A. Pulmonary edema is a condition in which fluid accumulates in the _____ of the lungs.

B. It is caused by inadequate pumping of the _____ _____ of the heart.

C. It can be chronic or can develop _____ and become life threatening.

D. Signs and symptoms of pulmonary edema

i. Shortness of breath brought on by _____

ii. Difficulty _____ in positions other than sitting upright

iii. Frothy bloody _____ containing pus

iv. Increased _____

v. Cold, clammy, cyanotic _____

vi. _____ swelling

vii. Decreased _____

viii. Increased _____

E. Treatment options for pulmonary edema

i. The goal of treatment is to remove _____ _____ from the lungs.

ii. Emergency _____ is required in severe cases.

iii. High levels of _____ can be administered while the patient sits in a(n) _____ position.

iv. _____ are often administered.

v. Medications to improve _____ _____ are also prescribed when heart failure is the underlying issue.

vi. The _____ cause must be treated to prevent further pulmonary complications.

16. Pulmonary Embolism

A. Pulmonary embolism is a(n) _____ _____ in the lung that occurs when a clot breaks away from the wall of a vein in the leg, _____, arm, or sometimes the _____ side of the heart and travels throughout the bloodstream.

B. The clot becomes lodged in a(n) _____ that is so narrow the clot cannot _____ through.

C. The wedged _____ prevents blood flow to a section of the lung, causing it to suffer infarction due to being deprived of _____.

D. Signs and symptoms of pulmonary embolism

   i. The most common symptom is _____ of _____.

   ii. Sharp, _____ pain occurs when the patient tries to take a deep breath or _____.

   iii. Other signs and symptoms include rapid _____ and rapid heart rate; anxiety or _____; dry _____ or coughing up mucus or blood; sweating; _____ lips and/or nailbeds; and low _____ _____, resulting in loss of consciousness.

E. Treatment options for pulmonary embolism

   i. Pulmonary embolism can be life threatening and is often treated in _____ _____ settings.

   ii. Thrombolytics are used to help _____ the embolus.

   iii. Blood-_____ medications help prevent formation of new clots.

   iv. _____ therapy is initiated to help with breathing.

   v. Medication to raise _____ _____ may be necessary.

17. Severe Acute Respiratory Syndrome (SARS)

A. SARS first infected people in parts of Asia, _____ _____, and Europe in early _____.

B. Experts believe that SARS first developed in _____ rather than _____.

C. This _____ contagious illness is spread via _____ droplets.

D. Signs and symptoms of SARS

   i. Shortness of _____

   ii. Dry _____

   iii. Difficulty _____

   iv. Fevers greater than _____°F

   v. _____ aches

   vi. Headaches, _____, and chills

E. Treatment options for SARS

   i. High doses of _____ reduce _____ of the lungs.

   ii. _____ therapy may be used.

      iii. A patient with SARS is placed in _____ during treatment to prevent _____ of the disease.

      iv. _____ medications are used to help with associated symptoms.

18. Sinusitis

    A. Sinusitis is an infection or inflammation of the _____ _____ that line the inside of the nose and the sinus cavities.

    B. Drainage of fluid from the sinuses into the _____ and _____ becomes blocked, which causes pressure and pain in the sinuses.

    C. Sinuses that do not drain properly are more vulnerable to _____ and _____ growth.

    D. Signs and symptoms of sinusitis

        i. Pain and _____ in the face surrounding the sinus _____

      ii. Stuffy or _____ nose and greenish or yellow nasal _____

      iii. Sore throat, _____ drip, and a cough that worsens at night

      iv. Bad _____, tooth _____, and a dulled sense of _____

    E. Treatment options for sinusitis

        i. A combination of medications, including antibiotics, _____, analgesics, _____, and mucolytics

      ii. Home remedies including moist _____ application to the face, _____ baths, increased _____ and fluid intake, and using a(n) _____ to eliminate dry air

19. Tuberculosis (TB)

    A. Tuberculosis is a contagious disease caused by the bacterium _____ _____.

    B. TB bacteria are spread when infected _____ are inhaled.

    C. Infected droplets are expelled through talking, _____, _____, coughing, sneezing, and _____.

    D. Signs and symptoms of tuberculosis

        i. Signs of active tuberculosis include a long-lasting _____, hemoptysis, and night _____.

      ii. Other signs and symptoms can include _____, chills, _____, pain when coughing and sometimes simply _____, and loss of appetite.

      iii. Those with advanced TB may have _____ of the fingers and toes.

E. Treatment options for tuberculosis

    i. Treatment is long _____ as it usually takes 9 to 12 _____ to eradicate the bacteria.

    ii. Patients may be ordered to practice _____ and stay homebound or _____ to prevent the spread of infection.

    iii. Four _____ that are taken at the same time are used to begin eradication of the bacteria.

    iv. After showing negative cultures, patients must continue _____ treatment for another 4 to 7 _____ to prevent the development of multidrug-resistant TB.

APPLIED PRACTICE

1. Label the structures of the respiratory system.

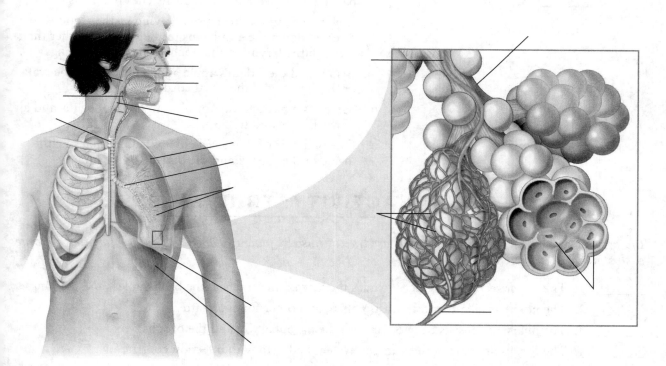

2. Match the structure of the respiratory tract with its correct function.

1. _____ Nose
2. _____ Mouth
3. _____ Paranasal sinuses
4. _____ Pharynx
5. _____ Larynx
6. _____ Trachea
7. _____ Bronchi
8. _____ Bronchioles
9. _____ Alveoli
10. _____ Epiglottis
11. _____ Pleura
12. _____ Thyroid cartilage
13. _____ Lungs
14. _____ Hilum
15. _____ Septum

a. Small air sacs in the lungs that support capillaries where the exchange of oxygen and carbon dioxide takes place.

b. Wedge-shaped area on the central portion of each lung where the primary bronchus, arteries, veins, and nerves enter and exit the lung.

c. Warms and moistens inhaled air.

d. Has two main branches, right and left, that are also considered primary.

e. A wall of cartilage that separates the two nasal cavities.

f. Serves the functions of respiration and voice.

g. The smallest branches of the bronchial tree.

h. Produces vocal sounds and is called the "voice box."

i. Cone-shaped organs located within the chest.

j. Decreases the weight of the skull and aids in phonation.

k. Also called the "windpipe" and serves as an open passageway through which air reaches the lungs.

l. Covers the larynx during swallowing so that food is directed down the esophagus to the stomach rather than through the larynx to the trachea and into the lungs.

m. Also called the Adam's apple and helps protect the walls of the larynx and the vocal cords.

n. Serves as a passageway for food to the esophagus and air to the larynx and trachea.

o. One of a pair of thin sheets of epithelium that line the inside of the thorax and the outside of the lungs.

LEARNING ACTIVITY: TRUE/FALSE

Indicate whether the following statements are true or false by placing a T or an F on the line that precedes each statement.

_____ 1. The upper respiratory tract includes the larynx, the trachea, the bronchioles, and the lungs.

_____ 2. The nose has cilia that trap dust, pollen, and other foreign matter.

_____ 3. The pharynx consists of two sections: the nasopharynx and the oropharynx.

_____ 4. The tonsils are part of the immune system and help with infection control.

_____ 5. The thyroid cartilage, or Adam's apple, is the smallest of the cartilage structures.

_____ 6. When the vocal cords are long and relaxed, high sounds are produced.

_____ 7. The respiratory rates in older adults may lower as the combined effects of pollution, smoking, and disease wear on the integrity of the tissues.

_____ 8. At birth, the lungs are pinkish in color, but as adulthood approaches, they turn a dark slate gray.

_____ 9. The right lung has three lobes, but the left lung has only two.

_____ 10. Asthma is related to the same process that causes allergic reactions.

CRITICAL THINKING

Answer the following questions to the best of your ability. Use the textbook as a reference.

1. Markus Barnes has a form of COPD that prevents him from fully exhaling the air from his lungs. He asks you why it is so hard for him to breathe. Briefly explain to the patient why he feels so short of breath.

   _____

   _____

   _____

   _____

2. Severe acute respiratory syndrome (SARS) was spread from China to North America by infected persons traveling by airplane. Is it possible to control the spread of disease from persons entering the country? If so, how? What should China have done to prevent the spread of the disease within and outside China?

   _____

   _____

   _____

   _____

   _____

RESEARCH ACTIVITY

Use Internet search engines to research the following topic and write a brief description of what you find. It is important to use reputable websites.

1. Visit www.lung.org. What information do you think will be most useful with regard to patient education? Explore the Lung Health and Diseases section. Which section do you find most interesting? Explain why.

   _____

   _____

   _____

   _____

CHAPTER 29

The Digestive System

STUDENT STUDY GUIDE

Use the following guide to assist in your learning of the concepts from the chapter.

I. Functions and Organs of the Digestive System

  1. The Digestive System

    A. The three main functions are _____, _____, and _____.

    B. List the four layers of the wall of the alimentary canal.

      i. _____

      ii. _____

      iii. _____

      iv. _____

  2. The Mouth

    A. Saliva produced during chewing _____ food and _____ digestion by chemically breaking down food.

    B. Food is formed into a(n) _____ for swallowing.

    C. The oral cavity (mouth) is formed by the _____, the _____ and _____, and the tongue.

    D. List the three distinct sections of the tongue.

      i. _____

      ii. _____

      iii. _____

  3. The Teeth

    A. List the deciduous teeth and how many of each a person has.

      i. _____

      ii. _____

      iii. _____

    B. List the permanent teeth and how many of each a person has.

      i. _____

      ii. _____

iii. _____

iv. _____

C. List the three main parts of the tooth.

    i. _____—The part above the gum

    ii. _____—Embedded in the gums

    iii. _____—The portion between the root and the crown

D. Describe the solid portions of the tooth.

    i. Dentin—_____

    ii. Enamel—_____

    iii. Cementum—_____

4. The Pharynx

A. The pharynx is the beginning of the _____ _____ of the digestive tract that leads to the stomach.

B. Once food is _____, the bolus passes through the pharynx into the

_____.

5. The Esophagus

A. The esophagus starts at the _____ and ends at the

_____.

B. Wave-like muscular contractions, called _____, move food to the

_____.

6. The Stomach

A. The stomach can hold _____ to _____ liters of food and fluid.

B. The stomach secretes _____ acid and _____ juices that convert food into _____.

C. The stomach has two sphincters.

    i. The _____ _____ opens and closes, allowing food and liquid to enter the stomach.

    ii. The _____ _____ facilitates passage of food and liquid out of the stomach.

7. The Small Intestine

A. The small intestine is a tube about _____ feet long and _____ inch(es) in diameter.

B. List the three sections of the small intestine.

    i. _____

    ii. _____

    iii. _____

C. _____ absorption takes place in the small intestine.

8. The Large Intestine

   A. The large intestine is about _____ feet long and 2.5 inches in diameter.

   B. The functions of the large intestine are to complete _____ and
      _____.

   C. List the sections of the large intestine.

      i. _____

      ii. _____

      iii. _____

      iv. _____

9. Accessory Organs of the Digestive System

   A. Salivary glands

      i. _____ glands are located on either side of the face, just below the ear.

      ii. _____ glands are located in the floor of the mouth.

      iii. _____ glands are below the tongue, forward of the submandibular
           gland.

   B. Liver

      i. The liver plays an essential role in the metabolism of _____, fats, and
         _____.

      ii. The liver produces four substances that are important to body functioning.

          a. _____—Digestive juice that emulsifies fats

          b. _____—Essential for blood clotting

          c. _____—Prevents the clotting of blood

          d. _____—Albumin and gamma globulin

      iii. The liver stores _____ and vitamins.

      iv. The liver produces _____ heat and _____
          substances.

   C. Gallbladder

      i. The gallbladder is a membranous sac in which _____ is stored and
         concentrated.

      ii. Components of bile can build up and form _____.

      iii. The gallbladder is not essential, and its _____ does not usually cause
           an interruption in the _____ _____.

   D. Pancreas

      i. The pancreas is about _____ to _____ inches long.

      ii. It contains cells that produce _____ enzymes.

iii. It also has cells that secrete the hormones _____ and

_____.

iv. It is considered to be a structure of both the digestive and _____

systems.

II. Common Pathology Associated with the Digestive System

1. Appendicitis

A. Appendicitis is a(n) _____ of the appendix.

B. It has no known _____, and its removal does not seem to cause a(n)

_____ in digestive function.

C. Signs and symptoms of appendicitis

i. Acute pain on the _____ point of the abdomen.

ii. Pain is often described as _____ and severe and can lead to nausea

and _____.

iii. Diarrhea, abdominal _____, constipation, and low-grade

_____ are also possible symptoms.

D. Treatment options for appendicitis

i. Emergency treatment is necessary and a(n) _____ is almost always

performed.

2. Cirrhosis

A. Cirrhosis is scarring of the _____ tissue.

B. After many years, scarring starts to replace _____ tissue.

C. Excessive _____ consumption, certain forms of viral

_____, and obesity can lead to cirrhosis.

D. Signs and symptoms of cirrhosis

i. Fluid buildup in the _____ (edema) and _____ (ascites)

ii. Fatigue

iii. Yellowing of the skin (_____)

iv. Itching

v. Nosebleeds

vi. _____ of the palms

vii. Easy _____

viii. _____ loss and _____ loss

ix. _____ pain

x. Frequent _____

xi. Confusion

E. Treatment options for cirrhosis

   i. _____

   ii. _____

   iii. _____

   iv. _____

3. Colitis

A. Colitis is an inflammation of the _____ intestine.

B. Symptoms of colitis

   i. _____ pain

   ii. Diarrhea

   iii. Dehydration

   iv. _____ and chills

   v. _____ bloating

   vi. Increased _____ _____

   vii. _____ stools

   viii. The constant urge to have a(n) _____ _____ (tenesmus)

C. Treatment options for colitis

   i. Treatment of the underlying cause—infection, _____, lack of _____ flow, or another cause

4. Colorectal Cancer

A. Colorectal cancer is the _____-leading cause of cancer-related deaths.

B. Colorectal cancer involves both _____ and _____ cancer occurring together.

C. Colon cancer develops when the cells of _____ _____ mutate and become cancerous.

D. Screenings can help prevent _____ to _____-stage cancer.

E. Signs and symptoms of colorectal cancer

   i. Change in _____ habits

   ii. _____ bleeding

   iii. Bloody _____

   iv. Long and _____ stool

   v. Persistent _____ cramping

   vi. _____ and abdominal pain

   vii. _____ loss and _____ loss

   viii. Excessive _____

F. Treatment options for colorectal cancer

    i. Three primary treatment options are _____, _____ and _____.

    ii. If part of the colon is removed, a(n) _____ is sometimes performed, and then stool does not leave the body through the rectum.

5. Crohn's Disease and Ulcerative Colitis

    A. Crohn's disease is a chronic _____ _____ of the _____.

    B. _____ _____ is closely linked to Crohn's disease but affects only the colon.

    C. When linked together, both are known as _____ _____ disease.

    D. Signs and symptoms of Crohn's disease and ulcerative colitis

        i. _____ pain

        ii. _____ and _____ with defecation

        iii. _____ bleeding

        iv. Bloody or watery _____

        v. _____ appetite

        vi. Weight _____

    E. Treatment options for Crohn's disease and ulcerative colitis

        i. There is _____ _____.

        ii. A large focus is placed on: the following.

            a. Eating a(n) _____ and _____ diet

            b. _____ plenty of fluids

            c. Limiting _____ products

            d. Avoiding high-_____ and high-_____ foods

        iii. Medications may include the following.

            a. _____

            b. _____

            c. _____

            d. _____

        iv. Severe Crohn's disease may eventually require a(n) _____.

6. Diverticulosis and Diverticulitis

    A. Diverticulosis involves having small _____ or sacs in wall of the _____.

B. Diverticulitis is a(n) _____ or _____ of the diverticula, possibly caused by stool becoming stuck and causing the formation of _____.

C. Signs and symptoms of diverticulosis and diverticulitis

    i. Diverticulosis generally has few or _____ symptoms.

    ii. Diverticulitis has a number of symptoms.

        a. _____

        b. _____

        c. _____

        d. _____

        e. _____

        f. _____

        g. _____

        h. _____

D. Treatment options for diverticulosis and diverticulitis

    i. Prevention of _____ formation is ideal and involves eating a(n) _____ diet, which can help maintain regular _____ _____.

    ii. Minor symptoms of diverticulitis may be treated with the following.

        a. _____ and increased _____ intake

        b. Application of _____

        c. _____ to treat infection

    iii. In serious cases, _____ and _____ may be necessary.

7. Gastroesophageal Reflux Disease (GERD)

A. GERD occurs when the _____ sphincter does not close completely or when it relaxes, causing _____ _____ to move back up into the _____.

B. This action is called _____.

C. Untreated, GERD can lead to the following.

    i. _____ esophagitis

    ii. _____ of the esophagus

    iii. Esophageal _____

    iv. Esophageal _____

    v. Esophageal _____

D. Signs and symptoms of GERD

    i. _____ that is worse when lying down, _____ over, and during the _____

    ii. Sore _____

    iii. _____ voice

    iv. Bad _____ in the mouth

    v. Feeling of food being _____ behind the _____

    vi. Belching

    vii. _____ of food

E. Treatment options for GERD

    i. Medications can block the production of _____ acid and protect the _____ of the esophagus.

    ii. Patients measures for treatment

        a. Avoiding _____ that cause symptoms

        b. Not _____ _____ until at least 3 hours after eating

        c. Losing _____

        d. Sleeping on a bed with the head elevated _____ _____

    iii. Over-the-counter _____ may also provide comfort.

    iv. Fundoplication can be performed if _____ and basic _____ do not work.

8. Hemorrhoids

A. A hemorrhoid is a dilated, or _____, vein in the walls of the _____ and sometimes the _____.

B. It is caused by increased _____ in the anus, usually because of _____ or occasionally chronic _____.

C. Signs and symptoms of hemorrhoids

    i. Bleeding after _____, particularly _____ _____ blood on toilet tissue or in the toilet bowl.

    ii. Itching and _____ in the anal region

    iii. _____ that cause intense discomfort

D. Treatment options for hemorrhoids

    i. Changing the _____ to prevent constipation

    ii. _____ softeners

    iii. Topical _____ creams

    iv. Corticosteroid creams that help reduce _____ and _____

9. Hiatal Hernia

   A. A hiatal hernia develops when a part of the _____ pushes upward and enters the _____ cavity through a weakened esophageal _____.

   B. Causes of hiatal hernia

      i. _____

      ii. _____

      iii. _____

      iv. _____

      v. _____

      vi. _____

      vii. _____

      viii. _____

   C. Signs and symptoms of hiatal hernia

      i. Some patients are _____

      ii. _____ and hiccups

      iii. Chest pain or _____

      iv. Difficulty _____

      v. Coughing

      vi. It is common to have both a hiatal hernia and _____.

      vii. Some patients are _____.

   D. Treatment options for hiatal hernia

      i. The only cure for a hernia is _____ repair.

      ii. Medications to treat _____ _____ may be used.

      iii. Activity changes, including the following, may reduce symptoms.

         a. Refraining from lifting _____ _____

         b. Improving _____

         c. Increasing _____

         d. Losing _____ _____

         e. Incorporating _____ after a meal rather than lying down

      iv. Dietary restrictions include avoiding the following.

         a. _____

         b. _____

         c. _____

         d. _____

10. Inguinal Hernia

   A. An inguinal hernia occurs at a weakened spot on the _____ _____ or groin that allows a portion of the intestine to push through, causing a bulge in the _____ or groin.

   B. An inguinal hernia can be the result of a(n) _____ muscular wall that stems from improper closing of muscular wall openings prior to _____.

   C. An inguinal hernia may also develop suddenly as a result of _____ _____.

   D. An incarcerated hernia is one that is _____ in the opening it came through and cannot be _____ through the opening by _____.

   E. Incarcerated hernias may become _____, which can be a life-threatening condition.

   F. Signs and symptoms of inguinal hernia

      i. Pain and _____ in the affected area that worsens when a person bends or _____ an object

      ii. Tugging or _____ sensations

      iii. A feeling of _____ in the area of the hernia, scrotum, or inner thigh

      iv. _____

      v. Nausea and _____ if the hernia becomes incarcerated

   G. Treatment options for inguinal hernia

      i. _____ is the only treatment and cure.

11. Irritable Bowel Syndrome (IBS)

   A. IBS is a common disorder that interferes with normal _____ _____.

   B. A leading factor related to IBS is the impact of _____ on the body and colon _____.

   C. _____ are twice as likely as _____ to suffer from IBS.

   D. Signs and symptoms of IBS

      i. Abdominal _____ and _____

      ii. _____, nausea, and a feeling of _____

      iii. Changes in _____ _____

      iv. Uncontrollable urge to _____

   E. Treatment options for IBS

      i. There is no _____.

ii. Dietary recommendations include the following.

a. _____

b. _____

c. _____

iii. Lifestyle changes include the following.

a. _____

b. _____

iv. Medications may also be _____ based on the patient's individual

_____.

12. Oral Cancer

A. Oral cancer can develop on the lips, _____ _____ gums,

under the _____, the front two-thirds of the tongue, the hard palate of the

_____, and the tissue located behind the _____

_____.

B. Risk factors for development of oral cancer

i. _____

ii. _____

iii. _____

iv. _____

v. _____

vi. _____

vii. _____

viii. _____

C. Signs and symptoms of oral cancer

i. Sores, _____, irritation, or _____ in the mouth

lasting more than _____ weeks

ii. _____ or _____ patches in the mouth

iii. Sore _____ and sores under _____

iv. Lump in the _____, tongue, or neck

v. Weight _____

vi. Unexplained _____ in the mouth

vii. Swollen _____ _____ in the neck

viii. Trouble chewing, _____, or speaking

D. Treatment options for oral cancer

   i. Treatment depends on the _____ and stage of the condition.

   ii. Surgery to remove part or all of the _____ and some surrounding _____ may be required.

   iii. _____ and _____ are other treatment options.

13. Pancreatic Cancer

A. The most common type of pancreatic cancer is _____ of the pancreas.

B. It is one of the _____ of all cancers.

C. Only ____ percent of pancreatic cancer patients will survive for _____ year(s) after diagnosis.

D. Signs and symptoms of pancreatic cancer

   i. Early signs of pancreatic cancer include the following.

     a. _____-colored stool

     b. _____ urine

     c. Jaundice or _____ of the skin

     d. Upper _____ pain or discomfort

     e. Weight _____

     f. Loss of _____

     g. Nausea and _____

   ii. Other signs and symptoms may include _____ pain, blood _____, diarrhea, and _____.

E. Treatment options for pancreatic cancer

   i. _____, chemotherapy, and _____ may be used, depending on the type and stage of the cancer.

   ii. Surgery to _____ remove the _____ _____ is the only known cure but is not an option for all forms of pancreatic cancer.

   iii. The _____ _____ is the most common surgery performed to remove pancreatic cancer.

14. Peptic Ulcer Disease (PUD)

A. PUD is characterized by a disruption in the lining of the _____, _____, or _____.

B. PUD most frequently occurs in the _____.

C. Most cases are caused by the bacterium _____ _____.

D. When the mucosal lining is damaged, _____ becomes exposed, and irritation may cause a(n) _____ to form.

E. Signs and symptoms of PUD

    i. _____

    ii. _____

    iii. _____

    iv. _____

F. Signs and symptoms of gastric ulcers

    i. _____ or a(n) _____ _____ in the upper abdomen and sometimes the lower chest

    ii. Pain that is made worse by _____

    iii. Difficulty _____ or regurgitation

    iv. Bloating, _____, and feeling sick, particularly after _____

    v. _____ and nausea

    vi. Loss of _____ and _____ loss

    vii. Blood in the stool, indicating that an ulcer is _____, which is a more _____ condition

G. Treatment options for PUD

    i. Avoiding _____ and alcohol

    ii. _____ to treat *H. pylori* infections

    iii. Changing _____ that may aggravate the condition

    iv. Medications that promote _____ and block the production of _____ (proton pump inhibitors)

    v. Medications (histamine blockers) to protect the _____ by decreasing or stopping the secretion of _____ _____

    vi. _____ if an ulcer doesn't respond to medications or other therapies

15. Pyloric Stenosis

A. Pyloric stenosis is a condition that develops in some _____ when the pylorus gradually _____ and _____, interfering with the flow of _____ into the _____.

B. Signs and symptoms of pyloric stenosis

    i. An infant may repeatedly _____ after feeding.

    ii. As the pylorus constricts, the vomiting becomes more _____ and more _____.

iii. The infant loses _____, develops symptoms of _____, is _____ than normal, and is very _____ when awake.

C. Treatment options for pyloric stenosis

i. Pyloric stenosis is always treated with _____ (pyloromyotomy).

APPLIED PRACTICE

1. Label the structures of the digestive system.

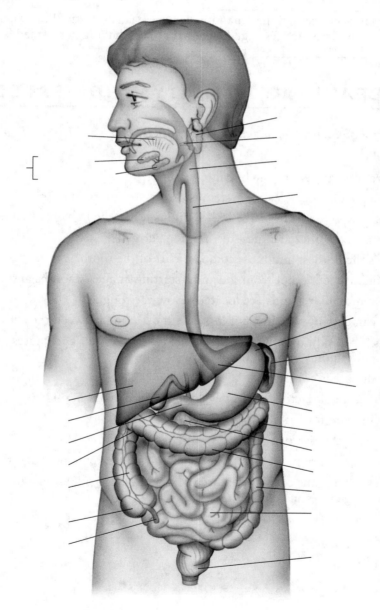

2. Evaluate your knowledge of diagnostic procedures related to the digestive system by answering the following questions. Refer to Table 29-3 in your textbook for assistance.

A. De'Shawn had to have his gallbladder removed. The procedure he had performed is a(n) _____.

B. Betty had to have a tissue sample removed from her esophagus. A flexible tube was placed down her throat for visualization. The procedure she had performed is a(n) _____.

C. Mariella suffered from gallstones and had a procedure completed in which the stones were crushed while they remained in the gallbladder. The procedure she had performed is _____.

D. Jamiel suffers from stomach ulcers. He is having a procedure to decrease the amount of acid secretion into his stomach by resectioning his vagus nerve. The procedure he is having performed is a(n) _____.

E. Juan's physician is concerned that Juan might have gastrointestinal bleeding. Juan will need to provide a fecal specimen for testing. The test that he is having performed is a(n) _____ test.

LEARNING ACTIVITY: TRUE/FALSE

Indicate whether the following statements are true or false by placing a T or an F on the line that precedes each statement.

_____ 1. There are three types of taste buds.

_____ 2. The main part of the digestive system is the gastrointestinal tract.

_____ 3. Humans have two sets of teeth: 25 deciduous teeth (the baby teeth) and 35 permanent teeth.

_____ 4. The incisor teeth are the largest teeth in the permanent set.

_____ 5. Enamel is the hardest and most compact part of the tooth.

_____ 6. All deciduous teeth erupt from the gums starting at age 7 months and end at 3 years.

_____ 7. The submandibular glands are located below the tongue.

_____ 8. Anyone can get appendicitis, but it occurs most often between the ages of 10 and 30.

_____ 9. Volvulus is a condition in which the bowel twists on itself and causes an obstruction that is painful and requires immediate surgery.

_____ 10. Crohn's disease is contagious.

_____ 11. Slouching is a risk factor for the development of a hiatal hernia.

_____ 12. There is no cure for irritable bowel syndrome.

_____ 13. Age increases the risk of oral cancer.

_____ 14. About 50 percent of pancreatic cancers can be surgically removed at the time of diagnosis.

_____ 15. The accessory organs of digestion are the mouth, pharynx, esophagus, stomach, small intestine, large intestine, and rectum.

CRITICAL THINKING

Answer the following questions to the best of your ability. Use the textbook as a reference.

1. Mr. McNeill is experiencing constipation and has called in for advice on how to deal with this. Try to recall what you have read in this chapter of your textbook and use your common sense to list a few things that may help. After you have done that, check the book and review the items that you may not have remembered.

   _____

   _____

   _____

   _____

2. Some digestive disorders, such as stomach ulcers, IBS, and GERD, may be associated with a person's lifestyle. As a member of the health care profession, what is your role when assisting in the care of these patients? What should you avoid doing when providing care?

   _____

   _____

   _____

   _____

   _____

RESEARCH ACTIVITY

Use Internet search engines to research the following topic and write a brief description of what you find. It is important to use reputable websites.

1. As a medical assistant, it will be your responsibility to instruct patients on how to prepare for certain types of diagnostic tests, such as a colonoscopy, endoscopy, or sigmoidoscopy. Select a condition from your textbook, research the types of tests performed for diagnosis, select one of the tests, and research the instructions that would be provided to patients. Write a short essay explaining the condition, the procedure, and the preparatory instructions that patients should be given prior to the procedure. Cite the Internet sources you use for your research.

   _____

   _____

   _____

   _____

CHAPTER 30
The Urinary System

STUDENT STUDY GUIDE

Use the following guide to assist in your learning of the concepts from the chapter.

I. Organs of the Urinary System

   1. The urinary system is sometimes called the _____ system.

   2. The main organs of the urinary system are the _____.

   3. Kidneys

     A. The kidneys are located at the back of the _____ cavity, against the muscles of the _____, and on either side of the _____ _____.

     B. Three capsules surround the kidney: the _____ capsule, the _____ capsule, and the _____ fascia.

     C. External structure of the kidney

       i. The _____ is the point of entry for the renal artery and vein, nerves, and lymphatic vessels.

       ii. The renal _____ is a small collecting area for _____ within the kidney.

     D. Internal structure of the kidney

       i. Two distinct parts of the internal portion of the kidney are the renal _____ and the renal _____.

     E. Nephrons

       i. Nephrons are the _____ units of the kidney.

       ii. Each kidney contains more than _____ _____ nephrons.

       iii. A nephron consists of a(n) _____ capsule and a renal _____.

   4. Ureters

     A. The ureters are two narrow and muscular _____.

     B. They carry the newly formed _____ from the renal pelvis in each kidney down to the _____ _____.

     C. They are about _____ to _____ inches long.

5. The Urinary Bladder

   A. The urinary bladder is a muscular _____ that serves as a(n) _____ for urine.

   B. The urinary bladder consists of four layers.

      i. _____

      ii. _____

      iii. _____

      iv. _____

   C. As the bladder fills with urine, it _____, and the walls become _____.

6. The Urethra

   A. The urethra is a tube of _____ and membrane extending from the _____ to the urinary _____.

   B. In males, the urethra is approximately _____ cm long.

   C. The male urethra has three sections: the _____, the _____, and the _____.

   D. The male urethra transports _____ and _____.

   E. In females, the urethra is approximately _____ cm long and transports only _____.

II. Urine

  1. Urine consists of about 95 percent _____ and 5 percent _____ _____.

  2. An adult feels the need to urinate when the bladder contains _____ to _____ mL of urine, but it can hold up to _____ mL.

  3. Physical Characteristics of Urine

   A. Deviances from normal ranges could indicate a(n) _____ or _____ of the urinary system.

   B. Normal urine has the following characteristics.

      i. Clear and not _____

      ii. _____ colored

      iii. A mildly _____ odor

      iv. A slightly acidic pH of _____

      v. A(n) _____ _____ of 1.003 to 1.030

III. Common Pathology Associated with the Urinary System

  1. Cystitis

   A. Cystitis is a(n) _____ of the bladder.

   B. It occurs when _____ infect the lower urinary tract.

C. It is most prevalent in _____ active women, ages _____ to _____.

D. In men, cystitis is usually secondary to another _____.

E. Signs and symptoms of cystitis

    i. The most common symptoms are _____ and _____ of urination.

    ii. Other common symptoms include _____, _____ urination, and urine that is dark, cloudy, or _____ tinged.

    iii. Urine may also have a(n) _____ odor.

    iv. If cystitis is left untreated, symptoms may include _____ and _____.

    v. _____ (burning or painful urination) may be the only symptom with chronic cystitis.

F. Treatment options for cystitis

    i. _____ to clear up infection

    ii. Medications to relieve the sense of _____, pain, or _____

    iii. Increasing _____ intake

2. Glomerulonephritis

A. Glomerulonephritis is an inflammation of the kidneys that primarily affects the _____.

B. It hinders the kidneys' ability to properly filter _____ and _____ from the blood.

C. It can be acute or _____.

D. It can lead to kidney _____.

E. Signs and symptoms of glomerulonephritis

    i. Signs and symptoms _____ depending on whether the patient suffers from the _____ or _____ form of this disease.

    ii. Urine may be _____ _____ in appearance because of the presence of _____ in the urine.

    iii. Other signs and symptoms of glomerulonephritis include the following.

        a. _____

        b. _____

        c. _____

        d. _____

        e. _____

        f. _____

        g. _____

F. Treatment options for glomerulonephritis

    i. Blood _____ control

    ii. _____ to reduce inflammation of renal tissue

    iii. Limitation of sodium, _____, fluids, and _____

3. Incontinence

  A. Incontinence occurs when the body is unable to _____ a(n) _____ flow of urine.

  B. It is commonly seen in women who have had _____.

  C. Signs and symptoms of incontinence (which vary based on type)

    i. _____ _____, the most common form, occurs with sneezing, _____, and _____.

    ii. _____ _____ occurs when misfired _____ signals tell the brain that urination is necessary. A sudden, _____ _____ to urinate precipitates a leaking or gushing of urine.

    iii. _____ _____ is a condition in which the bladder contracts without _____, and leakage occurs, if the patient is not able to respond to that need to void _____.

    iv. _____ _____ occurs when a(n) _____ prohibits complete emptying of the bladder.

    v. _____ _____ _____ is known as enuresis, or nocturnal enuresis. Enuresis is common in _____ _____; by age 8 years the _____ gland should be secreting antidiuretic hormone to stop bed-wetting at night.

    vi. _____ _____ is a temporary condition that is the result of an acute medical issue that _____ after the underlying cause has been treated.

  D. Treatment options for incontinence

    i. _____ that relax the bladder wall and reduce overactive _____

    ii. Surgery

    iii. _____ exercises to strengthen pelvic floor muscles

    iv. _____ modification training

    v. Antidiuretic hormone and medications to control the _____

4. Kidney Stones

  A. Kidney stones are also called _____ _____.

  B. Most kidney stones are a combination of _____ and _____.

  C. When renal calculi pass into the _____, they slow or _____ urine flow.

D. The stones have a(n) _____ surface; they irritate and scratch the _____, causing bleeding and _____ physical pain.

E. The bleeding and decreased urine flow _____ the kidney and cause _____.

F. Signs and symptoms of kidney stones

    i. Intense lower back, _____, or _____ pain

    ii. Possible nausea, vomiting, and _____ _____ output

    iii. _____ pain in the lower abdomen

    iv. _____ revealed by urinalysis

G. Treatment options for kidney stones

    i. Some _____ pass on their own.

    ii. _____ involves passing shock waves through the body to break down the physical _____ of a stone.

    iii. Surgical intervention to either _____ or disintegrate the stone may be necessary.

5. Polycystic Kidney Disease (PKD)

A. PKD is a disorder in which multiple _____ of cysts develop primarily _____ and on the _____ of the kidneys.

B. The cysts are _____, meaning noncancerous.

C. Polycystic conditions may be present in _____ systems and _____ other than the kidneys.

D. Developing high _____ _____ is the greatest risk for people with PKD.

E. Signs and symptoms of PKD

    i. High _____ _____

    ii. Back or _____ pain related to enlarged _____

    iii. _____ pain, particularly over the liver

    iv. _____ pain

    v. Drowsiness

    vi. Increase in the size of the _____

    vii. _____ in the urine

    viii. Excessive _____ _____ urination

    ix. _____ failure

    x. Kidney _____

    xi. Headache

F. Treatment options for PKD

    i. There is no _____ for this condition.

    ii. The focus is on _____ _____ and minimizing _____.

    iii. Cysts that are _____, intensely _____, causing a(n) _____, or _____ may need to be drained during a surgical procedure.

    iv. Complete _____ of cysts is not a feasible option.

6. Pyelonephritis

    A. Pyelonephritis is a urinary tract _____ that has progressed to the kidney and renal _____.

    B. It can be caused by bacteria or a(n) _____, but usually it is caused by the bacterium _____ _____.

    C. Signs and symptoms of pyelonephritis

        i. _____, _____, and groin pain

        ii. Urinary _____ and frequency

        iii. Pain and _____ during urination

        iv. Fever and _____

        v. _____ and vomiting

        vi. Concentrated and _____ urine, which may be _____ smelling

        vii. _____ in the urine

        viii. _____ in elderly patients

    D. Treatment options for pyelonephritis

        i. _____ may be prescribed.

        ii. If pyelonephritis is left untreated, _____ may result that could cause _____ kidney damage.

7. Acute Renal Failure

    A. Acute renal failure occurs when there is a change in the _____ function of the kidneys.

    B. Rapid onset of acute renal failure can occur in a matter of _____ or over the course of 2 _____.

    C. Signs and symptoms of acute renal failure

        i. Decreased urine _____, resulting in _____ of the legs, feet, and ankles

        ii. Ascites (fluid in the _____)

        iii. High _____ _____

        iv. _____ and vomiting

v. Seizures

vi. Shortness of _____

vii. _____ stools

viii. Fatigue

ix. Increased _____

x. A(n) _____ _____ in the mouth

D. Treatment options for acute renal failure

i. The focus is on addressing what has caused the _____ _____ and improving and restoring kidney _____.

ii. _____ to remove excess fluid from the body may be used.

iii. _____ are used to treat or prevent urinary infections.

iv. The patient may require _____.

8. Chronic Renal Failure

A. Chronic renal failure is a gradual and _____ loss of kidney function that transpires over the course of _____ to _____.

B. The final stages of chronic renal failure are referred to as _____ renal disease.

C. _____ and _____ are the two most common causes of chronic renal failure in the United States.

D. Signs and symptoms of chronic renal failure

i. Symptoms may be mild or nonexistent until at least _____ percent of kidney function is _____.

ii. Early signs and symptoms include the following.

a. _____

b. _____

c. _____

d. _____

e. _____

iii. End-stage signs and symptoms include the following.

a. _____

b. _____

c. _____

d. _____

e. _____

f. _____

g. _____

h. _____

E. Treatment options for chronic renal failure

    i. The goal of treatment is to identify, _____, and _____ what is causing the kidneys to fail.

    ii. The focus is on preventing excess _____ _____ while the kidneys have a chance to heal and resume their normal _____.

    iii. If normal function cannot be regained, _____ may be necessary.

F. Dialysis

    i. With hemodialysis, a machine _____ and _____ the blood outside the body.

    ii. Peritoneal dialysis is done through the tissues of the _____.

APPLIED PRACTICE

1. Label the various structures that comprise the kidneys.

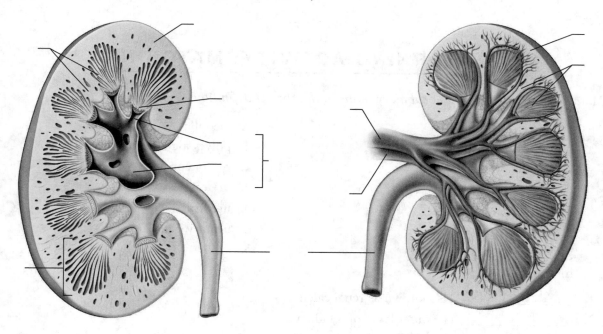

2. *Read the scenario and answer the questions that follow.*

Scenario A

Mr. Bai Feng, born 8-13-66, presents to the office today with a fever of 99.7°F, noticeable beads of sweat on his brow, and complaints of right-sided pain in his lower back. He states, "I am in so much pain I can't stand up straight, and I feel like I always have to urinate." A urine specimen is obtained for urinalysis and shows positive for blood in the urine, as well as other abnormalities. His urine specimen is sent to the laboratory for further testing.

A. Based on his urinalysis and symptoms, what would be a likely diagnosis? *(Medical assistants never make a diagnosis; this is a question about your knowledge of the signs and symptoms of various conditions that are presented in the textbook.)*

_____

_____

B. Draw a picture of the urinary system (kidneys, ureters, urinary bladder, and urethra). Circle the area of the urinary system that is likely to be the causative factor for Mr. Feng's pain.

LEARNING ACTIVITY: MATCHING

Match each of the selected vocabulary terms to the correct definition.

a. acute renal failure
b. cortex
c. frequency
d. glomerulonephritis
e. incontinence
f. cystitis
g. kidney stones
h. kidneys

i. medulla
j. polycystic kidney disease (PKD)
k. pyelonephritis
l. ureters
m. urethra
n. urinary bladder
o. void

1. _____ Also known as renal calculi.
2. _____ The outer layer of a kidney.
3. _____ A muscular sac in the pelvic cavity that serves as a reservoir for urine.
4. _____ A kidney disease that hinders the kidneys' ability to properly filter waste and fluids from the blood.
5. _____ The involuntary and unpredictable flow of urine.
6. _____ The middle portion of the kidney.
7. _____ Two muscular tubes that carry the newly formed urine from each kidney down to the bladder.
8. _____ The need to void often.
9. _____ An infection that has progressed to the kidney and renal pelvis.
10. _____ A musculomembranous tube extending from the bladder to the urinary meatus.

11. _____ Occurs when something causes a change in the filtering function of the kidneys.
12. _____ A pair of bean-shaped organs located at the back of the abdominal cavity.
13. _____ An inflammation of the bladder.
14. _____ To urinate.
15. _____ A disorder in which clusters of cysts develop primarily within the kidneys.

CRITICAL THINKING

Answer the following questions to the best of your ability. Use the textbook as a reference.

1. Pilar Lopez, age 68, has been hospitalized for dehydration. Why is Pilar more likely to develop dehydration at the age of 68 as opposed to when she was 28 years old?

_____

_____

_____

_____

_____

2. When discussing urinary issues with patients, what cultural considerations are important to consider?

_____

_____

_____

_____

_____

RESEARCH ACTIVITY

Use Internet search engines to research the following topic and write a brief description of what you find. It is important to use reputable websites.

1. Visit www.kidney.org. As you navigate through the site, what information do you find that would be helpful for a patient who is in need of a kidney transplant? What information would be helpful for medical assistants and other members of the health care team? How could this website be beneficial for a urology/nephrology office?

_____

_____

_____

_____

_____

CHAPTER 31
The Endocrine System

STUDENT STUDY GUIDE

Use the following guide to assist in your learning of the concepts from the chapter.

I. Introduction

    1. Glands that secrete substances are _____ glands.

    2. Glands that secrete substances to the outside of the body are _____ glands.

    3. Exocrine glands include the _____ glands, _____ glands, and _____ glands.

    4. Exocrine glands send their secretions to outer surfaces through _____.

    5. Endocrine glands secrete their hormones directly into the _____ or surrounding _____.

II. General Function of the Endocrine System

    1. The general and vital function of the endocrine system is the _____ and _____ of hormones.

    2. Many disorders of the endocrine system are associated with either the _____ (excessive secretion) or the _____ (insufficient secretion) of hormones.

    3. _____ _____ means that the body acts to reverse the direction of change to regain or maintain _____.

    4. _____ _____ encourages stimuli to continue or even _____, which also helps maintain homeostasis.

III. Specific Glands and Their Functions*

    1. Hypothalamus

        A. The hypothalamus is situated in the _____ of the brain.

        B. It secretes _____ and _____ hormones.

        C. Two hormones it produces are _____ hormone and _____.

        D. These hormones are produced by the hypothalamus but secreted by the _____ _____.

---

*Functions of the hormones secreted by endocrine glands will be covered in a separate activity, later in this chapter.

2. Pituitary Gland

   A. The pituitary gland is located near the _____ of the brain.

   B. It is considered the "_____ _____" because it regulates
      all other endocrine glands.

   C. It consists of the _____ and posterior lobes.

   D. List the hormones produced in the anterior lobe.

      i. _____

      ii. _____

      iii. _____

      iv. _____

      v. _____

      vi. _____

      vii. _____

   E. The posterior lobe is responsible for storing and secreting the _____

      _____ and _____, which are produced by the

      hypothalamus.

3. Pineal Gland

   A. The pineal gland secretes _____.

   B. Functions of melatonin

      i. It helps regulate the _____ rhythm.

      ii. It helps regulate the _____ system.

4. Thyroid Gland

   A. The thyroid gland is the _____ of all the endocrine glands.

   B. It is responsible for the body's _____.

   C. List the hormones the thyroid gland secretes.

      i. _____

      ii. _____

      iii. _____

5. Parathyroid Glands

   A. Each of these small glands is about the shape and size of a(n) _____ of

      _____.

   B. They secrete the _____ hormone, which regulates the amount of

      _____ stored and circulated within the body.

6. Pancreas

   A. The pancreas is considered to be both a(n) _____ and a(n)

      _____ gland.

B. The endocrine function is found within the _____ of _____.

   i. _____, _____, and _____ cells are the three main types of cells that make up the islets of Langerhans.

   ii. These cells play major roles in how the body balances _____ _____ levels.

7. Adrenal Glands

  A. The adrenal glands are located on the top of each _____.

  B. Each gland has a(n) _____ portion (the cortex) and a(n) _____ portion (the medulla).

  C. The adrenal cortex secretes _____ (cortisol and corticosterone), _____ (aldosterone), and _____.

  D. The adrenal medulla synthesizes, secretes, and stores _____, which are released into the bloodstream when a person is experiencing _____ or _____ stress.

8. Ovaries

  A. The ovaries are the primary _____ _____ of the female body.

  B. The ovaries produce the hormones _____ and _____.

9. Testes

  A. The testes are located in the male _____.

  B. They produce the hormone _____.

10. Placenta

  A. The placenta is a spongy structure that joins _____ and _____ and provides the blood supply between the two.

  B. It acts as an endocrine gland by producing the following.

   i. _____

   ii. _____

   iii. _____

11. Gastrointestinal Mucosa

  A. The mucosal lining of the _____ and _____ intestine contains endocrine cells that produce specific hormones that facilitate _____.

  B. Hormones secreted by the gastrointestinal mucosa include the following.

   i. _____

   ii. _____

   iii. _____

   iv. _____

12. Thymus Gland

    A. The thymus gland is located in the cavity of the _____.

    B. It has both _____ and endocrine functions.

    C. It secretes _____ and _____.

IV. Common Pathology Associated with the Endocrine System

  1. Acromegaly

    A. Acromegaly results from the overproduction of _____

        _____ by the _____ pituitary gland.

    B. Overproduction of growth hormone is often caused by a _____ tumor on the gland.

    C. _____ adults are most often affected.

    D. Signs and symptoms of acromegaly

      i. Acromegaly is commonly characterized by the abnormal growth of the _____ and _____.

      ii. Arthritis, _____ _____ syndrome, and weakness in the _____ are common related effects.

     iii. Facial changes

        a. The brow and lower jaw become more _____ and _____.

        b. The _____ bone becomes larger.

        c. Spacing between the teeth _____.

     iv. Other signs and symptoms

        a. A deeper _____

        b. Upper airway obstruction, resulting in _____ and _____ _____

        c. _____ changes

        d. Increased _____ and odor of the skin

        e. Weakness and _____

        f. In women, _____ and breast changes

        g. In men, _____

    E. Treatment options for acromegaly

      i. Treatment focuses on returning _____ _____ levels to a normal range.

      ii. Options include _____ removal of the tumor, _____ of the tumor, and _____ therapy to reduce the level of GH production.

2. Addison's Disease

   A. In Addison's disease, the cortex of the _____ _____ is damaged, _____ the production of adrenocortical hormones.

   B. It occurs at any _____ and affects men and women _____.

   C. Signs and symptoms of Addison's disease

      i. Weight loss as a result of _____ _____, chronic _____, chronic _____, and _____

      ii. Weakness and _____

      iii. Increased _____ of the skin and mucous membranes that produces a(n) _____ appearance

      iv. Changes in _____ pressure and _____ rate

      v. Paleness

      vi. Craving of _____ foods

      vii. _____ lesions

   D. Treatment options for Addison's disease

      i. The usual course of treatment is a lifelong replacement of _____ hormones and supplemental _____.

      ii. Patients may need to administer emergency _____ injections during _____ times.

3. Cushing's Disease

   A. Cushing's disease develops when a tumor on the _____ gland hypersecretes _____ hormone into the bloodstream.

   B. Signs and symptoms of Cushing's disease

      i. _____ weakness

      ii. Thinning of the _____

      iii. Easy _____

      iv. Rounding of _____ features

      v. _____ gain and fatigue

      vi. Acne

      vii. Backache (during _____ _____)

      viii. An excess of _____ collected between the _____ blades

      ix. In women, excessive _____ _____ and irregular _____ cycles

      x. In men, _____ and decreased sexual desire

C. Treatment options for Cushing's disease

    i. Treatment depends on the underlying _____.

    ii. Treatment options include surgical _____ or _____ of the pituitary tumor.

    iii. Medication may be prescribed to block the production of _____.

4. Diabetes Mellitus

  A. With diabetes mellitus, the body is unable to produce enough _____ to properly control _____ _____ levels or is unable to properly make use of the _____ that is produced.

  B. There are three types of diabetes mellitus.

    i. Type 1 diabetes

      a. Type 1 diabetes is typically diagnosed in _____, _____, and _____ adults.

      b. This form results when the body cannot produce sufficient _____ of insulin or produces _____ insulin at all.

      c. Careful _____ of type 1 diabetes is essential for proper insulin regulation.

    ii. Type 2 diabetes

      a. This is the _____ common form of the disease.

      b. It is typically associated with _____.

      c. It results from insulin _____ combined with insulin _____ that occurs as a person _____ weight and the body struggles to make enough _____ to keep blood _____ levels within the ideal, healthy range.

    iii. Gestational diabetes

      a. Gestational diabetes develops during _____ and results when the body is unable to make and use enough _____ to meet the requirements of both the _____ and the growing fetus.

      b. Most of the time, after the mother _____ _____ to the baby, diabetes _____.

  C. Signs and symptoms of diabetes mellitus

    i. _____ (frequent urination)

    ii. _____ (excessive thirst)

    iii. _____ (excessive hunger)

    iv. _____ vision

    v. Weakness

vi. Weight _____ (without trying)

vii. Lethargy and _____

viii. _____ skin

ix. Recurrent _____

x. Abdominal _____

xi. Vaginal _____ _____ in women

D. Treatment options for diabetes mellitus

   i. Type 1 diabetes

     a. _____ insulin treatment

     b. For some patients, an insulin _____

     c. Pancreatic _____

   ii. Type 2 diabetes

     a. Treatment begins with diet, exercise, and oral _____

       _____ to help control blood sugar levels.

     b. Many type 2 diabetics must also administer _____

       _____ in addition to taking oral medications.

     c. _____ surgery is often helpful to obese diabetic patients.

   iii. Gestational diabetes

     a. Closely monitor _____ and blood sugar levels.

   iv. Meet with an endocrinologist for a treatment plan, which may include daily

     _____ _____.

5. Dwarfism

A. Dwarfism refers to a group of conditions characterized by shorter-than-normal
_____ growth in the _____ and _____
or the trunk.

B. Those with dwarfism will not be taller than _____ feet _____ inches as a grown adult.

C. The most common form of dwarfism is _____.

D. Signs and symptoms of dwarfism

   i. Disproportionately _____ arms and _____ with a
trunk of normal length

   ii. _____ legs

   iii. Reduced joint _____ in the elbow

   iv. Loose ligaments that make other joints seem overly _____ or double
jointed

   v. Shortened _____ and feet

   vi. _____ head

vii. Prominent _____

viii. Flattened _____ of the nose

ix. Crowded _____

E. Treatment options for dwarfism

    i. There is no _____ for achondroplasia.

    ii. Focus is placed on the _____, management, and _____ of medical complications.

    iii. Surgery may be performed to relieve _____ on the nervous system, generally at the base of the skull and _____ back.

6. Gigantism

A. Gigantism is a rare disease that results from _____ secretion of _____ hormone during _____, before the closure of the bone growth _____.

B. Signs and symptoms of gigantism

    i. Overgrowth of the _____ bones and very tall _____

    ii. In children, _____ _____ for their age

    iii. Delayed _____

    iv. Increased _____

    v. _____ vision

    vi. Large _____ and feet

    vii. _____ fingers and toes

    viii. Muscle _____

    ix. Thickening of _____ features

C. Treatment options for gigantism

    i. If the underlying cause is a pituitary tumor, _____ _____ is ideal.

    ii. In other cases, medications that reduce the _____ of or _____ the effects of GH are prescribed.

    iii. _____ therapy to reduce GH levels is a last resort.

7. Hyperthyroidism

A. Hyperthyroidism is characterized by _____ thyroid hormone levels.

B. _____ _____, an autoimmune disorder, is the most common form of hyperthyroidism.

C. Signs and symptoms of hyperthyroidism

    i. _____ and restlessness

    ii. Heart _____

iii. Tremors

iv. Sweating

v. Frequent _____ movements

vi. In women, _____ changes

vii. Weight _____

viii. Changes in the _____ and hair

ix. Overall _____

x. _____ skin

xi. Hair _____

xii. High _____ pressure

xiii. _____, a condition in which the eyeballs protrude beyond their normal protective orbit

D. Treatment options for hyperthyroidism

i. _____ medications

ii. Radioactive _____ to destroy the thyroid

iii. _____ to remove the thyroid

8. Hypothyroidism

A. Hypothyroidism occurs when the thyroid produces _____ amounts of the thyroid hormones.

B. It is difficult to diagnose in its early stages because it develops _____, and symptoms are _____.

C. A goiter may develop as a result of _____ _____, an autoimmune _____ of the thyroid.

D. _____ is a rare, life-threatening condition that occurs when hypothyroidism is left _____ for a long period of time.

E. Signs and symptoms of hypothyroidism

i. Fatigue, decreased _____, intolerance to _____, constipation, loss of _____, muscle _____, stiffness, and weight _____.

ii. Other symptoms are _____ changes, decreased _____ desire, slowed _____ function, hair _____, dry _____, and _____ changes.

F. Treatment options for hypothyroidism

i. Typical treatment involves the _____ use of a(n) _____ thyroid hormone.

ii. This medication must be taken on a(n) _____ basis, usually for

_____.

iii. Hormone levels are monitored regularly with _____

_____, and the dosage should be _____ as

necessary.

APPLIED PRACTICE

1. Label the primary glands of the endocrine system on the image provided.

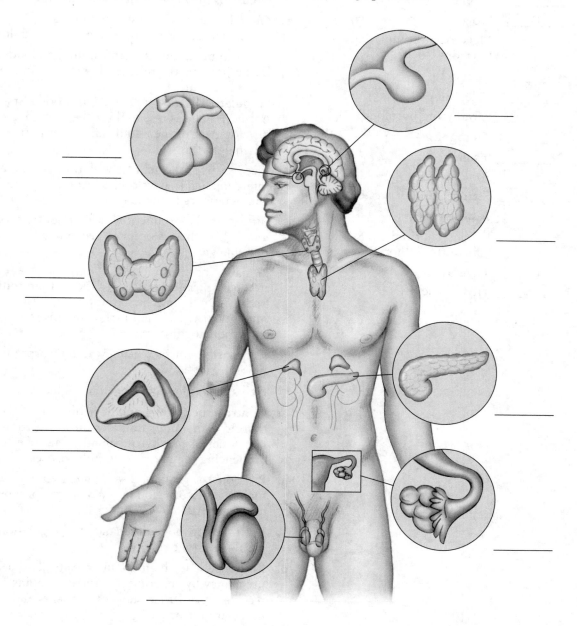

LEARNING ACTIVITY: MATCHING

1. _____ Antidiuretic hormone
2. _____ Oxytocin
3. _____ Growth hormone
4. _____ Adrenocorticotropic hormone
5. _____ Thyroid-stimulating hormone
6. _____ Follicle-stimulating hormone (FSH)
7. _____ Luteinizing hormone
8. _____ Prolactin
9. _____ Melanocyte-stimulating hormone
10. _____ T_3 and T_4
11. _____ Calcitonin
12. _____ Parathyroid hormone
13. _____ Glucagon
14. _____ Insulin
15. _____ Somatostatin
16. _____ Estrogen and progesterone
17. _____ Testosterone
18. _____ Human chorionic gonadotropin hormone
19. _____ Thymosin
20. _____ Thymopoietin

a. Plays a key role in childbirth and also influences our ability to trust and bond with others.

b. Gonadotropic hormone that stimulates the growth of ovarian follicles and eggs in females and the production of sperm in males.

c. Controls skin pigmentation in the epidermis.

d. Responsible for the amount of calcium that is stored in the bones and the amount of calcium that circulates throughout the bloodstream.

e. Gonadotropic hormone that stimulates the mammary glands to produce milk after childbirth.

f. Helps to maintain balance within the bloodstream by suppressing the release of glucagon and insulin when necessary.

g. Stimulates the adrenal cortex to produce its hormones and is essential for the growth and development of the middle and inner parts of the adrenal cortex.

h. Necessary for the act of copulation, or sexual intercourse, and developing secondary sexual characteristics in the male.

i. Influences the production of lymphocyte precursors and aids in their process of becoming T lymphocytes.

j. Gonadotropic hormone that plays an essential role in the maturation process of the ovarian follicles and in stimulating the development of the corpus luteum in the female. In the male it is responsible for producing testosterone.

k. Responsible for increasing water absorption in the blood by the kidneys.

l. Helps break down glycogen into glucose.

m. Controls the growth and development of the thyroid gland and stimulates the production of the hormones of the thyroid glands that are essential in influencing the body's metabolic processes.

n. Promote the growth, development, and maintenance of secondary female sex organs and characteristics.

o. Essential for the maintenance and regulation of the basal metabolic rate.

p. Responsible for maintaining a viable and healthy pregnancy by ensuring that the developing fetus is receiving proper amounts of nutrients and calories necessary for proper growth.

q. Promotes the maturation of T lymphocytes.
r. Essential for the growth and development of bones, muscles, and other organs in children and enhances bone and muscle mass and promotes the destruction of fats in adults.
s. Lowers blood sugar by allowing the body's cells to absorb glucose from the blood.
t. Influences bone and calcium metabolism.

LEARNING ACTIVITY: TRUE/FALSE

Indicate whether the following statements are true or false by placing a T or an F on the line that precedes each statement.

_____ 1. The hypothalamus acts as an on-and-off switch for hormone secretion.

_____ 2. Graves' disease results from a hyposecretion of T_3 and T_4.

_____ 3. Type 1 diabetes is very rare in children.

_____ 4. Addison's disease results from damage to the cortex of the adrenal gland.

_____ 5. Insulin and glucagon are secreted by the pancreas.

_____ 6. Hyposecretion of hormones from the adrenal cortex results in dwarfism.

_____ 7. Progesterone is a steroid hormone.

_____ 8. Copulation can occur without testosterone.

_____ 9. The thymus is also a part of the lymphatic/immune system.

_____ 10. Hormones that are secreted by the pancreas facilitate digestion.

CRITICAL THINKING

Answer the following questions to the best of your ability. Use the textbook as a resource.

1. Anya Mikovich is a 35-year-old patient who presents to the office complaining of restlessness, heart palpitations, tremors, and sweating. She states, "I am unable to relax and have been sweating a lot recently. I always feel hot." She is displaying exophthalmos and has lost 6 pounds since her last visit 3 months ago, although she claims she hasn't been trying to lose weight. Given her signs and symptoms, what endocrine disorder might the physician assume is afflicting this patient? Is this a condition that could be passed down to her children? What sign is unique to this condition as opposed to other endocrine disorders?

_____

_____

_____

_____

_____

2. A pregnant patient who is 9 days past her due date will need a hormone to induce labor and help stimulate the process of uterine contractions. What hormone may be given? What endocrine gland would produce this hormone naturally? What else does this hormone stimulate?

_____

_____

_____

_____

3. Why is it important to understand the laws of your state regarding individuals with diabetes who drive school buses and other forms of public transportation?

_____

_____

_____

_____

RESEARCH ACTIVITY

Use Internet search engines to research the following topic and write a brief description of what you find. It is important to use reputable websites.

1. Visit www.diabetes.org. Research information about how ethnicity and culture play roles in diabetes. What facts do you find most surprising regarding this topic? How prevalent is diabetes within your ethnic race or culture?

_____

_____

_____

_____

CHAPTER 32

The Reproductive System

STUDENT STUDY GUIDE

Use the following guide to assist in your learning of the concepts from the chapter.

I. The Female Reproductive System

  1. Ovaries

    A. The ovaries are _____-shaped structures that flank each side of the

    _____.

    B. The functions of the ovaries are to ovaries produce _____, or eggs, and

    _____.

    C. The ovaries have two microscopic divisions: the _____ and the

    _____.

    D. Ovulation occurs when a(n) _____ follicle ruptures on the

    _____ cortex and an ovum is released into the _____

    _____ and into one of the fallopian _____.

  2. Uterus

    A. The uterus is a(n) _____-shaped muscular organ with _____

    walls.

    B. The uterus has three distinct areas.

      i. The _____ portion, called the _____

      ii. The _____ portion, called the _____

      iii. The _____, called the _____

    C. The uterus has several functions.

      i. Shedding of the _____ during the monthly menstrual cycle

      ii. Providing _____ and supplying _____ to a growing fetus

      during pregnancy

      iii. Contracting during _____ to deliver the fetus from the uterus

  3. Fallopian Tubes

    A. The fallopian tubes extend along each side of the _____ and curve inward

    toward each _____.

    B. Their main function is to serve as _____ for _____ cells.

C. There are three layers of fallopian tubes.

   i. The _____ layer—Outermost and made of connective tissue

   ii. The _____ layer—Muscular and made of circular and longitudinal smooth muscle

   iii. The _____ layer—Innermost and consists of simple columnar epithelium

D. Each fallopian tube has three segments: _____, _____, and _____.

4. Vagina

   A. The vagina is typically _____ to _____ inches in length and is situated between the _____ and the rectum.

   B. It functions as the female organ of _____, as the pathway for menstrual _____, and as the pathway for the _____ of a fetus.

5. The Vulva

   A. List the five organs that make up the external female genitalia.

   i. _____

   ii. _____

   iii. _____

   iv. _____

   v. _____

6. Breasts

   A. Breasts are rounded structures made of _____, _____, and fibrous tissue that protrude from the chest.

   B. The _____ is the darkened area of circular skin in the center of each breast.

   C. The _____ is the elevated area in the center of the areola.

II. The Menstrual Cycle

   1. _____ occurs at the age of puberty.

   2. Four Phases of the Menstrual Cycle

   A. Menstruation phase

      i. This phase is characterized by the discharge of _____ _____ from the uterus as the _____ layer is shed.

      ii. The term _____ is commonly used to describe this phase of the menstrual cycle.

      iii. The length of this phase averages _____ to _____ days.

   B. Follicular phase

      i. This phase is characterized by the endometrial layer beginning to _____ and become _____.

ii. The _____ follicle begins to mature.

iii. This phase generally spans days 5 to _____ of the menstrual cycle.

C. Ovulation

i. This phase begins on the day the _____ is released from the _____ follicle.

ii. The body is preparing for a possible _____.

iii. This is when a woman is most _____ and able to _____.

D. Luteal phase

i. This phase is characterized by the _____ and continued thickening of the _____.

ii. While the _____ level is at its highest level, the _____ level continues decreasing.

iii. The _____ will die if fertilization does not occur during this phase.

iv. The onset of _____ marks the end of the luteal phase.

III. Pregnancy and Childbirth

1. _____ begins with conception and ends with the birthing process.

2. _____ occurs when a spermatozoa fertilizes an ovum during intercourse.

A. The ovum and the sperm contain _____ chromosomes each.

B. Their fusion results in a zygote containing _____ chromosomes.

3. Prenatal Care

A. It is important for mothers to receive _____ prenatal care from their _____.

B. A(n) _____-term, healthy pregnancy will last approximately _____ weeks.

C. These 40 weeks of pregnancy are divided into three _____.

D. First Trimester

i. The first trimester begins with _____ and ends around the _____ week of gestation.

ii. Important changes during the embryonic period (first 8 weeks)

a. _____

b. _____

c. _____

d. _____

e. _____

iii. The fetal period begins at week _____ and continues until birth.

E. Second Trimester

    i. The second trimester of pregnancy is between weeks _____ and _____.

    ii. Fetal _____ begin to be felt.

    iii. _____ hair forms on the shoulders, head, and back of the fetus.

    iv. List milestones in this trimester.

        a. _____

        b. _____

        c. _____

        d. _____

F. Third Trimester

    i. The third trimester lasts from the _____ week of pregnancy to _____.

    ii. The fetus is considered full term at _____ weeks and can at that point be born with very _____ complications.

4. The Process of Birth

A. _____ changes at the end of pregnancy allow for childbirth and _____ to begin.

B. Contractions occur within the _____ wall of the uterus and help with moving the fetus through the _____ _____.

C. _____ begins the childbirth process.

D. Three phases of labor

    i. Dilation

        a. This is the first and _____ stage of labor.

        b. The three phases of dilation are the _____, _____, and _____ phases.

    ii. Expulsion

        a. This phase is the actual _____ of the baby.

        b. It occurs when the cervix is fully dilated at _____ cm.

        c. The fetus begins to travel from the _____ into the _____ through very strong and forceful _____.

        d. The length of this stage can range from several _____ to several _____.

    iii. Placental stage

        a. This is the _____ stage of childbirth, and it begins after the baby has been born.

        b. The placenta is also known as the _____.

    c. This stage occurs approximately _____ minutes after the birth of the baby.

    d. The _____ begins to separate from the _____ wall and is expelled from the mother's body.

  E. Caesarian section

    i. A Caesarian section is performed when a mother is unable to _____ deliver a baby.

    ii. It is often performed to protect the _____ and _____ of the mother or baby.

    iii. It is commonly referred to as a(n) _____.

    iv. Reasons C-sections are performed

      a. The baby is in a(n) _____ position.

      b. There is a decrease in the supply of _____ to the _____ before birth.

      c. The baby is expected to weigh more than _____ pounds.

      d. Maternal _____ _____ make vaginal birth unsafe for either the mother or the baby.

      e. The mother has a previous history of _____ during pregnancy.

5. Contraception

  A. Contraception is also known as _____ _____.

  B. It reduces the risk of unwanted _____.

  C. List six methods of birth control.

    i. _____

    ii. _____

    iii. _____

    iv. _____

    v. _____

    vi. _____

6. Infertility

  A. The term infertility describes a situation in which a couple is unable to _____ a(n) _____.

  B. There are two types of infertility.

    i. Primary infertility—Diagnosed after _____ consecutive _____ of trying to conceive without success.

    ii. Secondary infertility—Diagnosed if the couple has had _____ pregnancy but has been unsuccessful at conceiving for a(n) _____ time after trying for _____ consecutive months.

C. Factors affecting infertility in women

    i. Being older than _____ years of age

    ii. _____ menstrual cycles, _____ of menstrual cycles, and lack of _____

    iii. Endometriosis

    iv. _____ ovarian syndrome and other issues related to _____ imbalances

    v. _____ of the reproductive organs as a result of _____ transmitted diseases

    vi. _____ issues with the reproductive organs

D. Factors affecting infertility in men

    i. Scarring of the _____ organs as a result of _____ transmitted diseases

    ii. Impotence and decreased _____ production

    iii. Low or nonexistent _____ count

    iv. Current or previous _____

    v. The use or overuse of certain _____ or _____

E. Common forms of treatment

    i. Surgery to repair scarred reproductive _____ or to remove _____

    ii. _____ therapies

    iii. Medications designed to increase _____

IV. Common Pathology Associated with the Female Reproductive System

  1. Breast Cancer

    A. Breast cancer is the development of _____ tumors within the breast tissue.

    B. The hormone _____ enables most cancerous tumors of the breast to grow and develop.

    C. Ductal Breast Cancer

      i. Ductal breast cancer develops in the _____ that transport milk to the _____.

      ii. It is the _____ _____ form of breast cancer.

      iii. It accounts for about _____ percent of breast cancer cases.

    D. Lobular Breast Cancer

      i. Lobular breast cancer develops in the _____ of the breast where milk is _____.

E. Inflammatory Breast Cancer

   i. Inflammatory breast cancer is a highly _____ cancer.

   ii. It accounts for _____ to _____ percent of breast cancer cases.

F. Signs and symptoms of breast cancer

   i. A(n) _____ or thickening of skin under the arm or above the

      _____ that does not go away

   ii. Breast _____, nipple _____, and changes in the

      _____ overlying the breasts

   iii. Changes in the skin of the breast such as _____, changes in

      _____, and _____

   iv. Signs and symptoms of inflammatory breast cancer

      a. Swelling and redness over _____ or more of the breast

      b. Burning or _____ of the breast

      c. Rapid growth or a feeling of _____

G. Treatment options for breast cancer

   i. _____ (removal of the lump) or _____ (removal of the

   entire breast) may be performed.

   ii. Chemotherapy and _____ are also available forms of treatment.

   iii. _____ therapy may also be implemented to block the effects of estrogen.

2. Cervical Cancer

A. Cervical cancer is the _____, uncontrolled growth of abnormal

   _____ on the cervix.

B. Regular _____ test screening is the single most important tool for

   _____ cervical cancer.

C. Most cases stem from risky _____ activity.

D. _____ percent of all cervical cancers result from the human papillomavirus.

E. Signs and symptoms of cervical cancer

   i. Abnormal changes in cervical cells _____ cause noticeable signs and

   symptoms.

   ii. List early signs and symptoms.

      a. _____

      b. _____

      c. _____

      d. _____

iii. List signs and symptoms that appear after cancer has progressed.

a. _____

b. _____

c. _____

d. _____

e. _____

F. Treatment options for cervical cancer

i. List three types of surgery to remove abnormal tissue and cells.

a. _____

b. _____

c. _____

ii. A(n) _____ (complete removal of the uterus) may be performed if cancer has spread to surrounding tissues.

iii. _____ and radiation may be options for advanced forms.

3. Cervicitis

A. Cervicitis is inflammation of the cervix that is usually caused by a(n) _____.

B. Most cases are caused by _____ _____ diseases.

C. Signs and symptoms of cervicitis

i. Vaginal discharge that is gray or _____ in color and possibly

_____

ii. Abnormal vaginal _____

iii. Pain that may be present during _____ as well as during

_____

D. Treatment options for cervicitis

i. It is important to treat the underlying _____ transmitted disease.

ii. _____ and antiviral medications may treat underlying infections.

iii. The patient's sexual _____ should also be treated.

iv. _____ should be maintained during the course of treatment.

4. Dysmenorrhea

A. Dysmenorrhea is painful _____ cramps during menstruation caused by muscular uterine _____.

B. Dysmenorrhea is usually referred to as _____.

C. _____ dysmenorrhea occurs when women experiences cramping and pain from the onset of their _____ cycles.

D. _____ dysmenorrhea occurs when pain and cramping accompany menstruation because of other _____ problems.

E. Signs and symptoms of dysmenorrhea

    i. Dull and _____ pain occurs in the lower abdomen.

    ii. Pain may also be felt in the lower _____ and _____.

    iii. Cramps usually last _____ or _____ days at the beginning of each menstrual period.

    iv. Some women may experience nausea and _____, diarrhea, _____, sweating, or _____.

F. Treatment options for dysmenorrhea

    i. Dysmenorrhea is often treated with the use of _____ antiinflammatory drugs (NSAIDs).

    ii. _____-strength NSAIDs may be given for more severe pain.

    iii. Other treatments to reduce pain and discomfort

        a. _____ therapy

        b. Meditation or _____

        c. Light circular _____ of the lower abdomen

        d. _____ certain dietary foods

    iv. In severe cases, _____ _____ pills may be prescribed to help thin the uterine lining.

5. Endometriosis

A. Endometriosis occurs when endometrial tissue is found outside the uterus, usually in the _____ or _____ cavity.

B. It reacts to changing levels of _____ but isn't sloughed with the _____ inside the uterus.

C. Endometriosis can cause scars and _____, which typically cause pain.

D. Signs and symptoms of endometriosis

    i. Infertility

    ii. _____ (painful intercourse)

    iii. Heavy _____ bleeding and very painful _____

    iv. Irregular _____

    v. _____ and vomiting

    vi. Pelvic pain after _____ or exercise

    vii. Dysmenorrhea

    viii. Decreasing symptoms after _____

E. Treatment options for endometriosis

    i. Hormone therapy, including high doses of _____ and oral _____

  ii. Medication for treating the _____

  iii. Surgery for _____ endometriosis

    a. Conservative surgery is aimed at restoring the _____ of the pelvic

     _____.

    b. Extensive surgery is performed on women with severe symptoms and

     no desire to _____ _____. Hysterectomy and

     _____ (removal of ovaries and fallopian tubes) are per-

     formed.

  iv. After the _____ are removed, hormone replacement must be

    _____.

6. Fibrocystic Breast Disease

 A. Fibrocystic breast disease presents as changes to the breast _____ that are

  considered to be common and _____.

 B. The hormone _____ seems to play a strong role as the changes tend to occur

  during ovulation and prior to menstruation.

 C. Signs and symptoms of fibrocystic breast disease

  i. A "cobblestone" consistency in the _____ _____

  ii. Irregularly _____ and _____ breast tissue

  iii. Breast _____ that may be persistent or intermittent

  iv. Feeling of _____ in the breasts

  v. _____ tenderness and swelling

  vi. Nipple _____, such as itching

 D. Treatment options for fibrocystic breast disease

  i. _____ modifications

  ii. Performing a monthly breast _____

  iii. Wearing a well-fitted _____ that provides good breast _____

  iv. Oral _____, which often decrease the symptoms

7. Ovarian Cancer

 A. Ovarian cancer begins with _____ cell changes in one or both ovaries.

 B. _____ _____ cancer occurs when cancer cells begin to grow on

  the outer covering of the ovary.

 C. A(n) _____ _____ tumor originates in the egg cells found within

  the ovary.

 D. A(n) _____ tumor originates in the ovarian cells that make up the

  _____ and _____ of the actual ovary.

E. Signs and symptoms of ovarian cancer
   i. Most often there are no _____ signs and symptoms and those that do occur may easily be _____ for other common illnesses.
   ii. Early-stage symptoms
      a. Mild _____ _____ or pain
      b. Abdominal _____
      c. Changes in _____ habits
      d. Feeling full after a(n) _____ _____
      e. Decreased _____
      f. Nausea and _____
      g. Chronic _____
      h. Pain in the lower _____ or _____
      i. Excessive _____ growth
      j. Abnormal menstrual or _____ bleeding
      k. More frequent _____
      l. Pain during _____
F. Treatment options for ovarian cancer
   i. Surgery, such as a bilateral or _____ salpingo-oophorectomy with or without a(n) _____
   ii. _____ therapy and chemotherapy
   iii. Complementary therapies such as _____
   iv. Alternative therapies such as traditional _____ _____ or special diets
8. Ovarian Cysts
   A. Ovarian cysts are pouches filled with liquid or a(n) _____ material that develops on or within the _____.
   B. Functional cysts are relatively _____ and usually disappear within _____ days without treatment.
   C. Other types of cysts that require treatment include true ovarian _____ and hormonal conditions such as _____ ovary syndrome.
   D. Signs and symptoms of ovarian cysts
      i. Often _____
      ii. Constant, _____ pelvic pain
      iii. Pelvic pain during _____, with _____, or after the beginning or end of a(n) _____ _____
      iv. Abdominal _____ or distention

E. Treatment options for ovarian cysts

    i. Oral _____ pills may be prescribed.

    ii. Surgical removal may be needed in cases of ovarian cysts that are not

       _____ cysts and cysts larger than _____ cm or persisting

       longer than _____ weeks.

9. Pelvic Inflammatory Disease (PID)

A. PID is the most _____ and _____ complication of untreated

    STDs.

B. PID is caused by disease-carrying organisms that migrate _____ from the

    urethra and _____ and infect the uterus, _____

    _____, and even ovaries.

C. List possible complications from untreated PID.

    i. _____

    ii. _____

    iii. _____

D. Signs and symptoms of PID

    i. Major signs and symptoms include lower _____ _____ and

       abnormal vaginal _____.

    ii. List other possible symptoms.

       a. _____

       b. _____

       c. _____

       d. _____

       e. _____

E. Treatment options for PID

    i. First, it is necessary to treat the primary source of _____.

    ii. Severe cases may require _____ and monitoring along

       with _____ _____ therapy.

    iii. Surgery may be indicated for extensive _____ of reproductive organs.

10. Premenstrual Syndrome (PMS)

A. PMS is a common condition associated with the _____ level of

    _____ produced during the menstrual cycle.

B. It affects approximately _____ percent of menstruating women.

C. Signs and symptoms of PMS

    i. _____

    ii. _____

iii. _____

iv. _____

v. _____

vi. _____

vii. _____

viii. _____

ix. _____

x. _____

xi. _____

xii. _____

xiii. _____

xiv. _____

xv. _____

xvi. _____

D. Treatment options for PMS

    i. Healthy _____

    ii. Regular _____ exercise

    iii. _____ therapy

    iv. Stress _____ techniques

    v. Certain herbal products, such as _____ and _____

    _____

    vi. Medications to aid physical symptoms

        a. _____ to reduce fluid retention

        b. _____ medication and _____ to help with anxiety and mood disorders

        c. Ibuprofen and _____ to help with aches and pains

11. Sexually Transmitted Diseases (STDs)

A. STD is a term that describes more than _____ types of _____.

B. STDs are transmitted by means of sexual contact and exchange of _____, _____, and other _____ fluids.

C. In the United States, about _____ percent of the population will experience an STD at some point.

D. List the most common STDs in the United States.

    i. _____

    ii. _____

    iii. _____

      iv. _____

       v. _____

      vi. _____

  E. Signs and symptoms of STDs

        i. Signs and symptoms _____ depending on the type of _____.

       ii. Signs and symptoms in women

          a. Bleeding not associated with _____

          b. Abnormal vaginal _____ with odor

          c. _____ burning and itching

          d. Pelvic pain during _____ _____

     iii. Signs and symptoms in men

          a. _____ discharge

          b. Lymph node swelling in the _____ area

     iv. Both men and women may experience painful and burning _____ and

        skin _____.

      v. General signs and symptoms

          a. _____

          b. _____

          c. _____

          d. _____

  F. Treatment options for STDs

        i. Medical intervention and treatment, sometimes including _____ or

        _____.

       ii. STDs caused by bacterium and treated with antibiotics include _____,

        _____, and _____.

     iii. STDs caused by viruses and treated with antivirals include _____

        _____.

     iv. The risk of contracting an STD can be _____ by adopting certain

        _____ behaviors.

12. Uterine Cancer

  A. Uterine cancer generally develops in the _____ _____ of the

    endometrium.

  B. Treatment can be very _____ if uterine cancer is detected and treated early.

  C. Signs and symptoms of uterine cancer

        i. Signs and symptoms that may be associated with other disorders include

        _____ between menstrual periods, _____ bleeding or

_____ during periods or after _____, and bleeding after
_____.

    ii. Other symptoms

       a. Cramping pain and pressure in the _____, pelvis, _____, or legs

       b. Difficulty _____

       c. Discomfort in the _____ area

D. Treatment options for uterine cancer

    i. The usual treatment is a total _____, which includes the removal of the uterus and _____.

    ii. _____ tubes and _____ are also usually removed.

    iii. _____ is a common treatment in early stages of cancer.

    iv. Later stages may require _____ or _____ therapy.

13. Uterine Fibroids

A. Uterine fibroids are found within the _____ of the uterus.

B. They are _____ tumors that can vary in size from a seed to a(n) _____ ball.

C. They are composed of _____ and muscle cells.

D. Signs and symptoms of uterine fibroids

    i. Heavy _____ or painful _____

    ii. Bleeding between _____

    iii. Feeling of _____ in the pelvic area

    iv. Frequent _____

    v. _____ during sex

    vi. Lower _____ pain

    vii. Reproductive problems, including _____ and early onset of _____

E. Treatment options for uterine fibroids

    i. Over-the-counter medications for relief of _____ and inflammation

    ii. A physician may prescribe _____-releasing _____ agonists to decrease the size of the fibroids.

    iii. List surgical procedures that may be used to treat moderate to severe cases.

       a. _____

       b. _____

       c. _____

       d. _____

14. Vaginitis
    A. Vaginitis is inflammation of the vagina commonly caused by bacterial vaginitis, trichomoniasis, and _____ _____.
    B. _____ vaginitis is a condition that is a result of menopause and decreased _____ levels.
    C. Signs and symptoms of vaginitis
        i. _____ and irritation
        ii. Vaginal discharge with a marked change in _____, _____, and _____
        iii. Pain and burning during _____
        iv. _____ bleeding
        v. Pain during _____
    D. Treatment options for vaginitis
        i. Vaginal _____ or creams may be prescribed for _____ vaginitis.
        ii. Yeast infections are usually treated with _____ creams or suppositories.
        iii. Trichomoniasis is frequently treated with _____.
        iv. Atrophic vaginitis is treated with _____.
V. The Male Reproductive System
    1. External Organs
        A. Scrotum
            i. The scrotum is a(n) _____ structure situated _____ to the penis.
            ii. It is suspended from the _____ region and is divided into two sacs by a(n) _____.
            iii. Each sac contains a(n) _____.
            iv. Testes are 1 degree _____ than the temperature of the body, which is ideal for _____ viability.
        B. Penis
            i. The penis is composed of longitudinal columns of _____ tissue covered by skin.
            ii. Three columns of erectile tissue
                a. Two columns are the _____ _____.
                b. The third column is the _____ _____.
            iii. The prepuce, or _____, covers the penis.
            iv. _____ is a procedure in which the foreskin is removed.
            v. The erectile state occurs with _____ stimulation.

vi. Functions of the penis

    a. It serves as the male organ for _____ or copulation.

    b. It is the site through which _____ and _____ are eliminated from the body.

2. Internal Organs (List seven internal male reproductive organs.)

  i. _____

  ii. _____

  iii. _____

  iv. _____

  v. _____

  vi. _____

  vii. _____

VI. Common Pathology Associated with the Male Reproductive System

1. Benign Prostatic Hyperplasia (BPH)

A. BPH is a condition marked by _____ of the prostate.

B. The _____ of the prostate gland may be due to changes in _____ levels including the hormones _____, _____, and _____.

C. The likelihood of developing BPH increases with _____.

D. A consequence of BPH is a change in _____ patterns.

E. Signs and symptoms of BPH

  i. Urinary urgency

  ii. _____ nocturia

  iii. Difficulty producing a urine _____

  iv. Straining of the _____

  v. _____ retention

  vi. Recurring _____

  vii. A feeling that the _____ is not empty

F. Treatment options for BPH

  i. Medications to _____ the size of the prostate or relax the smooth muscle of the prostate and the _____ neck to improve urine _____ and reduce bladder outlet _____

  ii. Surgery to _____ the size of the prostate and enlarge the _____ to allow for more adequate urine flow

2. Epididymitis

A. Epididymitis is inflammation or _____ of the epididymis.

B. It is the most common cause of _____ pain in adult men.

C. Causes of epididymitis

    i. The same organisms that cause some _____

    ii. _____ surgery

    iii. Accumulated _____ within the vas deferens, as a result of infection or

    _____

D. Signs and symptoms of epididymitis

    i. Sudden _____ and _____ of the scrotum

    ii. _____ and hardened inflamed testicle

    iii. Chills

    iv. _____ pain

    v. Pain with _____ or ejaculation

    vi. Acute _____

    vii. _____ _____ in the groin causing pain in the scrotum

E. Treatment options for epididymitis

    i. _____ therapy

    ii. Pain medications, either _____ or over-the-counter

    iii. Antiinflammatory drugs to reduce _____

3. Erectile Dysfunction

A. Erectile dysfunction is the inability to achieve or maintain a(n) _____ sufficient for sexual intercourse.

B. Diagnosis is made when the inability to achieve or maintain an erection until _____ occurs more than _____ percent of the time.

C. Erectile dysfunction can happen at _____ age for a number of various _____.

D. Chances for development increase _____ with _____.

E. Signs and symptoms of erectile dysfunction

    i. Inability to _____ an erection

    ii. Inability to _____ an erection

F. Treatment options for erectile dysfunction

    i. _____ therapy

    ii. Medication _____

    iii. _____ and _____ injection therapies

    iv. Surgery, including penile _____

4. Hydrocele

A. A hydrocele is a(n) _____-filled sac that surrounds one or both testicles.

B. It may be _____ and uncomfortable.

C. It is not _____ and generally not _____.

D. It is most common in _____ _____ and can be either congenital

or _____.

E. Signs and symptoms of hydrocele

   i. The main symptom is a painless, swollen _____ or _____

     area.

   ii. The scrotum may have a(n) _____ tinge or appear translucent.

   iii. The presence of _____ indicates that another medical condition is present

     and should be addressed by a physician.

F. Treatment options for hydrocele

   i. Hydroceles generally _____ on their own.

   ii. Medical intervention is initiated if a hydrocele becomes _____ or

     _____.

5. Prostate Cancer

A. Prostate cancer is a(n) _____ tumor that grows in the prostate gland.

B. Men under _____ are rarely at risk for this form of cancer.

C. Prostate cancer is the _____ cause of cancer-related death in men aged _____

and over.

D. Signs and symptoms of prostate cancer

   i. Dull pain in the lower _____ area, particularly _____ pain

   ii. Blood in the _____ or _____

   iii. _____ when urinating

   iv. _____ dysfunction

   v. Frequent urination, especially at _____

   vi. Painful urination or _____

   vii. Smaller stream of _____ or _____ need to urinate

   viii. Loss of _____ and weight

   ix. Persistent _____ pain, occasional _____ loss, or loss of

     _____ function when cancer has spread

E. Treatment options for prostate cancer

   i. Treatment depends on the patient's overall _____ and _____

     score.

   ii. Early stages of cancer may be treated with _____ therapy and

     _____.

   iii. More advanced stages may be treated with _____, additional

     _____, and _____ therapy.

APPLIED PRACTICE

1. Label the uterus, ovaries, and associated structures.

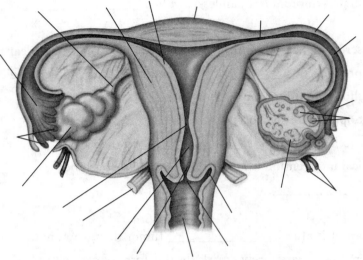

2. Label the structures of the male reproductive system.

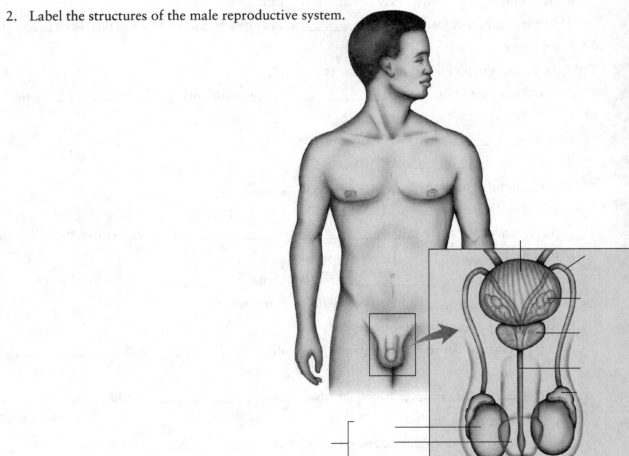

LEARNING ACTIVITY: FILL IN THE BLANK

Using words from the list below, fill in the blanks to complete the following statements.
Note: Not all of the words in the list will be used.

benign prostatic hyperplasia (BPH)
cervical cancer
circumcision
dysmenorrhea
endometriosis
hydrocele
hysterectomy
menarche
ovarian cancer

ovarian cysts
pelvic inflammatory disease (PID)
perineum
premenstrual syndrome (PMS)
scrotum
testes
urethritis
uterine fibroids
vaginitis

1. Phimosis is typically treated by performing a(n) _____.
2. Anorchism is a congenital absence of one or both _____.
3. _____ occurs at the age of puberty.
4. The main symptom of a(n) _____ is a swollen scrotum or groin area.
5. The _____ is between the vulva and the anus.
6. _____ is an enlargement of the prostate gland.
7. Symptoms of epididymitis include chills, fever, and acute _____.
8. The most important tool for preventing _____ is regular Pap testing.
9. Bacterial infections, trichomoniasis, and yeast infections can cause _____.
10. Typically, by the time _____ is diagnosed, the cancer is usually at an advanced stage.
11. _____ is defined as the symptoms that develop just prior to the onset of a menstrual period.
12. _____ are pouches filled with liquid or a semisolid material.
13. _____ is painful cramping associated with menstruation.
14. A(n) _____ involves the removal of the uterus.
15. _____ is the most common and serious complication of untreated STDs among women.

CRITICAL THINKING

Answer the following questions to the best of your ability. Use the textbook as a reference.

1. While working as a medical assistant at an OB/GYN office, you encounter a patient who recently found out that she will be having a baby boy. The mother asks you if you think that her infant son should be circumcised. How would you respond?

   _____

   _____

   _____

   _____

2. Leonard Olesnanik, 75 years old, is being seen for frequent nighttime urination, blood-tinged urine, and pain in his pelvic area. Mr. Olesnanik's medical history includes obesity, hypertension, and alcoholism. He is also a veteran of the Vietnam War. Dr. Wellington is concerned that Mr. Olesnanik may have prostate cancer, not only because of his symptoms but also because he is considered higher risk for developing the cancer. Which of the information provided places Mr. Olesnanik at high risk for prostate cancer? If a diagnosis of prostate cancer is made, what will determine his course of treatment?

   _____

   _____

   _____

   _____

   _____

RESEARCH ACTIVITY

Use Internet search engines to research the following topic and write a brief description of what you find. It is important to use reputable websites.

1. Visit www.cdc.gov/std. As you navigate through the site, what information do you find that would be helpful to provide to a patient who has a sexually transmitted disease?

   _____

   _____

   _____

   _____

CHAPTER 33
Infection Control

STUDENT STUDY GUIDE

Use the following guide to assist in your learning of the concepts from the chapter.

I. Microorganisms and Pathogens

1. Microorganisms are so small that they can only be seen with a(n) _____.

2. Disease-causing microorganisms are called _____.

3. List the four main types of microorganisms.

   A. _____

   B. _____

   C. _____

   D. _____

4. How Microorganisms Grow

   A. In order to grow, microorganisms need the following.

      i. _____

      ii. _____

      iii. _____

      iv. _____

   B. _____ bacteria require oxygen in order to live.

   C. _____ bacteria do not require oxygen to live.

5. Multidrug-Resistant Microorganisms (MDROs)

   A. MDROs are referred to as "_____" because they do not respond to traditional medications and treatments.

   B. MDROs have developed resistance to _____ drugs.

   C. List three examples of MDROs.

      i. _____

      ii. _____

      iii. _____

D. Methicillin-resistant *Staphylococcus aureus* (MRSA)

    i. MRSA is an organism that is highly resistant to _____.

    ii. Two forms include _____-associated MRSA and _____-based MRSA.

    iii. Symptoms of *Staphylococcus* infection include _____ formation, fever, _____, and _____ around the area of infection.

    iv. Diagnosis of *S. aureus* is established by culture from the _____ individual.

    v. Sensitivity tests determine which _____ are most effective in killing the organism.

E. Vancomycin-resistant Enterococci (VRE)

    i. Most species of enterococci are _____, but some are capable of causing serious _____.

    ii. Vancomycin is an antibiotic generally used after all other antibiotics have _____.

    iii. VRE are bacteria that have developed a(n) _____ to vancomycin.

    iv. Signs and symptoms of VRE vary, depending on the source of the _____.

    v. It is spread by _____ _____ from human to human, usually by caregivers who have not practiced proper _____.

II. Infections

  1. Chain of Infection

    A. The _____ _____ begins the chain of infection and harbors and nourishes a(n) _____.

    B. The _____ of _____ is how the pathogen leaves the reservoir host.

    C. There must be a means of _____ for the pathogen to spread to another person.

    D. The _____ of _____ is the means by which a pathogen enters the body.

    E. A(n) _____ _____ must be capable of being infected and is unable to fight off the infection.

    F. A susceptible host who is infected becomes the new _____ _____.

2. The Stages and Types of Infections

   A. List the stages of infection.

      i. _____ by the pathogen

     ii. _____ (reproduction) of the pathogen

    iii. A(n) _____ period

    iv. A(n) _____ period

     v. A(n) _____ period

    vi. The _____ period

   B. Acute infections

      i. Acute infections have a rapid transition from _____ of the pathogen to the _____ period.

     ii. The body is usually able to rid itself of the virus and recover within _____ to _____ weeks of onset.

   C. Chronic infections

      i. Some chronic infections are _____.

     ii. Transition of stages from invasion to the prodromal period _____ based on the _____ of infection.

   D. Latent infections

      i. A latent infection is characterized by periods of _____ and _____.

     ii. The main characteristic is that the virus lies _____ for extended periods of time and then the virus becomes _____ within the body again due to an external or internal trigger.

   E. Opportunistic infections

      i. Opportunistic infections occur when the host's immune system has already been _____ by another disease-causing _____.

     ii. The immune system has become _____ and more susceptible to other _____.

   F. Nosocomial infections

      i. A nosocomial infection is an infection acquired while in a(n) _____ facility.

     ii. List the most common types of nosocomial infections.

       a. _____

       b. _____

       c. _____

3. The Inflammatory Response to Infection

    A. The process includes the following.

        i. _____ of blood vessels to allow increased blood flow

        ii. Production of watery _____ and materials (exudates such as pus)

        iii. Invasion of _____ and monocytes into the injured tissues

    B. The inflammatory response can be local or _____.

    C. List the four cardinal signs of acute inflammation.

        i. _____

        ii. _____

        iii. _____

        iv. _____

III. The Body's Natural Barriers

    1. Prevention and Protection

      A. The largest natural barrier to infection is intact _____.

      B. _____ _____ lining the body's orifices and various

        tracts repel microorganisms.

      C. The lymphatic system and the blood

        i. The lymphatic system and the blood produce _____ to identify and

          destroy disease-causing _____ that enter the body.

        ii. _____ is the process of engulfing, digesting, and destroying

          pathogens.

      D. Antigen–antibody reaction

        i. Antibodies have the ability to _____ antigens or make them more

          susceptible to _____.

        ii. The antigen–antibody reaction occurs in response to an invasion of

          _____.

      E. Immunity

        i. Immunity is _____ to disease.

        ii. Immunity is either _____, _____, or

          _____.

IV. Infection Control: Precautions and Standards

    1. Several _____ _____ have developed guidelines, precautions,

      and standards to protect patients and health care workers from exposure to pathogens.

    2. Universal Precautions

      A. The Centers for Disease Control and Prevention established _____

        _____ in 1985.

B. Universal precautions serve to protect health care workers and patients from

_____, _____, and other bloodborne pathogens.

C. The idea behind universal precautions is to treat all _____ and

_____ fluids as if they are _____.

3. Standard Precautions

A. Standard precautions apply to all blood, _____ _____

secretions, and excretions except _____, whether blood is visible or

_____.

B. Original guidelines dealt with _____ and the use of personal

_____ equipment.

C. List the general topics covered by the current and complete set of standard precautions,
including updates from 2007.

   i. _____

   ii. _____

   iii. _____

   iv. _____

   v. _____

D. When practicing standard precautions, always take into consideration patients with a(n)

_____ sensitivity.

4. Transmission-Based Precautions

A. These precautions are used in addition to _____ _____

to further interrupt the spread of pathogens.

B. List the three categories of transmission-based precautions.

   i. _____

   ii. _____

   iii. _____

C. Airborne precautions often involve the following.

   i. _____ isolation

   ii. Required use of _____ and _____ by all health

   care personnel who come in contact with the patient

D. Droplet precautions

   i. Droplet precautions are used for patients suspected of being infected with organisms

   spread by droplets during _____, _____, and

   _____.

   ii. A mask should be worn if the health care worker is within _____

   _____ of an infected patient.

iii. _____ and _____ are worn if there is a chance of
   coming into contact with blood or body fluids of suspected patients.

E. Contact precautions
   i. Contact precautions specialized precautions used when infections are difficult to
      _____ and the likelihood of microorganism _____
      is high.
   ii. Precautions include the following.
       a. _____ patients and wearing _____ and gloves
       b. If there is a chance of coming in contact with body _____,
          wearing a mask and protective _____

F. Radiation isolation precautions
   i. Radiation isolation precautions are not specifically for _____
      _____.
   ii. _____ a patient who has had radiation from others who may be
       harmed by radioactivity.

5. Bloodborne Pathogen Standard
   A. _____ developed the bloodborne pathogen standard in
      _____.
   B. The aim of this standard is to minimize _____ of health care workers to
      harmful _____ pathogens.
   C. The standard was updated to reflect changes established by the _____
      Safety and Prevention _____.
   D. OSHA guidelines apply to facilities in which the employees could be "_____
      _____" to come into contact with potentially _____
      materials.
   E. List the topics that must be included in exposure control plans.
      i. _____
      ii. _____
      iii. _____
      iv. _____
      v. _____
      vi. _____

V. Infection Control: Physical and Chemical Barriers
   1. Medical Asepsis
      A. Medical asepsis refers to the destruction of organisms after they _____ the
         _____.

B. _____ _____ is considered the first step of infection control.

C. The following are suggested forms of practicing medical asepsis.

    i. Wash hands _____ and _____ any contact with patients or equipment.

    ii. Handle all _____ and materials as though they contain pathogens.

    iii. Use gloves for protection when handling contaminated _____ or _____.

    iv. Do not wear _____ that can attract and harbor bacteria.

    v. Use _____ equipment whenever possible and dispose of all equipment _____ after use.

    vi. Clean all _____ equipment as soon as possible after patient use, using an approved _____ and while wearing appropriate _____.

    vii. Use only clean or sterile _____ for each patient.

    viii. Use a protective covering over _____ if there is any danger of contaminated materials or supplies coming into contact with them.

    ix. _____ items that fall on the floor if they cannot be cleaned.

    x. Place all wet or damp _____ and _____ in a waterproof bag to protect the persons handling the _____ removal.

D. Hand hygiene

    i. Frequent and diligent hand hygiene provides the _____ _____ against the spread of disease.

    ii. _____ your hands to prevent cracking or breaks in the skin.

E. Alcohol-based hand rubs

    i. Alcohol-based hand rubs have the advantage of not requiring _____.

    ii. Many contain emollients that _____ and prevent _____ of the skin.

    iii. The CDC states that hands should always be washed with soap and water in the following instances.

        a. Every _____ time hand hygiene is performed

        b. If they are visibly soiled with _____ or _____ fluids

        c. Before _____

        d. After using the _____

    iv. _____ should be removed before using the hand rubs.

v. Approximately _____ to _____ ml of the gel should be placed in the palm of the hand.

vi. Spread hand rub over the surface of both hands up to _____ _____ above the wrist.

2. Protective Clothing and Personal Protective Equipment (PPE)

   A. Protective clothing and equipment are worn for two reasons.

      i. To protect the _____ from any microorganisms that might be present on the health care worker's _____

      ii. To protect the health care worker from carrying microorganisms _____ from the _____

   B. PPE should be chosen in consideration of the possibility of _____.

   C. The following is the correct order for removing PPE.

      i. Remove _____.

      ii. Remove _____ or _____ _____.

      iii. Remove _____.

      iv. Remove _____ or _____.

3. Surgical Asepsis

   A. Surgical asepsis refers to the techniques practiced to maintain a(n) _____ environment.

   B. It involves the destruction of organisms _____ they enter the _____.

   C. Sanitization

      i. Sanitation is a(n) _____ process that inhibits or inactivates pathogens through the careful cleaning of _____ and _____ to remove debris.

      ii. Items are rinsed and _____ using a brush and detergent with a(n) _____ pH.

      iii. Items are then rinsed in _____ water and air dried.

      iv. Thick _____ gloves are worn for protection.

      v. Sanitization does not destroy _____ and bacteria.

   D. Ultrasonic sanitization

      i. Instruments and equipment are placed into a(n) _____ _____.

      ii. Within the tank, _____ _____ vibrate to break up the contamination.

      iii. The articles are then _____ thoroughly.

E. Disinfection

    i. Disinfection destroys or inhibits the _____ of disease-causing organisms.

    ii. It does not always kill _____ or certain _____.

    iii. _____ _____ are used in the medical office for disinfection.

    iv. A 1:10 _____ solution is commonly used for disinfection.

    v. Completely immerse contaminated items in the _____ solution for the specified amount of time.

    vi. Rinse in _____ and then dry them.

    vii. Antiseptics

        a. Use antiseptics to disinfect a patient's _____ before performing invasive _____.

        b. Antiseptics used for patient skin include 70 percent _____ alcohol and povidone-_____ solutions.

4. Sterilization

A. Sterilization is a process that _____ all microorganisms.

B. Heat sterilization can kill _____, _____, and other microorganisms.

C. _____ _____ is used for sterilizing dense ointments.

D. _____ gloves must be used when touching sterilized items.

5. Autoclave

A. Most _____ _____ have an autoclave for sterilization.

B. List four types of autoclaving.

    i. _____

    ii. _____

    iii. _____

    iv. _____

C. High-heat and high-moisture sterilization require _____ pounds of pressure per square inch (PSI) and a temperature of _____°F to _____°F.

D. Heat is actually transferred to the items by way of the _____ condensation through the use of _____ _____.

E. Autoclave maintenance

    i. Read and follow the _____ instructions.

    ii. The autoclave should be cleaned on a(n) _____ _____.

  iii. The air exhaust valve should be cleaned before _____

    _____.

  iv. An outside _____ _____ should perform regulated

    checks on the autoclave to ensure proper functioning (at various intervals).

F. Autoclave wrapping materials and loading the autoclave

  i. Wrapping materials must be _____ and _____

    enough to hold together during the steam process.

  ii. List commonly used wrapping materials.

    a. _____

    b. _____

    c. _____

    d. _____

  iii. Autoclave _____ tape is used to secure packages and changes

    _____ to indicate exposure to high temperature.

  iv. Sterilization _____ strips are placed _____ the

    wrappers of packages, and color changes on the strip indicate that complete

    sterilization has occurred.

  v. Sterilization pouches are ideal for _____, lightweight instruments.

  vi. Each package requires proper labeling, including the following.

    a. _____

    b. _____

    c. _____

G. Record keeping and quality control

  i. Record keeping for quality control measures includes the following.

    a. _____

    b. _____

    c. _____

  ii. It is important not to _____ or cram items inside the autoclave chamber.

  iii. Consistent spacing is vital to allow the steam to properly _____ and

    _____ the packages.

  iv. Autoclaved packages are stored in _____ and

    _____-free shelves or drawers.

  v. The _____ dated packs are placed in front of the stack so that they

    can be used _____.

  vi. Instruments are considered sterile for _____ days in plastic bags and _____ days in

    muslin.

H. Chemical gas sterilization

    i. Chemical gas sterilization removes or kills life through the use of

      _____.

    ii. The _____ most commonly used for sterilization is ethylene oxide

      (EtO) at _____ temperature.

    iii. Various technologies are under _____ for use in health care facilities

      but have not yet been cleared by the _____.

I. Chemical liquid sterilization

    i. Chemical liquid sterilization sterilizes objects by using a chemical that is

      _____ to the microbes.

    ii. Instruments may be submerged in _____ chemicals rather than

      _____ to perform this procedure.

    iii. Proper sterilization by chemical liquid can take _____ to

      _____ to work effectively.

KEY TERMINOLOGY REVIEW

Use the key terms found at the beginning of the chapter to finish the following sentences. Key terms may be more than one word in length.

1. _____ is a process that kills all microorganisms, both pathogenic and nonpathogenic.

2. The body has a natural protective mechanism called _____.

3. Microorganisms that are normally found on the skin and in the urinary, gastrointestinal, and respiratory tracts are known as _____.

4. _____ destroys or inhibits the activity of disease-causing organisms, although it does not always kill spores or certain viruses.

5. _____ is the state of being free from germs.

APPLIED PRACTICE

Answer the questions related to the scenario below.

Scenario

Shandra Graham, CMA (AAMA), did not know that she was infected with the flu virus when she went to work at Peachtree Medical Center. She forgot to wash her hands after she had coughed just prior to assisting her patient, Adam Kenney, into the examination room. While she was checking Mr. Kenney's blood pressure, Shandra sneezed and, unfortunately, was unable to cover her mouth.

Two days later, Mr. Kenney developed some muscle aches that he at first attributed to his exercise regimen. By day 5 after his office visit, Mr. Kenney had a high fever, chills, and intense muscular aches.

1. Who, in this scenario, represents the reservoir host in the cycle of infection?

   _____

2. What is the portal of exit of the infectious pathogen?

   _____

3. What is the means of transmission of the pathogen?

   _____

4. Who is the susceptible host?

   _____

5. Explain the incubation period. In this scenario, when is the incubation period for the reservoir host?

   _____

   _____

   _____

6. What is the prodromal period for the person who became infected?

   _____

   _____

   _____

LEARNING ACTIVITY: MULTIPLE CHOICE

Circle the correct answer to each of the following questions.

1. In what decade did the United States experience an epidemic of HIV?

   a. 1960s
   b. 1970s
   c. 1980s
   d. 1990s

2. Which of the following were developed to reduce the transmission of certain diseases, such as TB, measles, or chickenpox?

   a. Hand hygiene guidelines
   b. Contact precautions
   c. Airborne precautions
   d. Droplet precautions

3. Waterless hand sanitizers kill _____ percent of common microorganisms in 15 seconds.

   a. 100
   b. 99.9
   c. 97.9
   d. 95.9

4. The ordinary hygiene habits of everyday life are a form of

   a. medical asepsis.
   b. surgical asepsis.
   c. bloodborne asepsis.
   d. universal precautions.

5. Which organization's guidelines apply to facilities in which the employees could be "reasonably anticipated" to come into contact with potentially infectious materials?

    a. CDC
    b. FDA
    c. DEA
    d. OSHA

6. How long is the incubation period for hepatitis B?

    a. 14–50 days
    b. 60–90 days
    c. 90–120 days
    d. 120–240 days

7. A patient with a(n) _____ allergy might have a cross-sensitivity to latex.

    a. chocolate
    b. peanut
    c. avocado
    d. milk

8. An exposure control program must be implemented in each facility and must include which of the following?

    a. Exposure determination
    b. Method of compliance
    c. Postexposure evaluation
    d. All of the above

9. When did the CDC develop the universal precautions?

    a. 1965
    b. 1974
    c. 1985
    d. 1991

10. Chemical germicides are used in

    a. disinfection.
    b. ultrasonic sanitization.
    c. hand hygiene.
    d. sterilization.

CRITICAL THINKING

Answer the following questions to the best of your ability. Use the textbook as a reference.

1. Miguel Rodriguez has been hospitalized for 2 weeks. He has an indwelling catheter and a feeding tube. While in the hospital, he acquired MRSA. Since he contracted MRSA in the hospital, how would his infection be classified? Given the information provided, what is the likely source of the infection? How would the patient's diagnosis of MRSA be obtained? What serious complications can arise if MRSA is left untreated?

_____

_____

_____

_____

_____

2. While working as a clinical medical assistant, Chloe notices that her coworker Rita never washes her hands and always uses alcohol-based hand sanitizers. When asked why she never washes her hands, Rita answers, "The soap in the office irritates my hands, and I know that hand sanitizer kills more germs than handwashing." If you were Chloe, how would you respond to Rita's answer?

_____

_____

_____

_____

RESEARCH ACTIVITY

Use Internet search engines to research the following topic and write a brief description of what you find. It is important to use reputable websites.

1. Visit the website for the Occupational Safety and Health Administration, www.osha.gov. Locate information on bloodborne pathogen training. What information is available from OSHA? Then, using a search engine, investigate online bloodborne pathogen training. Is there a specific training program that appeals to you? If so, explain why.

_____

_____

_____

_____

CHAPTER 34
Vital Signs

STUDENT STUDY GUIDE

Use the following guide to assist in your learning of the concepts from the chapter.

I. Measuring Height and Weight

   1. Weight and height are called _____ measurements.

   2. _____ is often obtained at each office visit, and _____ might only be measured during an annual physical.

   3. Weight

      A. It is important to be _____ and provide sufficient privacy when obtaining a patient's weight.

      B. _____ and outerwear should be removed prior to obtaining a patient's weight.

      C. Patients who can't stand may be weighed on a(n) _____ or _____ scale.

      D. When a patient refuses to get weighed, simply note "_____ _____" in the medical record.

   4. Height

      A. True height must be measured without _____.

      B. When measuring height, the patient stands with _____, _____, and _____ of head touching the measuring stick or bar.

      C. Height is measured in either _____ and _____ or _____.

II. Vital Signs

   1. Vital signs are indicators of the body's ability to maintain _____.

   2. List the vital signs.

      A. _____

      B. _____

      C. _____

      D. _____

3. Health care professionals are required to use _____

_____ to maintain infection control while measuring vital signs.

III. Temperature

1. Physiology of Body Temperature

A. Body temperature is regulated by _____ the amount of heat the body

_____ with the amount of heat the body _____.

B. The hypothalamus is able to adjust body temperature, as needed.

C. List four ways the body loses heat.

   i. _____

   ii. _____

   iii. _____

   iv. _____

2. Temperature: Normal Values and Terms

A. Temperature is recorded in either degrees _____ or degrees

_____.

B. The average body temperature is _____°F.

C. Medical assistants should always be alert to the _____ of

_____ in body temperature.

3. Fahrenheit and Celsius Conversions

A. _____ is used throughout the United States.

B. _____ is used by some physicians, hospitals, and medical facilities.

C. Fahrenheit degrees = (Celsius degrees × _____) + 32

D. Celsius degrees = (Fahrenheit degrees − _____) × 5/9

4. Abnormal Temperatures

A. Fever is also called _____.

B. A fever occurs when the body temperature is over _____°F.

C. List four common types of fevers.

   i. _____

   ii. _____

   iii. _____

   iv. _____

D. Hyperpyrexia and hyperthermia occur when the body temperature exceeds _____°F.

E. _____ results from a regulated rise in core body temperature, such as in

response to a(n) _____.

F. _____ results from an unregulated rise in core body temperature, as in

exposure to high _____ _____.

G. Hypothermia

    i. Hypothermia is defined as a body temperature below _____°F.

    ii. It commonly occurs in cases of _____ _____ to cool or cold temperatures and/or submersion in _____ _____.

    iii. A body temperature below _____°F is considered severe hypothermia and may be life threatening.

5. Sites for Measuring Body Temperature

A. List five sites where body temperature can be measured.

    i. _____

    ii. _____

    iii. _____

    iv. _____

    v. _____

B. List the normal body temperature for each site of measurement.

    i. Oral = _____°F

    ii. Rectal = _____°F

    iii. Axillary (under the arm) = _____°F

    iv. Aural (ear) = _____°F

    v. Temporal artery = _____°F

C. Oral

    i. The _____ common way to take a patient's temperature is orally.

    ii. The thermometer is placed under the _____ and on either side of the _____ _____.

    iii. Patients should not _____ during the procedure and should close the lips _____ around the thermometer.

    iv. Wait _____ _____ to obtain an oral temperature if the patient has recently smoked or has had anything to drink.

D. Aural (ear)/tympanic membrane

    i. Some thermometers are able to detect _____ _____ in the ear canal and calculate body temperature.

    ii. This method is sometimes preferred over the _____ method.

    iii. A tympanic thermometer should not be used if the patient has complaints of _____ _____ or has _____ _____.

E. Axillary

    i. This method has been proven to be the _____ accurate of the temperature measurement methods.

    ii. It is the recommended site for _____ _____ or for any patients unable to _____ _____ an oral thermometer in their mouths.

F. Rectal

    i. This is considered to be the _____ accurate and _____ method.

    ii. The rectal route is advised for the following patients.

        a. _____

        b. _____

        c. _____

    iii. A(n) _____ thermometer should be used for rectal readings so that the same one isn't used for taking a(n) _____ temperature.

G. Temporal artery

    i. This is a newer, _____ method of obtaining body temperature.

    ii. A temporal thermometer uses a(n) _____ scanning device that detects the temperature of the _____ as it is flowing through the _____ artery.

    iii. It is a(n) _____ and fairly _____ method of obtaining body temperature.

H. List the types of thermometers available.

    i. _____

    ii. _____

    iii. _____

    iv. _____

    v. _____

IV. Pulse

    1. Pulse rate is the number of times the heart _____ per _____.

    2. A normal resting heart rate for adults ranges from _____ to _____ beats a minute.

    3. To calculate your maximum heart rate, _____ your age from _____.

    4. Maximum heart rate is the _____ number of times your heart should beat per minute while _____.

    5. A resting heart rate above 100 bpm is termed _____.

6. A resting heart rate below 60 bpm is termed _____.

7. List eight factors that influence pulse rate.

    i. _____

    ii. _____

    iii. _____

    iv. _____

    v. _____

    vi. _____

    vii. _____

    viii. _____

8. Fill in normal pulse rates based on age in the table below.

Less than 1 year	_____–_____ bpm
2–6 years	_____–_____ bpm
6–10 years	_____–_____ bpm
11–16 years	_____–_____ bpm
Adult	_____–_____ bpm
Older adult	_____–_____ bpm

9. Characteristics of Pulse Rate

    A. _____ is the number of beats per minute.

    B. _____ refers to the strength of the pulse when the heart contracts.

        i. The most common volume characteristics are _____ and

        _____.

    C. _____ refers to the regularity, or equal spacing, of all the beats of the

    pulse.

        i. Irregular pulse rhythm is known as _____ or

        _____.

        ii. A(n) _____ _____ occurs when the heart

        occasionally skips a beat.

10. Pulse Sites (List all nine sites.)

    A. _____

    B. _____

    C. _____

    D. _____

    E. _____

    F. _____

G. _____

H. _____

I. _____

11. Apical Pulse Rate

A. The apical pulse rate is counted at the _____ of the heart.

B. A(n) _____ is used and placed over the apex.

C. This method is most often used for pulse measurements of _____ and

_____ children.

D. A(n) _____-_____ (A-R) pulse rate may be taken to

determine if there is a difference between the pulse rates at the two sites.

E. The _____ measurement is subtracted from the _____

measurement to determine the pulse _____.

F. A pulse deficit may indicate that the heart contractions are not _____

_____ to produce a(n) _____ radial pulse.

V. Respiration

1. The respiratory cycle consists of one _____ and one

_____.

2. Respiratory rate is a(n) _____ of how well _____ is being

provided to the tissues of the body.

3. Characteristics of Respiration

A. Do not measure respiration rate if the patient has recently experienced

_____.

B. Each _____ and _____ constitutes one complete

respiration.

C. Respiratory rate

i. Respiratory rate is the number of respirations per _____.

ii. The normal respiration rate for healthy adults at rest is _____ to _____ cycles per

minute.

iii. Fill in the table below to indicate average respiratory rates for various age groups.

Newborn	_____–_____ per minute
1–2 years old	_____–_____ per minute
3–8 years old	_____–_____ per minute
9–11 years old	_____–_____ per minute
12–Adult	_____–_____ per minute

iv. List five factors that affect respiratory rate.

a. _____

b. _____

c. _____

d. _____

e. _____

D. Respiratory rhythm

i. Respiratory rhythm refers to the _____ and

_____ spacing of breaths.

ii. With irregular breathing patterns, the _____ and amount of air

_____ and _____ and the rate of

_____ per minute will vary.

iii. When abnormalities in respiratory rhythm are detected, continue assessment and

measurement of breathing for _____ to _____ more minutes.

E. Respiration depth

i. Depth of respiration is the _____ of air that is inhaled and exhaled.

ii. _____ refers to deep and rapid respirations.

iii. _____ refers to shallow and slow respirations.

iv. The body becomes _____ of the amount of oxygen needed for

proper functioning when there isn't enough oxygen taken in during

_____.

F. Respiratory quality

i. Respiratory quality refers to normal and abnormal breathing _____.

ii. Normal respirations do not have any _____, _____.

iii. Describe the following abnormal breath sounds.

a. Stridor— _____

b. Stertor (stertorous breathing)— _____

c. Crackles (also called rales)— _____

d. Rhonchi— _____

e. Wheezes— _____

f. Cheyne-Stokes breathing— _____

VI. Blood Pressure

1. Blood pressure aids in _____ and _____, especially for

cardiovascular health.

2. Blood Pressure Readings
   A. Blood pressure is the amount of force _____ on the arterial _____ while the heart is pumping blood.
   B. Systolic blood pressure is the _____ pressure that occurs as the _____ ventricle of the heart is _____.
   C. Diastolic blood pressure is the _____ pressure level that occurs when the heart is _____ and the ventricle is at _____ and refilling with blood.
   D. Blood pressure is recorded much like a(n) _____, with the _____ reading over the _____ reading.
   E. _____ _____ is calculated by subtracting the diastolic reading from the systolic reading.
   F. Measuring blood pressure as a routine part of office visits starts with children aged _____ and over.
   G. "_____ coat syndrome," which is apprehension about visiting the physician, often results in _____ blood pressure.
   H. Blood pressure is measured while the patient is seated in a(n) _____ position with both _____ flat on the floor.
   I. Sitting with legs crossed at the knees can _____ blood pressure readings.
   J. High blood pressure readings (either systolic or diastolic) are known as _____.
   K. Low blood pressure is termed _____.
3. Korotkoff Sounds
   A. These are the _____, _____ sounds heard while taking blood pressure.
   B. There are _____ phases of Korotkoff sounds.
   C. _____ pressure is the measurement that is read when the first distinct clear tapping sound is heard as the cuff _____, which is in Phase _____.
   D. _____ pressure is the pressure measurement at which the last sound is heard, which occurs in either Phase _____ or _____.
4. Blood Pressure Guidelines
   A. Fill in the following table to indicate average normal blood pressure readings for various age groups.

Newborn	_____/_____
6–9 years of age	_____/_____
10–15 years of age	_____/_____
16 years to adulthood	_____/_____
Adult	_____/_____

5. Factors Affecting Blood Pressure

   A. List four physiological factors affecting blood pressure.

      i. _____

      ii. _____

      iii. _____

      iv. _____

   B. Women generally have _____ blood pressure than men.

   C. Blood pressure _____ as people age.

   D. Blood pressure is usually at its _____ early in the morning and just before _____.

   E. The blood pressure reading in the _____ arm is usually 3 to 4 mmHg higher than in the _____ arm.

   F. _____ _____ refers to a(n) _____ in blood pressure that occurs when a patient changes positions from lying down to standing.

6. Equipment for Measuring Blood Pressure

   A. The _____ is more commonly referred to as a blood pressure cuff.

   B. The stethoscope _____ sound and is used to detect sounds produced by blood pressure.

   C. Sphygmomanometer

      i. Components of a sphygmomanometer include a(n) _____, inflatable _____ _____, cuff, and _____.

      ii. Using the correct-size blood pressure cuff is _____ and will ensure a more _____ blood pressure reading.

      iii. A cuff that is too large may result in a(n) _____ reading.

      iv. A cuff that is too small might result in a(n) _____ reading.

      v. List the three types of sphygmomanometers.

         a. _____

         b. _____

         c. _____

D. Stethoscope

    i. List the parts of a stethoscope.

      a. _____

      b. _____

      c. _____

      d. _____

      e. _____

7. Measuring Blood Pressure

A. The patient should be _____ before obtaining a blood pressure reading.

B. Ask the patient if there is a history of _____ and if the patient is aware of his or her _____ blood pressure reading.

C. For new patient visits, a blood pressure reading should be obtained on each _____ and recorded in the _____ _____.

D. Errors in blood pressure measurements

    i. _____ is very important in measuring blood pressure.

    ii. List the three categories of common reasons for blood pressure errors (refer to Table 34-17).

      a. _____

      b. _____

      c. _____

VII. Oxygen Saturation

1. Oxygen saturation determines the _____ _____ in the blood.

2. A(n) _____ _____ measures oxygen concentration in arterial blood.

3. Oxygen saturation is reported as _____.

4. Normal oxygen saturation is _____ to _____ percent.

5. Readings below _____ percent indicate life-threatening situations.

6. Pulse oximeters are selected based on the patient's _____, _____, and _____.

7. The _____ pulse oximeter is generally used for adult patients.

KEY TERMINOLOGY REVIEW

Without using your textbook, write a sentence using each selected key term in the correct context.

1. *afebrile*

   _____

   _____

2. *sphygmomanometer*

   _____

   _____

3. *tachypnea*

   _____

   _____

4. *pulse deficit*

   _____

   _____

5. *syncope*

   _____

   _____

APPLIED PRACTICE

Follow the directions as instructed for each question.

1. A patient who has a normal baseline temperature of 98.6°F has had the following average body temperatures over the past 5 days: Day 1: 101.2°F, Day 2: 100.1°F, Day 3: 98.6°F, Day 4: 100.0°F, Day 5: 101.3°F. How would you describe this fever? Explain your answer.

   _____

   _____

   _____

   _____

2. Your patient is a 73-year-old female. Though she is 5′5″ tall, she is very frail and thin, weighing only 98 pounds. Due to her history of hypotension with syncope, it is essential to obtain an accurate blood pressure reading. What size cuff would be most appropriate for this patient? Why is cuff size important to consider when obtaining accurate BP readings?

   _____

   _____

   _____

   _____

   _____

3. You are preparing a new patient for a physical examination. Because the patient has recently moved from a European country, he would like the medical assistant to tell him his body temperature in Celsius rather than Fahrenheit. When obtaining his temperature, the thermometer reads 99.0°F. How does this convert to Celsius? What is the conversion formula?

_____

_____

_____

_____

LEARNING ACTIVITY: FILL IN THE BLANK

Using words from the list below, fill in the blanks to complete the following statements.

Note: Not all terms will be used to complete the activity.

anthropometric	heat waves	rhythm
anthropometry	Korotkoff sounds	sphygmomanometer
apnea	movement	symptom
arterial	orthostatic hypotension	tachypnea
blood pressure	pulse	tympanic membrane thermometer
bradypnea	rate	volume
core	rectal	walls
eupnea	respirations	

1. Oral and _____ temperatures measure the body's _____ temperature.

2. _____ are counted by watching, listening, or feeling the _____ of inspiration and expiration on the patient's back, stomach, or chest.

3. The three characteristics to note when taking a pulse are _____, _____, and _____.

4. The _____ are the sounds heard as the _____ wall distends during the compression of the blood pressure cuff.

5. _____ refers to the drop in _____ that occurs when a patient moves from lying down to a standing position.

6. The _____ is the instrument used for measuring the pressure that the blood exerts against the _____ of the artery.

7. The _____, or aural thermometer, is so named because it is able to detect _____ within the ear canal and near the eardrum.

8. A respiratory rate of below 12 (called _____) or above 20 (called _____) in an adult should be reported to the physician immediately.

9. _____ means the absence of breathing for longer than 19 seconds, and

_____ means normal breathing.

10. Weight and height are _____ measurements because they relate to

_____, the science of size, proportion, weight, and height.

CRITICAL THINKING

Answer the following questions to the best of your ability. Use the textbook as a reference.

1. Adam Sanchez is being seen for an earache and sore throat. The physician is running behind in his schedule, and Mr. Sanchez is visibly irritated by his prolonged wait time. When you call him back for his appointment, you notice that he throws an empty cup of coffee into the waste can. He says, "I was waiting for so long, I had to step out for a smoke. I just got back inside when you called me back." Considering the information in this scenario, how will you attempt to obtain a temperature reading on Mr. Sanchez?

_____

_____

_____

_____

_____

2. If a patient walks in without an appointment and presents as extremely short of breath (SOB) and appears weak, should you spend the time finding weight and height and taking vital signs before alerting the doctor about the patient's immediate condition? Explain your answer.

_____

_____

_____

_____

_____

RESEARCH ACTIVITY

Use Internet search engines to research the following topic and write a brief description of what you find. It is important to use reputable websites.

1. Choose a health condition related to a vital sign (e.g., hypertension, obesity). Research informational websites related to your chosen condition. What type of information is included in the informational websites? How can this information be useful for patients?

_____

_____

_____

_____

CHAPTER 35
Assisting with Physical Examinations

STUDENT STUDY GUIDE

Use the following guide to assist in your learning of the concepts from the chapter.

I. Introduction

  1. List the roles of the medical assistant in the physical exam.

    A. _____

    B. _____

    C. _____

    D. _____

    E. _____

    F. _____

II. The Examination Room

  1. Preparing the Examination Room

    A. At the beginning of the day, make sure that the room is adequately _____
    with _____ and that the _____ is properly functioning.

    B. Summarize the tasks involved in cleaning examination rooms between patients.

      i. _____
         _____

      ii. _____
         _____

      iii. _____
         _____

      iv. _____
         _____

      v. _____
         _____

    C. No _____ of any other _____ should remain when a new
    patient is taken into an examination room.

2. Examination Room Features

   A. A standard examination room is most often furnished with a(n) _____ table, a(n) _____, a footstool, a(n) _____ cupboard, a(n) _____ can, _____ waste and _____ containers, a(n) _____ stool, and a chair.

   B. _____ equipment for specialist physicians may be present.

   C. _____ and _____ should be readily available for the physician.

   D. Proper _____ ensures patient safety and prevents damage to equipment.

3. Examination Room Safety

   A. Examination rooms must conform to the standards established by the _____ with _____ Act.

   B. ADA standards address the following.

      i. The _____ of doorways and hallways

      ii. Placement of _____ handles, _____ bars, and handrails

      iii. Spatial accommodations for patients in _____

      iv. _____ surfaces

   C. Unsafe situations must be addressed _____.

   D. All electrical cords and cables must be secured to the _____ or _____.

   E. All furniture should be checked for proper _____.

4. Patient Comfort

   A. Most medical offices keep the thermostat around _____°F to _____°F.

   B. Keep extra _____ or _____ available for patients who may get too cold while waiting in the examination room.

   C. Examination rooms should smell both _____ and _____.

   D. Try to eliminate sources of offensive _____.

   E. Room _____ sprays and air _____ can be useful for removing odor that lingers in the air.

5. Patient Privacy

   A. Do the following before entering an examination room that is occupied by a patient.

      i. _____

      ii. _____ yourself

      iii. Ask for _____ to enter

   B. Don't enter the room until the _____ has expressed _____.

   C. Be sure that gowns of all _____ are available for patients.

   D. Properly _____ patients to protect their _____ is important to patients' comfort during an examination.

III. Review of Patient Communication and Documentation

1. A(n) _____ and _____ medical record is vital to the treatment and care of a patient.

2. Effective Communication

   A. The following steps are involved in interviewing a patient.

      i. Review the patient's _____ _____ before meeting the patient.

      ii. Greet the patient by using his or her _____ _____ and introduce yourself.

      iii. Maintain a(n) _____ and _____ demeanor.

      iv. Ask _____ to interview the patient.

      v. Make the patient feel as _____ as possible during the office visit.

      vi. Be aware of _____ and _____ cues as the patient answers questions and describes the reason for the visit.

      vii. Avoid making _____ responses. Be cautious about _____ expressions and body _____ when listening to the patient's responses.

      viii. Avoid providing medical _____. Treat sensitive topics with _____ and keep in mind the possible _____ and personal beliefs of the patient.

      ix. _____ important points the patient has made, giving the patient a chance to correct anything you may have _____.

      x. _____ the interview in the patient's medical record.

3. Correct Documentation

   A. Proper documentation in a patient's medical record will also help ensure _____ of _____.

   B. Medical records are considered _____ documents and can be _____ or used as evidence in court.

   C. Charting guidelines

      i. Record the _____ and _____ of every entry.

      ii. Use medical _____ and _____ that are accepted by the medical office or facility.

      iii. Use correct _____ and _____.

      iv. _____ each entry.

      v. Accurately document _____; record facts, not _____.

      vi. Document the proper _____ in which events occurred.

      vii. Document appropriate information concerning _____ and

                _____ given.

      viii. Be _____.

IV. Patient Health History

  1. A patient's health history can give helpful _____ into his or her current

      _____ status and _____.

  2. It also assists the physician in assessing the patient's general _____, aids in

      _____, and helps the physician develop a(n) _____

      _____ for the patient.

  3. Physicians' preferences vary in regard to _____ should obtain the specific

      _____ in the patient history.

  4. Chief Complaint (CC)

    A. The chief complaint is also referred to as the _____ _____, and

        it is the reason the patient made the office visit.

    B. The CC usually contains one or two _____ or _____.

    C. Signs are _____, and symptoms are _____.

    D. The CC is often stated in the medical record in the patient's _____

        _____ with _____ marks around them.

    E. Ask _____, when, and where to obtain a more complete patient interview.

    F. Avoid using _____ _____ when you record the chief complaint

        as only a physician can provide a diagnosis.

  5. Pain

    A. No _____ individuals experience pain in the _____ way.

    B. List common terms to describe pain.

      i. _____

      ii. _____

      iii. _____

      iv. _____

      v. _____

      vi. _____

      vii. _____

    C. Pain is described on a scale of _____ to _____.

      i. _____ means no pain

      ii. _____ means extreme pain

    D. Describe the types of pain.

      i. Acute—_____

    ii. Chronic—_____

    iii. Radiating—_____

    iv. Intractable—_____

    v. Phantom—_____

6. Present Illness (PI)

    A. The PI provides a more _____, expansive description of the chief complaint.

    B. The PI must contain a detailed description of the symptom, including the

    _____, _____, and _____.

7. Past Medical History

    A. The past medical history includes all _____ and _____

    problems the patient has experienced in the past.

    B. List the information included in the past medical history.

      i. _____

      ii. _____

      iii. _____

      iv. _____

      v. _____

      vi. _____

      vii. _____

      viii. _____

      ix. _____

    C. Remind patients that all types of _____ should be included in their

    medication list, including _____ and _____ supplements.

8. Family Medical History

    A. Family medical history is a record of the health problems of the patient's

    _____ relatives or any relatives related by _____.

    B. History may be limited to immediate family members, including _____ and

    _____.

    C. Information obtained includes the following.

      i. Current _____ status

      ii. _____ health problems

      iii. Cause of _____ and _____ at death

    D. Family medical histories focus on diseases that may be _____ or

    _____.

9. Social History

    A. Social history includes lifestyle _____ or _____ that could affect the health status of the patient.

    B. Information obtained includes the following.

        i. Smoking, _____, and the use of _____ drugs

        ii. The patient's _____, marital _____, and _____ preferences

        iii. _____ choices, frequency of _____, and _____ habits

        iv. The patient's previous _____

        v. Lifelong _____ or _____, which often provide helpful information

V. Equipment and Supplies Used for Physical Examinations

    1. List the equipment commonly used in patient examinations.

    A. _____

    B. _____

    C. _____

    D. _____

    E. _____

    F. _____

    G. _____

    H. _____

    I. _____

    2. Supplies

    A. Supplies are _____ _____ used for patient examination and treatment.

    B. List seven examples of supplies.

        i. _____

        ii. _____

        iii. _____

        iv. _____

        v. _____

        vi. _____

        vii. _____

    C. _____ supplies and _____ the exam rooms are important to the efficiency of _____ _____ and maintaining work flow.

D. Inventory supply systems should contain the following information.

    i. List of _____ used in the facility

    ii. _____ _____ for each supply item

    iii. Each supplier's _____, _____, telephone number, and _____ person

    iv. _____ of each supply used monthly

    v. Reordering _____

VI. Examination Methods Used by the Physician

  1. The physician's _____ are the primary tools used during the physical examination.

  2. Inspection

    A. An inspection involves _____ examining the exterior surface of the body.

    B. The physician is examining the patient's general state of _____, overall _____, mood, _____, and social _____.

    C. The physician will make note of anything that is unusual in _____, size, _____, position, or _____.

  3. Palpation

    A. Palpation is the process of using the _____ to feel the _____ and other parts of the body to examine for any _____.

    B. It is used to identify any unusual _____, size, _____, and texture on the body.

  4. Percussion

    A. Percussion is the process of using the _____ to tap the body with _____, _____ blows to gain information about the _____ and _____ of the underlying body parts.

    B. _____ fingers of one hand are placed on the patient's _____ and then struck with the _____ and middle _____ of the other hand.

    C. Standard sounds or _____ are produced.

      i. An alteration of this sound or vibration helps determine the presence of _____, _____, or _____ in a cavity or a(n) _____ mass under the skin.

    D. Another method of percussion is used with a percussion or _____ hammer.

  5. Auscultation

    A. Auscultation is the process of _____ to _____ within the body.

B. Sounds assessed for strength and rhythm include those made by the following parts of the body.

    i. _____

    ii. _____

    iii. _____

    iv. _____

6. Mensuration

   A. Mensuration is the use of special tools to measure the body or specific body parts.

   B. List examples of tools used in mensuration.

    i. _____

    ii. _____

    iii. _____

   C. A(n) _____ measures the range of motion of a(n) _____.

7. Manipulation

   A. This is the process of passively assessing the _____ of _____ of a joint.

VII. Adult Examination

  1. List four common reasons for medical visits.

   A. _____

   B. _____

   C. _____

   D. _____

  2. The purpose of a physical examination is to _____ as much of the body as possible to help _____ new diseases or to evaluate the _____ of established treatment plans from previously diagnosed disorders.

  3. Patients have a routine physical examination as part of their annual _____ _____.

  4. A(n) _____ _____ is a preliminary presumptive diagnosis made by a physician based on the _____ history and _____ examination.

  5. A(n) _____ diagnosis is made when the physician will have to distinguish a particular _____ or disorder from others with similar _____ and _____.

  6. Only the _____ may actually diagnose a condition.

  7. A(n) _____ is a prediction of the course of the condition and the probable _____ rate.

VIII. Assisting with the Physical Examination

1. A medical assistant may help the physician during a physical examination in the following ways:

   A. _____ and _____ the patient for examination.

   B. Hand _____, _____, and other medical supplies to the physician.

   C. Document and label _____.

   D. Offer _____ and comfort to the patient.

   E. Act as a witness to the _____ of the physician and the patient.

   F. Carry out _____ _____ as directed by the physician.

   G. Schedule _____ _____ as ordered by the physician.

2. Patient Preparation

   A. Prepare the patient for any _____ that will be performed during the _____.

   B. Explain the procedures in a(n) _____, _____, and _____ manner.

   C. Ask patients to _____ their _____ before undressing and give detailed instructions if a(n) _____ sample is required.

   D. A gown and _____ are required for all examinations.

      i. Explain which items of _____ should be _____ and whether the gown should be worn with the opening in the _____ or the _____.

   E. The medical assistant may need to assist the patient with _____ or with stepping up onto the _____ _____.

   F. Report unusual _____ or _____ to the physician.

   G. Draping the patient

      i. Drapes are _____ that are used to protect patient _____ and keep the patient _____.

      ii. Drapes cover all but the _____ _____ that is being examined.

      iii. The drape must not _____ the physician's vision or _____ with the examination.

      iv. _____ drapes may be used to protect the _____ area from contamination.

      v. They also provide a sterile surface for _____, _____ materials, and dressings.

3. Positioning the Patient*

   A. List the nine standard positions used for various medical and surgical examinations and procedures.

   i. _____

   ii. _____

   iii. _____

   iv. _____

   v. _____

   vi. _____

   vii. _____

   viii. _____

   ix. _____

   B. Patient communication

   i. Explain to the patient why he or she is being placed in a specific _____ and the purpose of the _____.

   ii. A medical assistant must be _____ at all times, _____ the patient, and minimizing _____ and _____ as much as possible.

   iii. Positions may be uncomfortable because of the patient's _____.

   iv. When you are aware of the patient's _____ _____, you can take steps to make the patient more _____.

   v. Effective communication will help establish a sense of _____ between the _____ and the medical assistant.

   C. Laboratory and diagnostic tests

   i. Some tests may be conducted in the _____ on the day of the _____, while others may be _____ by appointment with a separate _____ or diagnostic facility.

IX. Sequence of Events in a Complete Physical Examination

   1. Typically, the physician will discuss the _____ _____ history, _____ complaint, and history of the _____ _____ first and then do a(n) _____ of _____.

   2. Review of Systems (Briefly summarize the review of each system.)

   A. Skin— _____

   _____

   B. Hair— _____

   _____

---

*Patient positioning will also be covered in other activities within this chapter.

Assisting with Physical Examinations **409**

C. Nails—_____

_____

D. Head—_____

_____

E. Neck—_____

_____

F. Eyes—_____

_____

G. Ears—_____

_____

H. Nose—_____

_____

I. Mouth—_____

_____

J. Throat—_____

_____

K. Arms—_____

_____

L. Heart—_____

_____

M. Chest—_____

_____

N. Lungs—_____

_____

O. Breasts—_____

_____

P. Abdomen—_____

_____

Q. Genitalia—_____

_____

R. Rectum—_____

_____

S. Legs and feet—_____

_____

T. Neurological system—_____

_____

KEY TERMINOLOGY REVIEW

Write a sentence using each selected key term in the correct context.

1. *mensuration*

   _____

2. *ophthalmoscope*

   _____

   _____

3. *turgor*

   _____

   _____

4. *acute pain*

   _____

   _____

5. *prognosis*

   _____

   _____

   _____

APPLIED PRACTICE

Follow the directions for each question.

1. Identify the patient position shown.

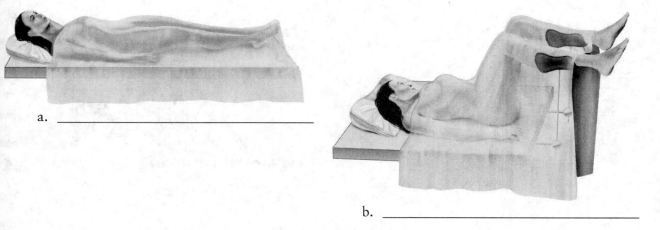

   a. _____

   b. _____

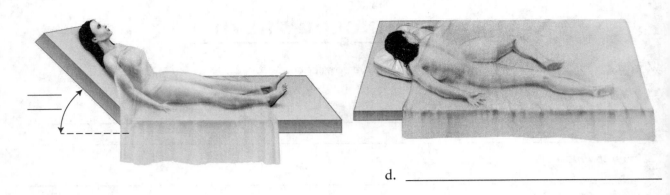

c. _____

d. _____

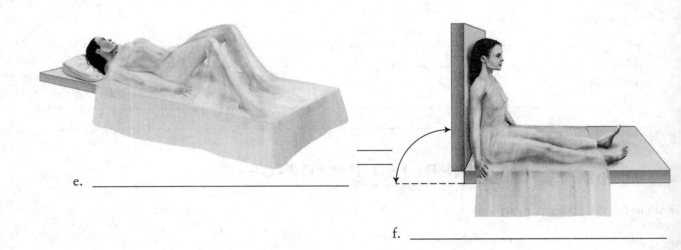

e. _____

f. _____

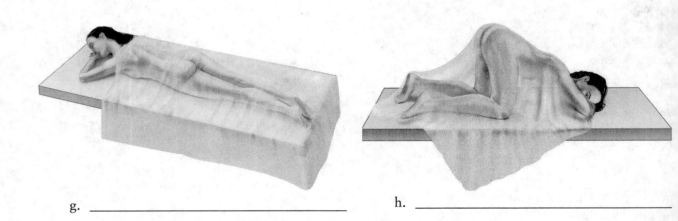

g. _____

h. _____

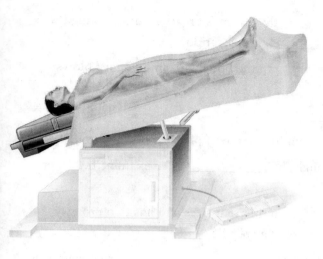

i. _____

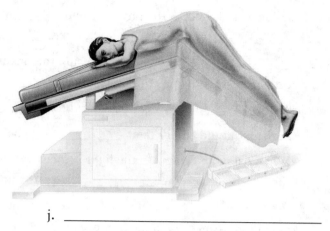

j. _____

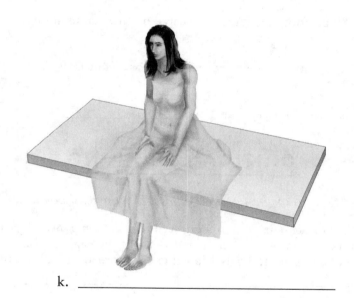

k. _____

LEARNING ACTIVITY: FILL IN THE BLANK

Using words from the following list, fill in the blanks to complete the following statements.
Note: Not all terms will be used, and some may be used more than one time.

auscultate	lithotomy	speculum
bladder	percussion	symmetry and texture
bowel sounds	90-degree angle	tuning fork
depth	rate	tympanic membrane
Fowler's	rhythm	underlying body parts
frequency	Snellen chart	vaginal examinations

Assisting with Physical Examinations **413**

1. Using a stethoscope, the physician will _____ the patient's breath sounds, noting the _____, _____, pitch, _____, and location.

2. _____ is the process of using the fingertips to tap the body with short, sharp blows in order to assess the position and size of _____.

3. The _____ position is used for _____.

4. Patients should empty their _____ before undressing for a physical examination.

5. When using an otoscope, the light is focused through the _____ to examine the outer ear, the ear canal, and the _____ (eardrum).

6. A(n) _____ is a metal instrument that comes in different sizes and has two prongs extending from the handle that are designed to vibrate at a specific _____.

7. Using a stethoscope, the physician will auscultate the patient's _____ for frequency, pitch, gurgling, and clicking sounds.

8. In the _____ position, the patient is seated on the examination table with the head of the table raised to a(n) _____.

9. A medical assistant will test the patient's visual acuity or distance vision by using a(n) _____.

10. The breasts will be assessed for size, shape, and _____.

CRITICAL THINKING

Answer the following questions to the best of your ability. Use the textbook as a reference.

1. Madeline is an 18-year-old female who is being seen for her first gynecological examination. She has come to her appointment alone and is very nervous about the vaginal examination. How can you show awareness of her concerns and help Madeline feel more at ease about the procedure?

    _____

    _____

    _____

    _____

    _____

2. Saina, a registered medical assistant, has just taken Sheldon Armstrong to an examination room and obtained his chief complaint. She notes his chief complaint as follows:

    Patient states "I have been having intense stomach pain."

    What other information should Saina obtain from the patient regarding his chief complaint?

    _____

    _____

    _____

    _____

    _____

RESEARCH ACTIVITY

Use Internet search engines to research the following topic and write a brief description of what you find. It is important to use reputable websites.

1. It is very important to be aware of the cultural norms of the patients seen in the medical office. Patients' culture can affect their approach to having physical examinations. Select a specific culture. Research this culture online or by interviewing individuals you know from this culture. Discuss the cultural differences and/or barriers that may affect the success of performing a physical examination.

_____

_____

_____

_____

_____

CHAPTER 36
Assisting with Medical Specialties

STUDENT STUDY GUIDE

Use the following guide to assist in your learning of the concepts from the chapter.

I. The Role of the Medical Assistant

    1. Medical assistants may work with primary care or internal _____ physicians, or they may work with physician _____.

    2. Primary care and internal medicine physicians are usually a patient's _____ _____ of contact for seeking medical treatment.

    3. A physician specialist is trained and _____ in a specific area or field and will perform more _____ diagnoses and intensive _____ and procedures.

    4. A medical assistant often has the most _____ to patients during their visit.

    5. A medical assistant will serve as a(n) "_____ coach" by helping patients understand their _____ and treatment and helping them adhere to the _____ plans.

    6. It is imperative that medical assistants have the ability to _____ effectively and display appropriate _____ to help patients in all circumstances.

II. Assisting with Allergy Care and Immunology

    1. A(n) _____ or _____ is a physician specialist who is trained in diagnosing, treating, and managing allergies, asthma, and other _____ system disorders.

    2. A clinical MA's tasks when working for an allergist/immunologist may include the following.

        A. Room patients and obtain _____ _____ and measurements.

        B. Record the patient's _____, including any specialized questionnaires pertaining to the patient's _____ or immunology history.

        C. Prepare the _____ _____ for specialty procedures, such as those associated with allergy testing.

        D. Administer _____ injections to patients and update shot records.

        E. Provide patient _____ and support based on the _____ protocol established by the physician.

3. Skin Tests

    A. All skin tests are usually performed on the patient's _____ or _____ and allow for the testing of different _____ at the same time.

    B. Briefly describe the three common types of skin tests.

        i. Scratch test—

        _____

        _____

        _____

        ii. Intradermal test—

        _____

        _____

        _____

        iii. Patch test—

        _____

        _____

        _____

    C. Radioallergosorbent test (RAST)

        i. This test measures levels of _____ to particular antigens in the blood.

        ii. The patient's blood sample is sent to a laboratory, where it is exposed to a variety of suspected _____.

        iii. This test doesn't directly expose the patient to any _____, which is important for patients who are at increased risk of a life-threatening _____ _____ occurring.

III. Assisting with Dermatology

    1. A dermatologist is a physician specialist who is trained in the _____ and _____ of disorders of the skin, or _____ system.

    2. A clinical MA's duties when working for a dermatologist may include the following.

    A. Room patients and obtain _____ _____ and measurements.

    B. _____ the patient's history, including any _____-related questionnaires established by the physician.

    C. _____ the exam room for specialty procedures, such as those associated with performing minor skin _____ and obtaining skin _____.

    D. Prepare the _____ and assist the physician with procedures related to _____ and _____ dermatology.

    E. Assist in the _____ of wounds and obtain wound _____.

    F. Provide patient _____ and support based on the treatment _____ established by the physician.

3. Medical assistants may also have special training to work as a(n) _____

_____.

   A. A Mohs technician assists the physician who performs the Mohs _____ to

remove _____ skin lesions and the surrounding _____ of skin.

4. Common Skin Disorders

   A. List the descriptive notes regarding lesions to enter into the patient's medical record.

      i. _____

      ii. _____

      iii. _____

      iv. _____

      v. _____

   B. Inflammatory skin disorders result in _____, _____, pain, and

often _____ over the affected site.

   C. List five types of inflammatory skin disorders.

      i. _____

      ii. _____

      iii. _____

      iv. _____

      v. _____

IV. Assisting with Cardiology

1. A(n) _____ is a physician specialist who is trained in the diagnosis, treatment, and

management of cardiovascular diseases and disorders.

2. A clinical MA's tasks when working for a cardiologist may include the following.

   A. _____ patients and obtain _____ _____ and

measurements.

   B. Record the patient's _____, including any _____-related

questionnaires.

   C. Schedule cardiovascular _____ in both inpatient and outpatient facilities.

   D. Provide patient _____ and support based on the treatment _____

established by the physician.

   E. Perform _____ and _____ monitoring.

3. A(n) _____ is only able to record a patient's heart activity for a few

_____ while the patient is hooked up to the machine.

4. A(n) _____ monitor is a small portable device that the patient wears usually for

_____ to _____ hours.

5. Cardiovascular Disease

   A. List four causes of cardiovascular diseases and disorders.

      i. _____

      ii. _____

      iii. _____

      iv. _____

   B. List six common signs and symptoms of cardiovascular disorders. Make sure to match these signs and symptoms with the descriptions provided.

      i. _____—Chest pain (crushing or stabbing type of pain)

      ii. _____—Irregular heartbeat

      iii. _____—Bluish skin color caused by lack of oxygen in the tissues

      iv. _____—Excessive sweating

      v. _____—Difficulty breathing

      vi. _____—Swelling, particularly of the extremities

6. Risk Factors for Cardiovascular Disease

   A. List the risk factors for cardiovascular disease that a(n) _____ medical assistant will recognize.

      i. _____

      ii. _____

      iii. _____

      iv. _____

      v. _____

      vi. _____

      vii. _____

V. Assisting with Endocrinology

   1. An endocrinologist is a physician specialist who is trained in the _____, _____, and _____ of diseases and disorders associated with the endocrine system.

   2. A clinical MA's tasks when working for an endocrinologist may include the following.

      A. Room patients and obtain _____ _____ and _____.

      B. Record the patient's _____ history and complete _____ system–related questionnaires.

      C. Perform frequent _____.

      D. Perform _____ monitoring and education related to proper use of glucose monitoring equipment, including _____, test strips, and lancets.

E. Provide _____ _____ and support based on the treatment _____ established by the physician for endocrine system–related diseases and disorders.

F. Assist the physician by helping maintain accurate _____ records.

G. Provide patient _____ and _____ regarding routinely scheduled diagnostic tests and procedures.

3. Hormones

A. Hormones are _____ _____ produced by the endocrine glands and transported to target tissue by the _____.

B. Hormones are able to regulate _____ and metabolism, _____ development, and mood, and they help maintain _____.

C. Medical assistants will recognize that the majority of endocrine disorders result from _____ _____.

4. Treatments Using Hormones

A. Many conditions are treated with hormones, many of which are _____ synthetically in _____.

B. List examples of hormones created synthetically (summarized in this section in the textbook).

   i. _____

   ii. _____

   iii. _____

5. Diabetes Mellitus (DM)

A. More than _____ million people, or _____ percent of the U.S. population, have diabetes mellitus.

B. DM is characterized by _____, which results from a lack of insulin or a(n) _____ to the effects of insulin.

C. List the primary symptoms of DM.

   i. _____

   ii. _____

   iii. _____

D. Additional signs and symptoms include rapid _____ loss, _____, itching, and _____ infections.

E. List seven life-threatening conditions that may occur if DM is left untreated.

   i. _____

   ii. _____

   iii. _____

iv. _____

v. _____

vi. _____

vii. _____

F. A critical part of managing diabetes is routine and _____ monitoring of blood _____ levels.

VI. Assisting with Gastroenterology

1. A(n) _____ is a physician specialist who is trained in the diagnosis, treatment, and management of diseases related to the digestive system and its associated structures.

2. A(n) _____ is a physician who specializes in proctology, which is a subspecialty of gastroenterology and treats disorders of the _____ and _____.

3. A clinical MA's tasks when working for a gastroenterologist/proctologist may include the following.

A. Room patients and obtain _____ _____ and measurements.

B. Record the patient's medical _____ and complete _____ system–related questionnaires.

C. Instruct patients regarding the proper method of obtaining _____ _____ and performing _____ on the samples obtained.

D. Prepare the examination room and assist with specialized procedures, such as _____.

E. Provide patients with _____ and _____ instructions regarding proper preparation for gastrointestinal procedures.

F. Provide patient _____ and support based on the treatment _____ established by the physician.

4. The medical assistant must be prepared to _____ and _____ the patient before, during, and after procedures.

5. Testing for Occult Blood

A. A(n) _____ _____ _____ test (FOBT) may be requested by the physician to check a patient's stool for _____ (hidden) blood.

B. A patient's stool is tested using special _____ that contain _____ on which the stool sample is placed.

C. The patient's stool can be tested either at _____ or in the _____ _____.

D. FOBT instructions for patients include the following.

    i. Drink plenty of _____.

    ii. Do not collect samples during _____.

    iii. Avoid eating _____ meats, liver, and _____ meats.

    iv. Avoid eating turnips, _____, _____, and melons.

    v. Avoid taking _____, _____ supplements, and large doses of vitamin C for _____ days before collecting specimens.

    vi. Eat a(n) _____-fiber diet.

    vii. Store slides at _____ _____, away from sun and heat.

6. Sigmoidoscopy

A. A(n) _____ is a(n) _____ of the interior of the sigmoid colon for _____ purposes.

B. A sigmoidoscopy may be performed to detect _____, _____, or _____ cancer or to investigate the source of _____ in the lower intestinal tract.

C. The patient may be placed in the _____ position or on a(n) _____ examination table.

D. A sigmoidoscopy is scheduled in _____ to allow for adequate patient _____.

E. Provide the patient with _____ instructions, usually in a(n) _____-by-_____ format, to ensure compliance and _____ the instructions with the patient to be sure they are understood.

F. Improper bowel preparation may result in the need to _____ the procedure.

G. The medical assistant can make the _____ discomfort easier for patients by instructing them to concentrate on _____ _____ through the mouth while relaxing the _____ muscles.

7. Colonoscopy

A. A colonoscopy may be performed so that the physician can see more of the _____ _____.

B. A colonoscopy is often performed in a(n) _____ or outpatient setting because an IV _____ is administered before the procedure.

C. The medical assistant working for a(n) _____ or a(n) _____ testing center may assist with the actual procedure.

D. A medical assistant working for a primary care physician may be responsible only for _____ the test and helping to _____ the patient for the procedure.

E. Similar to a sigmoidoscope, a colonoscope is a(n) _____ black _____ tube with a camera and a(n) _____ at the end.

F. The physician should have specific _____ _____ or a(n) _____ of information that can be provided to the patient on how to prepare for the colonoscopy.

VII. Assisting with Orthopedics

1. A(n) _____ is a physician who specializes in orthopedics, which is the medical field concerned with the diagnosis and treatment of conditions related to the _____ system.

2. Osteopathic physicians are doctors of _____ _____.

3. Osteopathic physicians receive specialized training in musculoskeletal _____.

4. A(n) _____ specializes in managing patients with joint inflammations and patients with _____ disorders.

5. A clinical MA's tasks when working for an orthopedist may include the following.

   A. _____ patients and obtain vital signs and _____.

   B. Record the patient's _____ history and complete appropriate forms and documentation related to the patient's _____ _____.

   C. Schedule appropriate _____ tests and _____ related to the musculoskeletal system and provide the patient with _____ specific to each test.

   D. Work closely with other allied health professionals, such as _____ therapists and occupational _____.

   E. Provide patient education and support based on the treatment _____ established by the physician.

   F. Apply therapeutic _____ as necessary.

   G. Perform or _____ X-rays and other _____ images to aid the physician in diagnosis and treatment of the patient's condition.

6. Caring for Patients with Musculoskeletal Problems

   A. In addition to bones and muscles, the musculoskeletal system includes all the connective tissue, such as _____, _____, and _____.

   B. The medical assistant's role includes _____ carefully to the patient's _____ of the problem.

   C. Examples of engaging, open-ended questions include the following.

      i. When did the problem _____?

      ii. What were you doing _____ the problem started?

      iii. What was done to _____ the problem?

      iv. What are your most pressing _____ _____?

D. Carefully note the exact location of the _____.

E. Ask the patient to quantify it on a scale of _____ to _____, with _____ being the greatest amount of pain.

F. Offer to _____ the patient to the examination room and provide a(n) _____, if necessary.

G. Make necessary _____ in the examination room to ensure that the patient is comfortable.

H. Observe the patient's _____ and the range of _____ of the affected area.

VIII. Assisting with Neurology

1. A(n) _____ specializes in treating and diagnosing conditions of the nervous system.

2. A(n) _____ performs surgical procedures on the nervous system.

3. A(n) _____ is a physician who specializes in diagnosing and treating mental health and emotional problems that may affect _____.

4. A clinical MA's tasks when working in neurology may include the following.

A. Room _____ and obtain vital signs and _____.

B. Record the patient's _____ history and complete appropriate forms and documentation related to the _____ _____.

C. Schedule appropriate _____ tests and procedures related to the nervous system and provide the patient with _____ specific to preparing for each test.

D. Provide patient _____ and _____ based on the treatment protocol established by the physician.

5. Assisting with Neurological Examinations

A. List nine major areas on which a neurological examination focuses.

   i. _____

   ii. _____

   iii. _____

   iv. _____

   v. _____

   vi. _____

   vii. _____

   viii. _____

   ix. _____

B. The MA's role in a neurological examination is to do the following.

    i. Ensure that necessary _____ are ready for use by the physician.

    ii. Provide _____ and _____ to patients.

    iii. Assist in _____ the patient as needed.

C. If asked to check the patient's pupils, the MA will check the pupils for the following.

    i. Equal _____

    ii. Equal _____ in both eyes in darkness or dim light

    iii. Rapid _____ to light in both eyes

    iv. Equal _____ to light

    v. _____ to objects near or far

D. When the pupil check is normal, _____ is documented in the patient's medical record.

E. PERRLA stands for pupils _____, _____, _____ to light and _____.

KEY TERMINOLOGY REVIEW

Use the key terms found at the beginning of the chapter to finish the following sentences. Key terms may be more than one word in length.

1. Hidden, or _____, blood in stool may be an indication of bleeding in the gastrointestinal tract.

2. _____ simply means excessive sweating.

3. A(n) _____ _____ helps a surgeon during surgery to remove cancerous skin lesions and surrounding layers of skin.

4. A(n) _____ specializes in a subspecialty of gastroenterology and treats disorders of the rectum and anus.

5. Noncancerous tumors are termed _____.

APPLIED PRACTICE

1. Complete the table below by providing descriptions of both benign and malignant dermatological neoplasms.

Benign (Noncancerous) Neoplasms	Description
Dermatofibroma	
Hemangioma	
Keloid	
Keratosis	
Leukoplakia	
Lipoma	
Nevus	
Malignant (Cancerous) Neoplasms	**Description**
Basal cell carcinoma	
Kaposi's sarcoma	
Malignant melanoma	
Squamous cell carcinoma	

2. Match each common allergy with its description below.

   a. allergic rhinitis   d. eczema
   b. asthma   e. urticaria
   c. contact dermatitis

   1. _____ Characterized by skin eruptions of pale reddish wheals with severe itching. It is also called hives.

   2. _____ Inflammation of the nasal mucosa that results in nasal congestion, rhinorrhea (runny nose), sneezing, and itching of the nose. Children suffering from this type of allergy may rub their nose in an upward movement, called the "allergic salute."

   3. _____ The major symptoms are wheezing, coughing, and dyspnea. The patient's airway is affected by constriction of the bronchial passages. This condition is most frequently seen in childhood.

   4. _____ Inflammation and irritation of the skin caused by contact with an irritating substance. Treatment consists of topical and systemic medications to relieve symptoms and removal of the causative allergen.

   5. _____ Superficial dermatitis accompanied by papules, vesicles, and crusting. The condition can be acute or chronic.

LEARNING ACTIVITY: MULTIPLE CHOICE

Circle the correct answer to each of the following questions.

1. Which of the following methods of diagnostic allergy testing requires bloodwork?
   a. RAST
   b. Scratch test
   c. Intradermal test
   d. Patch test

2. Which of the following is *not* a sign or symptom of diabetes mellitus?
   a. Increased urination
   b. Itching
   c. Weight gain
   d. Increased thirst

3. A patient with lupus would likely be seen by which physician specialist?
   a. An endocrinologist
   b. A rheumatologist
   c. A neurologist
   d. A gastroenterologist

4. Which of the following is *not* included in the supplies and equipment used for a neurology examination?
   a. Ophthalmoscope
   b. Percussion hammer
   c. Tuning fork
   d. Speculum

5. For very high-risk patients, the new goal is to have an LDL
   a. under 130 mg/dL.
   b. below 100 mg/dL.
   c. below 93 mg/dL.
   d. below 190 mg/dL.

CRITICAL THINKING

Answer the following questions to the best of your ability. Use the textbook as a reference.

1. Caroline works as a clinical medical assistant for an endocrinology practice. She receives a phone call from a patient who was recently diagnosed with diabetes. The patient is upset because she thinks the glucometer she uses to test her blood sugar at home is not recording accurate results. How could Caroline help the patient feel more confident about the accuracy of her test results?

   _____

   _____

   _____

   _____

   _____

2. Mr. Edwin has recently been diagnosed with high cholesterol and cardiovascular disease. The physician has asked you, the medical assistant, to review some educational pamphlets regarding dietary changes with Mr. Edwin. The physician would also like you to schedule an appointment for Mr. Edwin with a nutritionist to further discuss dietary changes and modifications. When you begin to review the pamphlets with Mr. Edwin, he refuses to participate and says, "I'm going to throw these away as soon as you leave, and there is no way I am going to see a nutritionist." How will you handle Mr. Edwin's refusal to participate in the physician's prescribed treatment plan?

_____

_____

_____

_____

_____

RESEARCH ACTIVITY

Use Internet search engines to research the following topic and write a brief description of what you find. It is important to use reputable websites.

1. Select one or two of the procedures/diagnostic tests discussed in the chapter. Research the procedure/diagnostic test on the Internet. Why might the test be performed, how is the test performed, and what are the outcomes that are expected from the test? Write an essay on your findings. Be sure to cite your sources.

_____

_____

_____

_____

_____

CHAPTER 37
Assisting with Reproductive Specialties

STUDENT STUDY GUIDE

Use the following guide to assist in your learning of the concepts from the chapter.

I. An Overview of the Reproductive Systems

1. List the parts of the male reproductive system.

   A. _____

   B. _____

   C. _____

   D. _____

   E. _____

2. These organs work together to produce _____ and the other components in semen to help in the _____ of an ovum in the female.

3. List the parts of the female reproductive system.

   A. _____

   B. _____

   C. _____

   D. _____

   E. _____

   F. _____

   G. _____

4. These organs are involved in the production and transportation of the _____ and the production of _____ hormones necessary to sustain _____.

5. The female reproductive system supports the development of the _____.

II. Female Reproductive Medical Issues

1. _____ deals with the health of and with the diseases and disorders of the female reproductive system.

2. _____ is concerned with the management of women during pregnancy, _____, and the period of time immediately after childbirth.

3. List two common procedures performed as a part of a woman's routine health screening.

    i. _____

    ii. _____

4. Assisting the Obstetrics and Gynecology Patient

    A. An important job responsibility of the medical assistant is to take a thorough patient _____ to identify the patient's _____ and provide information to aid the physician with _____ and treatment.

    B. A challenge is that some patients may feel shame or _____ about the reason for their visit and may withhold important _____ information.

    C. List breast cancer screening and early detection methods.

        i. _____

        ii. _____

        iii. _____

        iv. _____

    D. The medical assistant may have the responsibility of _____ and _____ the correct procedure for the BSE.

    E. Often during a routine _____ exam, the physician will perform a clinical breast exam (CBE).

    F. The physician _____ the breast using his or her _____ in a circular fashion around all the breast tissue to search for lumps, _____, or _____.

    G. A more effective test for breast cancer screening than SBE or CBE is a(n) _____.

    H. A(n) _____ is more sensitive and more effective in detecting breast cancer than a mammogram.

5. The Pelvic Examination

    A. A pelvic examination allows the physician to _____ and _____ assess a patient's reproductive organs.

    B. A pelvic exam is usually part of a routine physical examination or is performed if a patient complains of having symptoms, such as unusual _____ _____ or _____ pain.

C. When taking a gynecological history, ask the patient about the following.

    i. Her _____ cycle

    ii. Past _____

    iii. Any _____ during sexual intercourse

D. Also ask the patient about her _____ status and screen for any signs of _____ or abuse in the relationship.

E. For _____ reasons, a female medical assistant must be present to assist with a(n) _____ examination.

F. The size of the speculum selected will depend on the _____ maturity and _____ state of the patient.

G. Warming the speculum in _____ _____ or keeping it warm in a drawer equipped with a(n) _____ _____ will make the examination more comfortable for the patient.

6. Pap Test and Cervical Cancer

A. The Pap test is one of the most common screening tools for _____ and has reduced _____ cancer incidence and mortality rates in the United States by more than _____ percent.

B. The most common risk factor for cervical cancer is infection with _____ _____ (HPV).

C. The Pap test looks for changes in _____ _____ caused by HPV infection.

D. _____ is a new vaccine to prevent infection from the four types of HPV.

E. _____ is another available vaccine for cervical cancer.

7. Pap Test Procedure

A. A thin scraping of exfoliated cells is taken from the _____, _____, and endocervical canal using a cervical _____ and cervical brush or _____.

B. Briefly explain the two methods of conducting a Pap test.

    i. Dry method—

_____

_____

_____

_____

    ii. Liquid method—

_____

_____

_____

_____

C. When sending the samples, the laboratory _____ form has a specific field that requires the medical assistant to enter the first day of the patient's _____ _____ (_____).

D. When scheduling a Pap test, advise the patient of the following.

    i. Do not douche _____ to _____ hours before the examination. Doing so may wash away cervical cells that should be obtained during a Pap smear.

    ii. Avoid _____ _____ for at least 48 hours before the examination.

E. Do not schedule a Pap test when the patient may be _____.

F. After specimens are collected, the physician performs a(n) _____ pelvic examination.

    i. By this method, the physician can detect the _____, _____, and _____ of the uterus and ovaries and can identify any lumps or other abnormalities.

G. The medical assistant should be ready to assist the physician by doing the following.

    i. Providing new _____ before each procedure

    ii. _____ the physician's gloved finger

    iii. Assisting in handing the physician any _____ or _____ needed during the procedures

    iv. Monitoring the patient's _____ level and trying to reduce her _____ during the procedures

8. Grading of Pap Specimens

A. If a Pap test is positive or has _____ dysplasia, the patient is determined to have _____ intraepithelial lesion.

    i. This is not diagnostic of precancer or cancer but requires _____ _____.

B. A colposcopy procedure will view the _____, _____, and _____, and it allows for a(n) _____ from the cervix to be taken.

C. Once the cervical _____ is found to have dysplasia, the patient is determined to have cervical intraepithelial neoplasia, which is considered _____.

D. CIN grading system

   i. CIN I (1) is _____ (low-grade) dysplasia.

   ii. CIN II (2) is _____ to moderately _____ dysplasia.

   iii. CIN III (3) indicates _____ in _____, which is considered early-stage cancer.

9. Prenatal Care

A. Prenatal care is health care provided to _____ women before _____ that includes a series of visits and specific tests to monitor and promote the health of both mother and fetus.

B. The first trimester includes the period of time from implantation of the _____ in the uterus through the _____ week.

   i. This is the most _____ stage of fetal life.

C. The second trimester begins at the end of the _____ week and continues to the end of the _____ month.

   i. During this period, refinement of all the baby's _____ takes place.

   ii. Fetal _____ may be felt.

   iii. The baby's _____ can be determined.

D. The third trimester is the period from the end of the _____ month to _____.

   i. It is marked by an increase in the _____ and _____ of the fetus.

   ii. The fetus usually assumes a(n) _____-down position.

   iii. The fetus is said to have reached the age of _____ at 7 months.

10. First Prenatal Visit

A. The first prenatal visit requires more _____ than follow-up visits because a full _____ and prenatal _____ must be done.

B. List what is completed and ordered during the first prenatal visit.

   i. A complete _____ examination

   ii. Pelvic examination, including a(n) _____ _____

   iii. A complete _____ _____ test

   iv. A(n) _____ test

   v. A serology test for _____

   vi. A(n) _____ titer

   vii. Blood _____ and complete _____ analysis

C. The _____ _____ measurement is taken on the initial visit and is used as a guideline for all subsequent visits.

11. Prenatal History

    A. The patient's menstrual history includes the following.

        i. The patient's _____

        ii. Menstrual _____ cycle

        iii. Duration of _____

        iv. Amount of _____

        v. Menstrual cycle _____

        vi. Types of currently or previously used _____

    B. Past obstetrical history includes the following.

        i. _____—Total number of pregnancies

        ii. _____—Births after 20 weeks gestation, regardless of whether the infant is born dead or alive

        iii. _____—Number of fetuses that did not reach the age of viability, usually under 20 weeks gestation

        iv. This information should be charted using _____ _____.

    C. List the questions asked to determine present pregnancy information.

        i. _____

        ii. _____

        iii. _____

        iv. _____

        v. _____

    D. A(n) _____ _____ may be used to predict the estimated date of childbirth.

12. Prenatal Patient Education

    A. Information given to the patient includes the following.

        i. What to _____ during each _____ of pregnancy

        ii. _____ guidelines

        iii. Vitamin and _____ requirements

        iv. _____ to be avoided

    B. Be sure to remind patients of the _____ of prenatal visits when you schedule the _____ and follow-up visits.

13. Follow-Up Prenatal Visits

    A. Patients return for follow-up visits at the following intervals.

        i. Every _____ weeks through the 28th week

        ii. Every _____ weeks up to the 36th week

        iii. Every _____ until childbirth

B. The MA's role in follow-up prenatal visits includes the following.

   i. Setting up the _____ room

   ii. Obtaining a(n) _____ specimen from the patient

   iii. _____ the patient

   iv. Obtaining the patient's _____ _____

   v. Asking the patient if she has any _____ or issues

   vi. Charting all _____ in the patient's medical record

   vii. Assisting the patient onto the _____ table

   viii. _____ the patient appropriately

C. At 10 to 12 weeks, the fetal _____ _____ is audible with the use of a Doppler fetal monitor.

14. Screening Tests

   A. List screening tests that are commonly performed.*

   *These will be further addressed in an activity later in this chapter.

    i. _____

    ii. _____

    iii. _____

    iv. _____

    v. _____

    vi. _____

    vii. _____

    viii. _____

15. Childbirth

   A. _____, or birth, occurs anytime from week _____ to _____ under normal circumstances.

   B. Delivery before _____ weeks is considered a preterm or premature birth.

   C. The first stage of labor varies in length and ends with complete _____ and _____.

   D. Stage two, the _____ stage of labor, is the period from complete dilation and effacement through the _____ of the fetus.

   E. Stage three is the period from the birth of the fetus to the expulsion of the _____.

16. Postpartum Visit

   A. The _____ is the period after childbirth during which the patient's body slowly returns to its pre-pregnant state.

B. _____, vaginal discharge, may occur for _____ to _____ weeks after childbirth.

C. The patient should be instructed to call the physician if, at any time, the discharge becomes _____ or _____ smelling.

D. Menstruation should resume after about _____ week(s) in a non-nursing mother and _____ month(s) in a nursing mother.

E. A postpartum visit should be scheduled approximately _____ _____ after childbirth, during which the overall health status of the _____ is evaluated.

17. Complications During Pregnancy

A. _____ _____ is a complication in which the placenta develops in the lower portion of the uterus, blocking the opening in the cervix.

B. Abruptio placentae is a complication that occurs when the placenta tears away from the _____ wall, resulting in _____ and fetal _____.

C. Preeclampsia

i. Preeclampsia develops in approximately _____ percent of pregnant women and usually occurs after the _____ week of pregnancy.

ii. Symptoms include agitation and _____, changes in _____ status, decreased _____ output, _____, nausea and _____, pain in the upper-_____ quadrant, shortness of _____, sudden weight gain, swelling of the _____ or hands, and _____ impairment.

iii. If preeclampsia is uncontrolled and seizures develop, the patient is diagnosed with _____.

18. Methods of Contraception

A. Barrier methods work by preventing _____ from reaching the egg. List seven types of barrier methods.

i. _____

ii. _____

iii. _____

iv. _____

v. _____

vi. _____

vii. _____

B. Hormonal methods of birth control use hormones to change the levels of female hormones in the body to prevent _____ or _____ of the fertilized ovum. List eight types of hormonal methods.

    i. _____

    ii. _____

    iii. _____

    iv. _____

    v. _____

    vi. _____

    vii. _____

C. A(n) _____ _____ (_____) is a small device with progestin that is placed in the uterus by the physician.

D. Natural family planning is based on avoiding _____ around the time of ovulation.

    i. It is also known as the _____ method but has more recently been called _____ _____–based birth control.

E. _____ _____ is the withdrawal of the male's penis before ejaculating into the vagina.

F. Sterilization

    i. Since the _____, sterilization has become more common as a(n) _____ method of birth control.

    ii. _____ is a permanent method of birth control.

       a. The physician places tiny _____ coils in the _____ tubes.

       b. _____ _____ forms over these coils and blocks the tubes, thus preventing sperm from reaching the ovum.

    iii. _____ _____ is a permanent method of birth control that is effective 99 percent of the time.

       a. A small incision is made near the _____, and a laparoscope is inserted.

       b. Instruments are inserted to seal the tubes by _____ or closing them with _____ or rings.

III. Male Reproductive Medical Issues

  1. The prostate is a(n) _____-sized gland located between the bladder and the penis.

  2. Aging causes the prostate gland to _____, which eventually restricts _____ flow.

3. Enlargement of the prostate gland is called _____ _____ hyperplasia.

4. _____ and other _____ treatments are available that may relieve the symptoms in some men.

5. Prostate cancer is the _____ most common form of cancer in men.

6. Because of its _____ rate of growth, prostate cancer can be detected and treated in its _____ stages.

7. The following are symptoms of prostate cancer.

   i. _____ stream of urine

   ii. _____ in the urine

   iii. _____ dysfunction

   iv. Nocturia (frequency of urination at _____)

   v. Pelvic or _____ pain

8. Prostate cancer screening includes the following.

   i. A digital _____ examination

   ii. A(n) _____-specific _____ blood test

9. The American Cancer Society recommends screening for prostate cancer based on the results of the PSA blood test.

   i. Men with a PSA of less than 2.5 ng/mL may only need to be retested every _____ year(s).

   ii. Screening should be done every _____ year(s) for men whose PSA level is 2.5 ng/mL or higher.

10. List the additional tests that a physician may recommend based on elevated PSA levels.

   i. _____

   ii. _____

   iii. _____

11. A prostate _____ may be needed.

12. Circumcision

   A. Circumcision is the surgical removal of the _____.

   B. More than _____ percent of males in the United States are circumcised.

   C. Health benefits of circumcision include the following.

      i. Promoting _____ and easier _____

      ii. Decreased risk of _____ _____ infections

      iii. Decreased risk of _____ _____ infections

      iv. Decreased risk of _____ cancer

   D. Complications include _____ and _____.

   E. Circumcision may decrease sensitivity during _____ and may reduce a male's overall _____ satisfaction.

13. Testicular Examination

   A. Testicular cancer is a disease of young and middle-aged men.

      i. Some men in the _____ stages experience symptoms such as a(n) _____ on the testicle.

      ii. The testicle may be _____ or larger than normal, without a(n) _____.

   B. Screening for testicular cancer should be part of a general _____ exam.

   C. A regular testicular _____ to check for lumps or other abnormalities may be done monthly after _____.

14. Vasectomy

   A. _____ is a surgery to render the male sterile.

      i. It involves cutting the _____ _____ and tying off the ends to prevent sperm from being transported out of the _____.

   B. The procedures is performed in the _____ office, and the patient can return home _____ after the procedure.

IV. Sexually Transmitted Infections

1. Sexually transmitted infections can occur in males and females of any _____ and are transmitted by sexual contact from _____ to _____ or _____ to _____.

2. Patients often seek medical attention when they have symptoms, such as _____, _____, _____, and _____.

3. When left untreated, STIs cause a number of problems.

   i. Women may develop _____ _____ disease.

   ii. Men may have profuse _____ from the penis, _____ and pain in the testicles, and _____ urination.

4. STI Education

   A. Treating and preventing the spread of STIs begins with proper _____ and _____ sexual partners who may have been _____.

   B. List the strategies to reduce the chance of exposure to STIs.

      i. Use a(n) _____ _____ with spermicide during every act of sexual intercourse.

      ii. Limit the _____ of sexual partners.

      iii. Know your sexual _____ and their _____ of sexual partners.

      iv. Seek prompt _____ of any suspected STI.

      v. Complete all courses of _____ and comply with follow-up testing.

      vi. Cooperate in _____ sexual contacts.

C. The medical assistant should feel _____ with the facts about STIs and their

mode of _____ and be able to discuss them in a(n) _____,

nonjudgmental manner.

D. _____ is extremely important when dealing with sensitive information such

as testing _____ for an STI.

5. Reporting STIs

A. The medical assistant should be aware of the _____ requirements of

reporting patients with STIs to the proper _____ and _____

agencies.

B. In all 50 states, confirmed cases of _____/_____ are reportable conditions.

C. Gonorrhea and _____ are also reportable diseases in most states.

6. Types of Sexually Transmitted Infections

Complete the following table regarding STIs.

STI	Signs/Symptoms	Treatment
Bacterial vaginosis		
Chlamydia infection		
Genital herpes		
Genital HPV infection		
Gonorrhea		
Lymphogranuloma venereum		
PID		

STI	Signs/Symptoms	Treatment
Syphilis		
Trichomoniasis		

KEY TERMINOLOGY REVIEW

Write a sentence using each of the selected key terms in the correct context.

1. *amenorrhea*

_____

_____

2. *gravida*

_____

_____

3. *dysplasia*

_____

_____

4. *lochia*

_____

_____

5. *quickening*

_____

_____

APPLIED PRACTICE

Match the screening test with its description.

a. carrier testing (genetic)　　　　　b. chorionic villus sampling

c. nuchal translucency screening　　d. alpha-fetoprotein (AFP)

e. amniocentesis　　　　　　　　　　f. ultrasound

g. glucose tolerance testing　　　　　h. group B Streptococcus

1. _____ A special ultrasound test of the fetus to screen for the risk of Down syndrome and other chromosomal abnormalities. It is performed between 11 and 14 weeks and measures the thickness of the fluid buildup at the back of the fetus's neck.

2. _____ Performed between 24 and 28 weeks of pregnancy to test for gestational diabetes.

3. _____ Performed between weeks 15 and 20 to assess fetal sex, maturity, and development. It is recommended that women over age 35 and women who have a family history of genetic defects have this test.

4. _____ A procedure in which a small sample of cells is taken from the placenta and examined for chromosomal abnormalities. It is performed between 10 and 13 weeks of pregnancy.

5. _____ An infection that can be passed to an infant during delivery and is tested for using a vaginal culture at 35 to 37 weeks.

6. _____ Testing that is recommended if there is a family history of certain diseases, such as cystic fibrosis or hemophilia. It can be performed on the mother and/or father and done before or during the pregnancy.

7. _____ Testing that is used to determine the age, growth rate, and position of the fetus, as well as obvious birth defects. It is generally performed at 16 to 20 weeks and is generally painless.

8. _____ A blood test taken between the 15th and 18th week of pregnancy to detect neural tube defects, which are birth defects of the brain, spine, or spinal cord.

LEARNING ACTIVITY: FILL IN THE BLANK

Using your text as necessary, fill in the blanks in the following questions.

1. The ACS recommends that women who are 45 to 54 years of age begin having routine _____.

2. Females develop breast cancer 100 times more frequently than males, most likely due to the effects of _____ and _____.

3. Prior to the patient scheduling a Pap test, the medical assistant should advise her not to douche for _____ to _____ hours before the examination.

4. The pelvic examination begins with an examination of the _____.

5. Women who become sexually active at an early age, as well as those who have multiple partners, are at _____ risk of infection from HPV.

6. Essure sterilization is _____ percent effective.

7. The third trimester is the period from the end of the _____ month to birth.

8. The normal FHT is _____ to _____ beats per minute.

9. Condoms have an effectiveness rate of about _____ percent.

10. Women are fertile for about _____ years of their adult lives.

11. An alternative birth control method should be used for _____ to _____ weeks after a vasectomy or until a sample confirms the absence of sperm.

12. The symptoms of gonorrhea may not appear in females until _____ months after exposure.

13. _____ has no known cause and is the most common vaginal infection in women of childbearing age.

14. Untreated, gonorrhea can cause _____ in both males and females and, in rare circumstances, can spread to the blood or joints.

15. Benign prostate hyperplasia (BPH) is an enlargement of the prostate gland and is one of the most common conditions in men over _____ years.

CRITICAL THINKING

Answer the following questions to the best of your ability. Use the textbook as a reference.

1. Consider the following scenario: You are a female. You have completed your externship and have been hired by a urology clinic for your first full-time medical assistant position. You are directed by the physician to instruct a patient in how to perform a testicular self-exam. You are suddenly nervous about doing this with a real patient, even though you have practiced it in your medical assisting program with other students. Describe what you would do to calm yourself to bolster your own comfort and confidence.

_____

_____

_____

_____

_____

2. A patient, 18-year-old Maria Riojas, has come to the office with a chief complaint of bleeding between her periods. This will be her third GYN visit since menarche, and she is still quite apprehensive about the examination and getting undressed. She says that she hopes the doctor won't have to do a pelvic examination today; she just wants a stronger or different birth control pill. What would you, the medical assistant, say to the patient regarding her concerns?

_____

_____

_____

_____

_____

3. While assisting the physician with a pelvic examination and Pap test, you realize that the vaginal speculum about to be used was not properly sterilized. Use critical thinking skills to determine how you would handle this situation in regard to patient care, considering that both the physician and patient are unaware of the situation.

_____

_____

_____

_____

RESEARCH ACTIVITY

Use Internet search engines to research the following topic and write a brief description of what you find. It is important to use reputable websites.

1. Choose one of the STIs discussed in the chapter. Conduct research to further expand upon the information presented in the chapter. Research statistics related to the STI and other information that you find interesting. Write a paragraph that summarizes your findings and cite your sources.

_____

_____

_____

_____

CHAPTER 38

Assisting with Care of the Eye, Ear, Nose, and Throat

STUDENT STUDY GUIDE

Use the following guide to assist in your learning of the concepts from the chapter.

I. Introduction

1. The role of the medical assistant is to do the following tasks.

    A. Assist the physician during special _____ and procedures.

    B. _____ the patient before, during, and after procedures.

    C. Learn the procedures to perform visual and auditory _____ testing.

    D. _____, or put in, eye and ear medications.

    E. _____, or rinse, both eyes and ears.

2. Special instruments used for examinations include the following.

    A. The _____ is used to examine the tympanum, or

    _____.

    B. The _____ is used to view inner parts of the eye.

    C. Disposable _____ and _____ specula are used to examine the tympanic membrane and nose.

II. Study and Care of the Eye

1. A(n) _____ is a medical doctor who can do the following.

    A. Perform eye _____ and eye surgery.

    B. Prescribe _____, eyeglasses, and _____ lenses.

2. A(n) _____ can perform eye examinations, prescribe medications, and write prescriptions for eyeglasses and contact lenses.

3. A(n) _____ is a technician who specializes in grinding lenses and preparing _____ and contact lenses.

4. Eye Examination

    A. Before eye examinations, the overall _____ of the eye is evaluated for symptoms such as _____, pus-like discharge, and _____ tearing.

    B. The physician evaluates the patient's _____

5. Visual Acuity and Refractive Errors
   A. Normal visual acuity is referred to as _____ vision.
   B. Myopia, or _____, means that the eye sees _____ objects well, but _____ objects appear blurry.
   C. Hyperopia, or _____, means that the eyes see _____ objects well, but near objects are _____.
   D. _____ is the term associated with farsightedness that occurs with aging.
   E. Astigmatism is a refractive disorder in which irregularities in the _____ of the _____ cause light not to focus on the retina but to spread out over an area, causing overall _____ of vision.
   F. Strabismus is an eye disorder caused by _____ in the external eye muscles, often resulting in the eyes looking in _____ directions.

6. Assessing Visual Acuity
   A. Distance visual acuity
      i. Distance visual acuity is measured using the _____ _____, on which the largest symbols are on the top line, and each line after that is of decreasing size.
      ii. A result of 20/20 vision means that a person with _____ distance acuity could read that line at a distance of _____ feet.
      iii. The abbreviation for the right eye is _____.
      iv. The abbreviation for the left eye it is _____.
      v. The abbreviation for both eyes is _____.
      vi. Preschool children and other patients who are illiterate or have a language barrier use the _____ E, the _____ C, or _____ charts.
   B. Near visual acuity
      i. Testing for near visual acuity is done to test for hyperopia or _____.
      ii. Testing for near visual acuity is done by using the _____ card.
         a. The patient reads a card held at normal _____ distance (_____ to _____ inches).
         b. The card has a series of paragraphs _____ in size of print, with a(n) _____ above each.
         c. The patient's result is the number _____ the last paragraph he or she can read _____.

C. Color vision impairment

    i. Color vision impairment is the inability to distinctly _____ colors of the _____.

    ii. The ability to distinguish colors depends on the _____ of the retina.

    iii. The most common type of color vision defect is the inability to distinguish _____ and _____.

    iv. The _____ _____ is printed in either card or booklet form, with a single color-dot illustration containing a number or curved lines and shapes.

        a. The patient is shown _____ color plates or pages and must correctly identify _____ of them to be considered to have color vision within _____ limits.

D. Contrast sensitivity

    i. Contrast sensitivity measures the patient's ability to _____ faint differences in shades of _____.

    ii. It has been determined that contrast sensitivity is affected by most major _____ _____.

7. Irrigation of the Eye

A. Irrigation, or _____, of the eye is necessary to remove _____ substances or _____.

B. Eye irrigation requires the use of _____ technique and _____.

C. Never try to remove a foreign object from the eye using a(n) _____ stick because doing so may cause _____ abrasions.

8. Instillation of Eye Medication

A. Only _____ or _____ medications can be used in the eye, and they must be _____.

B. Encourage patients to _____ eye medications when the prescribed treatment time has been _____.

C. Eye medications should never be _____ with others or even used in the _____ eye if treatment is needed.

9. Eye Safety Guidelines

A. Having an eye examination every _____ to _____ years is important for monitoring changing conditions in the patient's vision.

B. It is important to wear _____ to protect eyes from ultraviolet rays, which can damage the cornea.

C. For minor eye problems, tell patients to avoid _____ and to apply _____ compresses.

D. It is important to wear _____ _____ when using tools or machinery that can cause flying objects.

E. If _____ splash in the eye, a patient should flood the eye with water for _____ minutes and seek immediate medical attention.

10. Changes in the Aging Eye

A. The aging eye may impair vision, and care must be taken to instruct elderly patients on _____ _____.

B. Decreasing _____ perception and difficulty seeing at _____ make elderly people more vulnerable to falling.

11. Assisting the Visually Impaired Patient

A. Blindness can be due to _____, birth _____, injury, or _____.

B. To be declared legally blind, a person must be able to see at _____ feet what a normal person would see at _____ feet.

C. Special _____ may be needed to help a visually impaired person function adequately.

D. _____ animals can help those who are visually impaired.

E. As a medical assistant, you should keep a list of _____ _____ for people with disabilities to best serve those with impairments.

III. Study and Care of the Ear

1. Physicians who specialize in the ear are _____, or otorhinolaryngologists, or ENT (_____, _____, and _____) doctors.

2. Ear Examination

A. The instruments used in the office for ear examinations are the _____, _____ fork, and _____.

B. A healthy eardrum should be _____ gray and _____.

C. An infected eardrum appears _____, swollen, and bulging.

3. Irrigation of the Ear

A. Irrigation of the ear is necessary to remove impacted _____ or _____ matter from the ear.

B. Patients may be apprehensive about the _____ of the procedure, and it is your responsibility to put them at _____ as much as possible.

4. Hearing Acuity

   A. There are many _____ of hearing loss.

   B. Two main categories of hearing loss are _____ hearing loss and _____ hearing loss.

      i. Sensorineural hearing loss—_____ _____ results from damage to the organ of _____ or damage to the _____ nerve.

      ii. Conduction hearing loss is caused by _____ of _____ waves; thus, the sound waves never reach the organ of Corti.

      iii. List four causes of conduction hearing loss.

         a. _____

         b. _____

         c. _____

         d. _____

   C. Various tests measure hearing _____, or sharpness of hearing.

   D. The abbreviations _____ is used for right ear.

   E. The abbreviation _____ is used for left ear.

   F. The abbreviation _____ is used for both ears.

   G. A(n) _____ test can help determine the need for more in-depth testing of hearing _____.

5. Hearing Assessment

   A. Tuning fork

      i. A tuning fork is a(n) _____, forked-shaped instrument that produces _____ when struck.

      ii. The vibrating instrument is held near the patient's _____ or placed on various locations on the head to give a(n) _____ hearing assessment.

   B. Audiometer

      i. An audiometer is a(n) _____ instrument that measures both frequencies and _____ of sound.

      ii. A(n) _____ records the patient responses and is used by the physician to evaluate hearing.

C. Pure tone audiometry

    i. Pure tone audiometry is performed in a(n) _____ room.

    ii. The patient usually wears _____.

    iii. The patient indicates when tones are heard by _____ a(n) _____ on the side where the tone is heard.

D. The medical assistant may be asked to perform a(n) _____ test and may do so with the _____ training.

E. The _____ will interpret the results and inform the patient of the outcome.

6. Additional Diagnostic Tests Related to the Ear

A. Tympanometry estimates the _____ in the middle ear.

B. The _____ is a special examination that evaluates balance through measurement of the movement of the eyes.

    i. It is used to evaluate patients with _____ and other disorders that affect hearing and _____.

C. Tonometry measures _____ pressure.

    i. Normal eye pressure has historically been considered to be less than _____ mm Hg, but this normal _____ limit may vary in different _____.

D. Visual field tests, known as _____ tests, measure the _____ and _____ vision of the patient.

    i. These tests can determine if the patient might have _____, _____ disease, possible optic _____ disease, or ptosis.

7. Assisting the Hearing-Impaired Patient

A. Provide for the _____ level of the hearing-impaired patient.

    i. Have available _____ with hearing amplifiers.

    ii. Don't lose _____ with a patient who is having difficulty hearing your _____.

B. Remember to _____ the patient when speaking.

    i. Do not to speak with _____ or hands over your face.

    ii. Speak clearly, without _____ your voice.

C. _____ patients may be reluctant to admit that they are having hearing problems.

D. List three indications that hearing loss has occurred.

    i. _____

    ii. _____

    iii. _____

E. A medical assistant is responsible for acting in the patient's _____

_____ and speaking to the _____ about concerns.

F. List other signs of aging related to the ears.

    i. _____

    ii. _____

    iii. _____

    iv. _____

8. Ear Safety Guidelines

A. Remind patients never to put anything in the _____

_____.

B. Patients must understand the connection between repetitive _____ to loud noise and _____.

C. Patients who are hearing impaired and cannot use devices such as _____ _____ may need other strategies to help increase their awareness of their _____ at home.

IV. Examination and Treatment of the Nose and Throat

1. The physician will use a nasal _____ to inspect the mucous lining of the nose for signs of _____ and infection.

2. A(n) _____ _____ is used to examine the throat for signs of infection, enlarged tonsils, and abnormalities of the tongue or oral cavity.

3. A throat _____ may be ordered if signs of infection are present.

4. List signs and symptoms of nasal problems.

A. _____

B. _____

C. _____

D. _____

KEY TERMINOLOGY REVIEW

Match the each of the following vocabulary terms to the correct definition.

a. astigmatism

b. frequencies

c. myopia

d. myringa

e. strabismus

1. _____ The medical term for the eardrum.

2. _____ An eye disorder caused by weakness in the external eye muscles, resulting in the eyes looking in different directions.

3. _____ A refractive disorder in which irregularities in the curvature of the cornea cause light not to focus on the retina but instead to spread out over an area, causing overall blurring of vision.

4. _____ Also known as nearsightedness.

5. _____ Number of fluctuations per second of energy in the form of sound waves.

APPLIED PRACTICE

Read the scenario and answer the questions that follow.

Scenario

Shawn Collins, RMA, is working as a medical assistant at a local family practice. Rajan Avuri, a 17-year-old patient, is being seen for a driver's license eye examination. As part of the exam, Shawn tests Rajan's vision with a Snellen eye chart similar to the Snellen eye chart below. Shawn asks Rajan to cover his right eye and read line 8. Rajan reads the following letters from left to right: "D, E, F, P, O, T, E, C." Shawn asks Rajan to continue on and read line 9. Rajan reads the following letters from left to right: "L, E, P, O, D, R, O, T."

Shawn then asks Rajan to uncover his right eye and cover his left eye for assessment. Beginning with line 8, Rajan reads the following letters from left to right: "D, E, F, R, O, T, E, C." Rajan is not able to distinguish any letters on the lines below line 8.

Tech-Med

NO. 3050

E

$\frac{20}{200}$ 200 FT.
61 m   **1**

F P

$\frac{20}{100}$ 100 FT.
30.5 m   **2**

T O Z

$\frac{20}{70}$ 70 FT.
21.3 m   **3**

L P E D

$\frac{20}{50}$ 50 FT.
15.2 m   **4**

P E C F D

$\frac{20}{40}$ 40 FT.
12.2 m   **5**

E D F C Z P

$\frac{20}{30}$ 30 FT.
9.14 m   **6**

F E L O P Z D

$\frac{20}{25}$ 25 FT.
7.62 m   **7**

D E F P O T E C

$\frac{20}{20}$ 20 FT.
6.10 m   **8**

L E F O D P C T

$\frac{20}{15}$ 15 FT.
4.57 m   **9**

F D P L T C E O

$\frac{20}{13}$ 13 FT.
3.96 m   **10**

P E Z O L C F T D

$\frac{20}{10}$ 10 FT.
3.05 m   **11**

    Assisting with Care of the Eye, Ear, Nose, and Throat   **453**

1. How should Shawn record Rajan's vision in his left eye? Explain your answer.

_____

_____

_____

2. How should Shawn record Rajan's vision in his right eye? Explain your answer.

_____

_____

_____

LEARNING ACTIVITY: MULTIPLE CHOICE

Circle the correct answer to each of the following questions.

1. Which of the following specialists is *not* a medical doctor?

   a. Ophthalmologist
   b. Otorhinolaryngologist
   c. Optometrist
   d. ENT

2. Which test measures pressure in the middle ear?

   a. Perimetry
   b. Tympanometry
   c. Tonometry
   d. Electronystagmograph

3. The ability to distinguish colors depends on the cones of the _____, which react to light and permit us to see shades of red, green, and blue.

   a. choroid
   b. iris
   c. cornea
   d. retina

4. With hyperopia, the eyeball is too _____ or the lens is too _____.

   a. short; thin
   b. short; thick
   c. long; thin
   d. long; thick

5. To be declared legally blind, a person must only be able to see at _____ feet what a normal person would see at 200 feet.

   a. 20
   b. 40
   c. 50
   d. 100

6. The most common type of color vision defect, which is inherited, is the inability to distinguish

   a. blue and yellow.
   b. red and green.
   c. blue and black.
   d. shades of gravy.

7. What does the abbreviation AD (*aurus dextra*) mean?
   a. Both ears
   b. Left ear
   c. Right ear
   d. None of the above

8. Which of the following instrument(s) is used in the office for ear examinations?
   a. Otoscope
   b. Tuning fork
   c. Audiometer
   d. All of the above

9. Sensorineural hearing loss is due to which of the following?
   a. Nerve damage
   b. Obstruction of sound waves
   c. Old age
   d. Infection

10. When instilling ear medication into a child's ear, which direction should the ear be pulled?
    a. Up and back
    b. Down and back
    c. Up
    d. Down

CRITICAL THINKING

Answer the following questions to the best of your ability. Use the textbook as a reference.

1. You need to perform a Snellen visual acuity test and an Ishihara color vision test per the physician's orders. You do not have an occluder or the Ishihara plates. Which of the tests, if any, could you still perform using a different item(s), and what replacement item(s) can you use?

   _____

   _____

   _____

   _____

2. Ellen, a CMA (AAMA), has physician's orders to instill eyedrops in a 13-year-old's right eye. Ellen employs sterile techniques as she prepares to instill the eyedrops. Just as she is about to place the drops in the patient's eye, the patient sneezes, and it happens so quickly that she is unable to cover her nose and mouth. The sterile gloves and medication bottle containing the eyedrops have been contaminated. How should Ellen proceed?

   _____

   _____

   _____

   _____

RESEARCH ACTIVITY

Use Internet search engines to research the following topic and write a brief description of what you find. It is important to use reputable websites.

1. Visit two or more different websites that deal with advocacy and support for those with vision and hearing loss. What information did you find that could be used to help families dealing with vision and hearing deficiencies? What websites did you find to be most useful, and why? Be sure to cite your sources.

   _____

   _____

   _____

   _____

   _____

CHAPTER 39
Assisting with Life Span Specialties: Pediatrics

STUDENT STUDY GUIDE

Use the following guide to assist in your learning of the concepts from the chapter.

I. Assisting in Pediatrics

1. Pediatrics deals with the _____ and care of children and the diagnosis and treatment of childhood _____.

2. A(n) _____ treats patients from birth to 20 years of age.

3. _____ care physicians may also care for pediatric patients.

4. Communicating with Pediatric Patients

   A. Children have a way of sensing and _____ to those who are _____ being around them.

   B. List five suggestions for communicating with a pediatric patient.

      i. _____

      ii. _____

      iii. _____

      iv. _____

      v. _____

II. The Pediatric Office

1. Office Reception Room

   A. The reception room should be _____, _____, and interesting to the child.

   B. The most practical and safest toys are _____-to-_____ plastic toys _____ tiny pieces or sharp edges.

   C. Infectious or sick children should be taken directly to a(n) _____ room, if possible.

   D. _____ should be picked up and put away throughout the day and sanitized at the end of each _____.

2. Patient Safety

    A. Children should never be left alone anyplace there is the possible danger of _____ or other injury.

    B. Place a protective _____ on an infant to keep him/her from _____ or falling.

3. Carrying an Infant

    A. When carrying an infant, try to mimic the way the _____ holds the child.

    B. List three positions for carrying infants.

       i. _____

       ii. _____

       iii. _____

    C. Supporting the infant's _____ should be foremost in your mind.

4. Wrapping an Infant

    A. _____ movements of an infant or a child may be necessary for a procedure or an evaluation to be performed.

    B. Wrapping or swaddling can be done using a small _____ or _____ blanket.

III. The Pediatric Patient

1. Development refers to the motor, _____, and _____ progress a child achieves.

2. The pediatrician looks for markers to detect abnormalities in _____, social, _____, and _____ development.

3. Apgar Scoring

    A. Apgar scoring is a method of evaluating a(n) _____ condition at 1 and 5 minutes after _____.

    B. Newborns scoring ____ to ____ are considered out of immediate danger.

    C. Newborns scoring ____ to ____ are considered moderately depressed.

    D. Newborns scoring ____ to ____ are severely depressed.

IV. Pediatric Office Visits

1. Well-Child Visits

    A. _____ and _____ are measured.

    B. _____ are given.

    C. _____ information is provided.

2. Growth

A. By _____ month(s), an infant's weight has doubled.

B. At 1 year of age, usually the child's length has _____ and weight has

_____.

C. By _____ years old, the child reaches half his/her adult height.

D. Adult proportions will not be reached until about _____ years.

E. Failure to thrive (FTT)

   i. FTT occurs when an infant doesn't gain a sufficient amount of _____,

      according to the standardized baby _____ _____.

   ii. If an infant's growth is considerably under the goal for his/her age,

      _____ _____ could be affected.

   iii. The most frequent cause of FTT is inadequate _____.

   iv. FTT may occur as a result of medical problems such as _____,

      _____, and _____ issues.

3. Measurements

A. The physician will examine the patient from _____ to _____.

B. List the vital signs obtained during a well-child visit.

   i. _____

   ii. _____

   iii. _____

   iv. _____

C. Weight–height and chest measurements

   i. For the most accurate weight, infants should be weighed either without a(n)

      _____ or with a completely _____ diaper.

   ii. The length of an infant is measured on the _____ table until the child

      can stand reasonably still on the _____ _____.

   iii. Measurement of the circumference of the head is also part of each well-child office visit

      until age _____ _____.

   iv. Chest circumference may be performed if the physician suspects over- or

      underdevelopment of the _____ or _____.

D. Growth charts

   i. A copy of the National Center for Health Statistics growth chart is part of every child's

      permanent _____ _____.

   ii. Individual growth charts are available for _____ and

      _____ aged birth to 36 months and _____ to _____ years.

iii. After the measurements are obtained, the medical assistant charts the information in both the _____ _____ and the _____ _____.

iv. When paper medical records are used, the plotting of measurements requires _____ and _____.

v. When using electronic medical records, the software program automatically _____ the child's growth and _____ range.

4. Sick-Child Visits

A. Pediatric offices have time blocked off in the _____ _____ to allow for sick-child visits.

B. Children develop sickness quite often because their bodies do not have a fully developed _____ system.

C. It is important to teach children the importance of breaking the cycle of infection—particularly hand _____ and covering their nose and mouth when they _____ or _____.

D. It is helpful to place a sick patient in a(n) _____ _____ as quickly as possible to help reduce the possibility of _____ infection.

5. Collecting a Urine Sample

A. If a child is toilet trained and over _____ to _____ years old, it is easiest and recommended that the _____ or caregiver collect the specimen.

B. Instructions must be given regarding proper cleansing of the _____ _____ prior to collecting a specimen.

C. A pediatric _____ _____ device is applied to patients who are too young or too ill to obtain a urine specimen otherwise.

D. Urine samples reflect the _____ _____ of many systems in the body and are an important _____ tool.

V. Pediatric Diseases and Disorders

1. Upper Respiratory Diseases and Disorders

A. The common cold is caused by more than _____ varieties of the rhinovirus.

B. During their first 2 years, children may have _____ to _____ colds a year.

C. Most upper respiratory infections are spread easily by _____ from the nose, throat, or _____ items handled by the infected person.

D. _____ is the best approach when dealing with upper respiratory infections.

E. List six respiratory disorders discussed in the textbook.*

---

*These conditions will be expanded upon in another workbook activity in this chapter.

i. _____

ii. _____

iii. _____

iv. _____

v. _____

vi. _____

2. Gastrointestinal Disorders

A. Diarrhea

   i. Diarrhea may be caused by _____, _____, and _____ infections; food allergies; and _____.

   ii. Diarrhea in infants and small children can rapidly lead to _____.

   iii. Diarrhea may also cause _____, or painful chafing or rawness of the skin in the diaper area.

   iv. Pediatricians often recommend using the _____ diet and avoiding _____ products until diarrhea subsides.

B. Colic

   i. Colic is severe gastrointestinal _____ that occurs in both breastfed and formula-fed infants.

   ii. Symptoms include intense _____, irritability, _____, distended abdomen, and _____.

   iii. As a medical assistant, your ability to _____ with the caregiver can ease frustration.

   iv. Over-the-counter _____ _____ drops can be helpful in reducing the infant's discomfort.

   v. Some babies find relief from being held in the _____ position.

3. Other Disorders

A. Autism

   i. Autism is a disorder that is marked by the brain's abnormal development of _____ and _____ skills.

   ii. Various forms are diagnosed within the autism _____ disorder.

   iii. Besides genetics, other possible causes of autism include the following.

     a. Exposure to _____ _____ during pregnancy

     b. Exposure to pesticides

     c. Exposure to flame-retardant _____

     d. Prenatal or postnatal _____

     e. Exposure to _____ _____

iv. Symptoms of autism

    a. Failure to make _____ _____

    b. Engaging in _____ behavior

    c. Delayed _____ skills

    d. Preference for _____ activities

    e. Upset by _____ in routine

    f. _____ to people

v. There is no cure, but early _____ by specialists could be helpful.

B. Sudden Infant Death Syndrome (SIDS)

    i. SIDS is the death of an apparently _____ infant, usually before age _____ year(s), with no known cause.

    ii. SIDS happens more frequently in _____ and is more prevalent among _____.

    iii. List factors that increase the risk of SIDS.

        a. _____

        b. _____

        c. _____

        d. _____

        e. _____

        f. _____

    iv. Possible prevention techniques

        a. Having the infant sleep on his/her _____ or in a(n) _____ position for at least the first 6 months

        b. Using _____ monitors

C. Febrile seizures

    i. Some children suffer febrile seizures, with high _____ following a rapid spike in _____ _____.

    ii. Seizures can involve jerking _____ and _____, loss of _____, and stiffening of the child's _____.

    iii. During a seizure, a child should be placed on his/her _____ in an area free of _____ _____.

    iv. The only treatment is to _____ the _____.

D. Obesity

    i. Obesity is defined as being _____ percent above the patient's ideal weight, with a body mass index over _____.

ii. Causes of obesity in children

    a. _____ tendencies

    b. Family patterns of _____

    c. Poor _____ choices

    d. Lack of _____

iii. Rarely is childhood obesity caused by a(n) _____ disorder.

iv. Obesity carries serious consequences to _____ in the short and long terms and may cause damage to a child's _____.

E. Fifth disease

    i. Fifth disease is a mildly contagious viral disease that occurs during

    _____.

    ii. List symptoms of Fifth disease.

        a. _____

        b. _____

        c. _____

    iii. Symptoms last about _____ _____.

    iv. It is important for children who are diagnosed with Fifth disease not to come in contact with _____ _____.

F. Roseola

    i. Roseola is characterized by a sudden _____ _____, which can last about _____ day(s), followed by a rash of tiny _____ _____ on the head and trunk.

    ii. List treatment options for roseola.

        a. _____

        b. _____

G. Hand, foot, and mouth disease

    i. With hand, foot, and mouth disease, a virus causes _____ to appear in the mouth, on hands, and on feet.

    ii. It commonly occurs in _____ and early _____.

    iii. Caused by the Coxsackie virus, it is spread by the _____–_____ route, saliva, or direct contact with _____.

    iv. Treatments include _____ fever with over-the-counter medications, rinsing the mouth with _____ _____ water, and increasing _____ intake.

VI. Adolescence and Puberty
   1. Two Stages of Adolescence
      i. Early adolescence—ages _____ to _____ years
      ii. Middle adolescence—ages _____ to _____ years
   2. Adolescence is a time of dramatic _____, _____, and _____ changes.
   3. Early Adolescence
      A. Puberty marks the beginning of the development of _____ _____ characteristics.
      B. Adolescents begin to make their own _____.
      C. _____ _____ to use drugs, have sex, and drink alcohol increases.
      D. Emotional changes
         i. Early adolescents become very concerned with _____ _____, clothes, and how _____ view them.
         ii. Early adolescents become more self-centered, _____, less affectionate toward _____, and more influenced by _____ _____.
         iii. _____ taking is common.
   4. Middle Adolescence
      A. Girls are often physically _____, whereas boys may still be _____.
      B. _____ image is often a primary concern.
      C. Middle teens may be developing more individual _____ and a definite, unique _____.
      D. They develop a more clear sense of _____ and may not be as strongly influenced by _____.
      E. Emotional changes
         i. Conflicts with _____ may decrease.
         ii. These adolescents exhibit greater _____ and a greater interest in the _____ _____.
         iii. Acceptance by _____ is incredibly important.
         iv. Some teens experience _____.
   5. Eating Disorders
      A. Eating disorders are prevalent among _____ and _____.
      B. Eating disorders are marked by extreme problems with _____ _____.

C. Some _____ and _____ treatments are effective for some eating disorders.

D. No specific treatment is available for _____ cases.

6. Anorexia Nervosa

A. Anorexia nervosa is associated with a(n) _____ sense of body image and the persistent quest for _____.

B. List seven signs of anorexia nervosa.

   i. _____

   ii. _____

   iii. _____

   iv. _____

   v. _____

   vi. _____

   vii. _____

C. Treatment includes _____, including family therapy and intensive _____ or _____ therapy.

7. Bulimia Nervosa

A. Bulimia nervosa is characterized by _____ eating and then use of any or all of the following.

   i. _____

   ii. _____

   iii. _____

B. Symptoms of bulimia include the following.

   i. Chronic _____ _____ from vomiting stomach acids

   ii. Worn _____ on teeth from stomach acids

   iii. Dehydration

   iv. Gastrointestinal _____ _____

   v. Intestinal irritation from _____ use

   vi. Swollen _____ glands

C. Treatment for bulimic patients includes _____ and _____ counseling.

8. Binge Eating Disorder

A. Binge eating disorder is characterized by binge eating episodes that happen all throughout the _____.

B. It is often associated with feelings of _____, _____,

_____ and other coexisting psychological disorders.

C. Treatment includes _____, _____, behavior

_____ techniques, and the possible use of _____ suppressants.

9. Other Specified Feeding or Eating Disorder (OSFED)

A. OSFED is a newer diagnosis that has replaced the more previous diagnosis

_____ _____ not otherwise _____.

B. List the five distinct subtypes of OSFEDs.

i. _____

ii. _____

iii. _____

iv. _____

v. _____

KEY TERMINOLOGY REVIEW

Match each of the following key terms to the correct definition.

a. excoriation
b. failure to thrive (FTT)
c. hydrocephalous
d. meatus
e. stridor

1. _____ Excessive fluid around the brain.

2. _____ A high-pitched sound heard during respiration.

3. _____ Painful chafing or rawness of the skin.

4. _____ The urinary tract opening.

5. _____ A syndrome identified when an infant gains insufficient weight according to the standardized baby growth charts.

APPLIED PRACTICE

Read the scenario below and answer the questions that follow.

Scenario

Sandra Norwood has brought her daughter, Maya, to the office for her 6-month well-baby visit. Austin Shwartz is the medical assistant working with Ms. Norwood and Maya. (Maya's chart entry for today's visit appears below.)

Norwood, Maya
DOB: 04-23-20XX
DATE: 10/30/20XX, 9:30 a.m.
Weight: 21 lb., length: 27″
Head Circumference: 17½″, Chest Circumference: 18″
CC: Mother states, "Maya is here for her 6-month checkup and shots."
A. Shwartz, RMA

Activity 1

1. Using the growth chart in the textbook and the information noted above in the chart, determine the percentiles for Maya's length for age and weight for age:

    a. Length-for-age percentile: _____

    b. Weight-for-age percentile: _____

Activity 2

Match each common childhood respiratory disorder with the correct description below.

   a. strep throat   d. otitis media

   b. croup   e. bronchiolitis

   c. respiratory syncytial virus   f. asthma

1. _____ An inflammation of the larynx and trachea that leads to a distinctive barking cough and hoarseness. Two types are spasmodic and viral.

2. _____ An infection of the middle ear caused by cold, allergies, or other respiratory infections. Fluid accumulates, applying pressure to the eardrum, causing pain, irritability, and sometimes fever.

3. _____ Inflammation and spasms of the bronchi, increased mucous secretions, and narrowing of the airways make it difficult to exhale and inhale for patients suffering from this disorder.

4. _____ Caused by a highly infectious bacteria, which may lead to other problems when left untreated, such as scarlet fever and rheumatic fever, which can damage heart valves.

5. _____ A highly contagious virus that affects the upper and lower respiratory tracts. It normally occurs in winter and early spring and is the most common cause of bronchiolitis.

6. _____ This is more common in children under 2 years old who have upper respiratory tract infections. Children with asthma and those exposed to secondhand smoke are at increased risk for developing this disorder.

LEARNING ACTIVITY: TRUE/FALSE

Indicate whether the following statements are true or false by placing a T or an F on the line that precedes each statement.

_____ 1. Injuries are the number-one cause of death in children within the first year of life.

_____ 2. A towering position creates both physical and emotional barriers and indicates a domineering role.

_____ 3. Toys in a reception area should be cleaned and disinfected daily.

_____ 4. Children mature at consistent rates; however, the stages that they pass through are variable.

_____ 5. By 5 years old, a child reaches half his or her adult height.

_____ 6. Eating disorders are prevalent among adolescents and teens.

_____ 7. Exposing a child to cool, moist night air is frequently effective to combat the effects of RSV.

_____ 8. Most upper respiratory infections are spread easily by droplets from the nose or throat or by contaminated items handled by the infected person.

_____ 9. A CDC survey found that 28 percent of high school students had suicidal thoughts, and 8.3 percent had attempted suicide.

_____ 10. A patient with roseola should not come in contact with a pregnant woman.

CRITICAL THINKING

Answer the following questions to the best of your ability. Use the textbook as a reference.

1. Javier is a 9-year-old boy who is slightly behind on his immunization schedule. Javier needs to receive two immunizations today in order to be considered up-to-date, which is a requirement for starting classes at his new school. He is a very smart boy and is incredibly agitated at the thought of receiving two shots. How would you explain the importance of receiving immunizations to Javier?

   _____

   _____

   _____

   _____

2. Natalie, a 4-year-old patient, is extremely nervous about her well-child checkup. The doctor has asked you, the medical assistant, to include a blood pressure measurement when her vital signs are obtained. As soon as Natalie sees the blood pressure cuff and stethoscope, she begins to whimper and cry. How could you explain the procedure of obtaining vital signs to Natalie in order to help put her at ease?

   _____

   _____

   _____

   _____

   _____

RESEARCH ACTIVITY

Use Internet search engines to research the following topic and write a brief description of what you find. It is important to use reputable websites.

1. To learn more about eating disorders and how they are treated, go online or use resources from your school or local library. Conduct research and then write a brief essay on your findings and what you learned. Be sure to cite your sources.

   _____

   _____

   _____

   _____

   _____

CHAPTER 40
Assisting with Life Span Specialties: Geriatrics

STUDENT STUDY GUIDE

Use the following guide to assist in your learning of the concepts from the chapter.

I. Introduction

1. _____ is the field of medicine specializing in the treatment and care of elderly patients.

2. A(n) _____ is a physician who diagnoses and treats diseases and conditions that predominantly affect elderly patients.

3. Geriatrics generally refers to people who are _____ years of age or older.

II. The Medical Assistant's Role in Geriatrics

1. The elderly have _____ acute illnesses than younger age groups.

2. _____ illness is the predominant issue for the geriatric population.

3. When reviewing medication lists, allot _____ _____ for a patient with extensive medication needs.

4. Because geriatric patients may have decreased _____ and instability, the MA may need to provide additional assistance to them.

5. It is important not to make assumptions about or _____ elderly patients.

6. Effective Communication

A. Have a(n) _____, relaxed, and _____ communication and interaction with geriatric patients.

B. List the basic principles of patient communication.

i. _____

ii. _____

iii. _____

iv. _____

III. The Aging Population

1. Every _____ has its own traditions and ways it views and treats the elderly.

2. The Social Security Act of _____ established a system of federal benefits to assist marginalized groups, including the _____.

3. In _____, two amendments were made to the Social Security Act to meet the needs of the _____ population as well as low-income individuals and families.

   A. _____—A medical insurance system to meet the needs of Americans aged 65 and older, as well as others with special health conditions.

   B. _____—A medical insurance program to finance health care for low-income individuals or those close to the public assistance level.

4. _____ and elderly adults living on small _____ incomes may be eligible for both Medicare and Medicaid.

5. A(n) _____ insurance policy is a supplemental insurance policy offered by a(n) _____ company to offset the health care costs that Medicare doesn't cover.

6. Life Expectancy

   A. By 2050, the estimated population of the elderly will be more than _____ million.

   B. Factors related to increased life expectancy

      i. Better living _____ and _____

      ii. _____ advances

      iii. New _____

      iv. Changes in _____ behaviors

   C. Types of elderly housing options

      i. _____-_____ facilities—Group settings designed for residents who cannot live independently but do not require _____-_____ care.

      ii. _____-_____ facilities—Facilities that provide 24-hour specialized care for residents who require a(n) _____ _____ of medical care and assistance for complex medical conditions and/or treatment.

7. The Baby Boomer Generation

   A. When servicemen returned from World War II, there was a significant _____ in the birth rate, and more babies were born in _____ than ever before.

   B. The baby boomer generation includes those born between _____ and _____.

   C. By _____ all surviving baby boomers will have reached senior citizen status.

   D. Considerations for the baby boomer generation

      i. Those without the _____ _____ net of grown children may receive less assistance from family members as they age.

      ii. Many baby boomers are facing the reality of caring for a(n) _____ and a young _____ at the same time.

      iii. _____ hardship, advancing age, and deterioration of _____ will put increased strain on _____ resources for health care.

IV. The Aging Process: Physical Changes

1. Factors That Affect How the Body Ages

   A. _____

   B. _____ choices

   C. _____ hazards

   D. _____ choices

   E. Health care _____

   F. An individual's _____ and _____ environment

2. Ageism is a(n) _____ against and incorrect _____ about an individual or individuals because of their age.

3. Physical Changes

   A. Integumentary system changes

      i. The skin becomes less _____, _____, and more fragile.

      ii. Wrinkles and sagging as well as "_____ spots" or "_____ spots" appear in areas that have had excessive exposure to the _____.

      iii. When preparing an elderly patient for examination, pay particular attention to _____ and signs of _____.

   B. Nervous system changes

      i. Nervous system function begins to _____ _____, and reaction times are _____.

      ii. Slower responses to changes in _____ can make an elderly patient more prone to _____ and injuries.

      iii. Offer your _____ to patients when walking and assist them on and off the _____ table.

      iv. Elderly people may wake up more often in the _____ of the night and get less _____ sleep.

   C. Sensory changes

      i. _____ and _____ reduce elderly patients' ability to interact with the environment around them.

      ii. Be alert for both _____ and _____ communication cues when asking elderly patients questions that might call into questions their independence.

      iii. At age 80 approximately half the sense of _____ has been lost.

      iv. _____ depends mostly on smell, so often the patient's appetite _____, and interest in food _____.

      v. Engage elderly patients in a discussion of _____ _____ and what they normally eat each day.

D. Musculoskeletal system changes
   i. The aging musculoskeletal system is characterized by the following.
      a. A decrease in muscle _____ and muscle _____
      b. A loss of _____
      c. Bone _____ loss
   ii. Cartilage can deteriorate, limiting _____ movement.
   iii. Changes in posture can lead to gait and stability problems, which increase the risk of _____ and _____ fractures.
   iv. _____ is the most common cause of bone loss in the elderly.
      a. Bone becomes _____ and _____ and may break from minor falls or _____ or even simple actions.
   v. Compared to men, women have _____ times the risk of developing osteoporosis.
   vi. Osteoporosis is often called _____ because bone loss is gradual and occurs without _____.
   vii. Healthy _____ choices can help prevent further bone loss and reduce the risk of fractures.
   viii. Encourage the use of _____ devices as needed.
   ix. Review _____ _____ with caregivers and family members.
E. Respiratory system changes
   i. Respiratory system aging is characterized by loss of _____ in the alveoli and _____.
   ii. Respiratory _____ become weaker, making it more _____ to move air into and out of the lungs.
   iii. Breathing _____ can be taught to help the elderly increase the depth of breathing and exercise _____ muscles.
F. Urinary system changes
   i. Aging of the urinary system involves decreased _____ mass and renal _____.
   ii. The kidneys' slower rate of _____ _____ may affect the excretion of drugs from the body.
   iii. The elderly have decreased bladder _____ _____ and an inability to empty the bladder completely, placing them at increased risk for _____ _____ _____.
   iv. Increased frequency of _____ and increased _____ may both become problems for many elderly people.

v. Patients may decrease fluid intake to reduce these problems, but there are dangers related to doing so. (List the dangers.)

a. _____

b. _____

c. _____

G. Digestive system changes

i. The passage of food throughout the digestive tract is _____, with less absorption of food, _____, and _____.

ii. There is an increase in _____ and _____.

iii. Liver function _____.

iv. Esophageal motility is _____, and the esophagus tends to become slightly _____.

v. Proper _____ education can be helpful.

H. Cardiovascular system changes

i. Lifestyle habits such as _____, high-_____ diets, and lack of _____ take a toll on the cardiovascular system.

ii. Cardiac _____ and the amount of _____ supplied to organs of the body decrease as a result of the heart _____ aging and other conditions.

iii. _____ hypotension occurs in some elderly patients.

a. Dizziness can increase an elderly patient's risk of _____ and injury.

I. Endocrine system changes

i. Aging of the endocrine system is characterized by decreasing levels of _____, thyroid _____, and _____ resistance.

ii. Elderly patients should have routine _____ _____ performed to screen for endocrine system dysfunctions.

J. Reproductive system changes

i. _____ activity patterns and _____ tend to be consistent over the lifespan, including during _____ age.

ii. Male patients may struggle with _____ dysfunction.

iii. Problems for women may include vaginal _____ and _____.

iv. _____ health should be discussed with patients.

v. The medical assistant must be ready to discuss these issues _____ and without _____.

V. The Aging Process: Mental Changes

1. Brain function _____ with aging.

2. Many _____ may have an impact on a patient's mental status.

3. Cognitive Ability

   A. List five factors that alter the psychologic status of the mind.

      i. _____

      ii. _____

      iii. _____

      iv. _____

      v. _____

   B. _____ is not altered by aging, though more time may be needed for _____ solving.

   C. Keeping the brain active with mentally _____ _____ can help maintain memory retrieval.

4. Memory

   A. List the three types of memory that correspond to the following descriptions.

      i. _____ _____—Things that can be recalled for about 30 seconds or so that will fade from memory if not repeated multiple times

      ii. _____ _____—Memories that have been activated multiple times and committed to the brain

      iii. _____ _____—Information gained through the senses that lasts a few seconds

   B. Medical assistants should encourage patients to exercise both their _____ _____ and their _____.

   C. List four common areas of struggle for people with memory loss.

      i. _____

      ii. _____

      iii. _____

      iv. _____

5. Effects of Medication on Mental Abilities

   A. Guidelines to help patients with daily medications

      i. Provide the patient with a pill _____.

      ii. Provide a(n) _____ _____ of medications the patient is currently taking.

      iii. Explain to the patient _____ he or she is taking each of the medications.

      iv. Provide verbal and written warnings about possible _____ and _____ interactions.

      v. _____ should be provided with these aids if the patient is not competent.

6. Confusion

   A. Confusion is a(n) _____ consequence of aging.

   B. _____ confusion lasts less than 3 months.

   C. _____ confusion lasts more than 3 months.

   D. List the three categories of confusion.

      i. _____

      ii. _____

      iii. _____

   E. The most common cause of acute-onset confusion in the elderly is _____

      _____ _____.

   F. Sundowner syndrome

      i. Sundowner syndrome occurs in patients with _____ disease or other forms of

         _____, and its symptoms appear after sundown or at night.

      ii. The following factors increase the incidence of this syndrome.

         a. Disruption of _____

         b. Disturbance in _____ patterns

         c. Use of _____

         d. Excessive _____ stimulation

      iii. Symptoms of confusion subside in the _____.

7. Depression

   A. Depression is defined as "an abnormal and persistent mood characterized by

      _____, _____, slowed mental processes, and changes in _____

      and sleeping habits."

   B. Depression is often overlooked in the elderly or _____ as part of another problem,

      such as _____.

   C. Many medical providers use the geriatric _____ _____ form to aid in

      the diagnosis of depression.

8. Dementia

   A. Dementia is a syndrome marked by progressive loss of _____ and decline in

      _____ abilities that interferes with daily life.

   B. More than _____ types of dementia are currently defined.

   C. Causes of dementia

      i. _____

      ii. _____

      iii. _____

      iv. _____

      v. _____

     vi. _____

   vii. _____

D. Signs and symptoms of dementia

      i. The patient may exhibit _____ regarding recent events or places.

     ii. The patient may forget what he or she is doing while in the middle of a(n) _____.

   iii. The patient may show a lack of _____ or have mood _____.

   iv. Patients become unable to follow _____, unable to perform _____ of daily living, and eventually become _____ as the brain shuts down.

E. Treatment options for dementia

      i. The underlying _____ or disorder must be treated first.

     ii. List three types of medications used to treat behavior-related issues.

        a. _____

        b. _____

        c. _____

9. Alzheimer's Disease (AD)

A. Alzheimer's disease is a progressive disorder of the _____ _____ _____ that eventually destroys mental capacities.

B. Abnormal changes to the brain in patients with AD include _____ (deposits of protein fragments) and _____ (twisted protein fibers).

C. Caring for a family member with AD can be _____, _____, and _____ devastating.

D. Signs and symptoms of Alzheimer's disease

      i. Warning signs of Alzheimer's (summarized from Box 40-3)

        a. Memory loss that disrupts _____ _____

        b. Difficulty performing _____ tasks

        c. Problems with _____

        d. Disorientation to _____ and _____

        e. Poor or decreased _____

        f. Problems with _____ thinking or problem solving

        g. Difficulty with spatial and _____ relationships

        h. Changes in _____

        i. Loss of _____

     ii. The following symptoms occur in people with Alzheimer's disease.

        a. Forgetting _____ experiences

        b. Rarely _____ later

    c. Becoming unable to _____ written/spoken directions

    d. Becoming unable to use notes as _____

    e. Becoming unable to _____ for self

E. Treatment options for Alzheimer's disease

    i. There is no _____ for AD.

    ii. Medications have been able to lessen the _____, such as memory loss and confusion, for a(n) _____ of time.

    iii. Patients should not drink _____ as it can worsen symptoms.

    iv. Depressed patients may benefit from taking _____ in the early stages.

    v. It is helpful to reduce _____ for AD patients.

    vi. Helping caregivers obtain _____ care allows time for relaxation and can be of great assistance.

VI. Legal and Medical Decisions

1. It is the professional responsibility of _____ and family _____ to provide guidance to caregivers when making difficult decisions regarding the declining health of elderly family members.

2. Advance Directives

A. An advance directive provides _____ or directives formulated by the _____, while he or she is still _____ to do so, that express his or her desires about _____ care.

B. Besides resuscitation, other directives may include the following.

    i. Withholding _____, with the exception of _____ relief

    ii. Withholding _____ and _____, particularly if nutrition is the only factor that would keep the patient alive

    iii. Desire for _____ donation

    iv. Desire for _____

C. A legal document called a Do Not Resuscitate order indicates that a patient does not wish to be resuscitated in the case of _____ or _____ arrest.

D. A(n) _____ power of _____ names the patient's health care representative, also called an agent, who can make medical decisions and carry out the advance directives if the patient is unable to do so.

E. The patient's _____ and _____ should be included in advising, drafting, and executing a legal advance directive and making sure that the patient's _____ and the _____ have copies of the _____ on file.

VII. Safety Guidelines for the Elderly Population
   1. The risk for personal injury increases after age _____.
   2. Provide a few examples of how safety can be improved in the following areas.
      A. Bathroom—

      _____

      _____

      B. Electrical cords—

      _____

      _____

      C. Emergency numbers—

      _____

      _____

      D. Floor wax—

      _____

      _____

      E. Furniture—

      _____

      _____

      F. Lighting—

      _____

      _____

      G. Rugs—

      _____

      _____

KEY TERMINOLOGY REVIEW

Match each of the following vocabulary terms to the correct definition.

a. ageism	d. extended-care facilities
b. assisted-living facilities	e. respite care
c. cognitive ability	

1. _____ Prejudice against and incorrect assumptions about an individual or individuals because of their age.

2. _____ The ability to think clearly, reason, and perceive that is affected by many factors.

3. _____ Temporary relief to individuals or families caring for a family member with a chronic condition, allowing time for relaxation.

4. _____ Facilities designed for residents who cannot live independently but do not require 24-hour care.

5. _____ Provides 24-hour specialized care for residents who require a high level of medical care and assistance for complex medical conditions and/or treatment.

APPLIED PRACTICE

Read the scenario and answer the questions that follow.

Scenario

Fredrick Alamar, age 73, presents to your office today for a physical and a flu vaccination. His daughter, Joyce, accompanies him to the appointment. Joyce mentions that her father has displayed increased confusion over the past 2 months. She is worried because dementia tends to "run in the family," and Mr. Alamar hasn't been the same since her mother, Mr. Alamar's wife of over 40 years, passed away unexpectedly. You, as a medical assistant, make notations of all of Joyce's concerns in the medical record. During the examination, Dr. Jensen asks Mr. Alamar and Joyce if the confusion tends to get worse at night. While Mr. Alamar is obviously uncomfortable about discussing his struggles with confusion, his daughter informs the physician that the confusion isn't worse at any particular time of the day.

1. Would Mr. Alamar's confusion be considered acute or chronic? Explain your answer.

_____

_____

_____

2. Considering the information provided, what other classification of confusion might apply to the patient's condition? Explain your answer.

_____

_____

_____

3. Why do you think Dr. Jensen asked if the confusion is worse at night?

_____

_____

_____

LEARNING ACTIVITY: MULTIPLE CHOICE

Circle the correct answer to each of the following questions.

1. By _____, all surviving baby boomers will have reached senior citizen status.
   a. 2019
   b. 2021
   c. 2025
   d. 2029

2. Which of the following is *not* an assistive device to aid older individuals?

   a. Handrails and grab bars
   b. Throw rugs
   c. Cane
   d. Bedside commode

3. Life expectancy is increasing due to which of the following?

   a. Better living conditions
   b. New medications
   c. Better nutrition
   d. All of the above

4. Factors that affect how we age include all except which of the following?

   a. Race
   b. Genetics
   c. Occupational hazards
   d. Lifestyle choices

5. Musculoskeletal system aging is characterized by

   a. increased muscle strength.
   b. liver spots.
   c. loss of flexibility.
   d. senile tremors.

6. Which of the following is a true statement concerning aging?

   a. Changes in sensorimotor abilities improve how the elderly interact with their environment.
   b. The loss of hearing, taste, smell, and mobility can lead to depression.
   c. The nervous system begins to speed up.
   d. All of the above

7. Urinary system changes that can occur with aging include

   a. decreased ability to concentrate urine.
   b. thyroid hypofunction.
   c. faster waste removal by the kidneys.
   d. orthostatic hypotension.

8. Which of the following is a controllable risk factor that plays a part in developing osteoporosis?

   a. Age
   b. Smoking
   c. Gender
   d. History of broken bones

9. The ability to think clearly, reason, and perceive is known as

   a. mental health.
   b. learning ability.
   c. cognitive ability.
   d. All of the above

10. Which of the following is *not* considered a normal, age-related memory change?

    a. Ability to follow written/spoken directions
    b. Using notes as reminders
    c. Forgetting entire experiences
    d. Ability to care for one's self

CRITICAL THINKING

Answer the following questions to the best of your ability. Use the textbook as a reference.

1. Explain how you can demonstrate respect to an elderly patient while communicating during patient care. How does ageism relate to this topic?

   _____

   _____

   _____

   _____

2. A 68-year-old patient named Mrs. Royer has come in today because she says she is depressed. Her family thinks she has the early stages of dementia, but she doesn't agree with them. Explain the diagnosing criteria used to evaluate depression. How might a physician determine if Mrs. Royer is truly depressed?

   _____

   _____

   _____

   _____

   _____

RESEARCH ACTIVITY

Use Internet search engines to research the following topic and write a brief description of what you find. It is important to use reputable websites.

1. In addition to what is mentioned in your textbook, research assistive aids that can help elderly patients with their daily activities. What aids do you think might be the most helpful? Which would you be most likely to recommend to future patients? Why?

   _____

   _____

   _____

   _____

CHAPTER 41
Assisting with Minor Surgery

STUDENT STUDY GUIDE

Use the following guide to assist in your learning of the concepts from the chapter.

I. The Medical Assistant's Role in Minor Surgery

  1. Administrative Duties Performed Prior to Surgery

    A. Completing _____ forms

    B. Obtaining _____ forms

    C. Meeting with the _____ to answer _____ related to the procedure

  2. Prior to Beginning Surgery

    A. Setting up the _____ _____ with the instruments and equipment necessary for the specific procedure

  3. During Procedure/Surgery

    A. Adding _____ to the sterile field

    B. Handing _____ _____ the provider (provided that the MA has properly scrubbed and is wearing sterile gloves)

  4. After Procedure/Surgery

    A. Providing _____ instructions to the patient

    B. Cleaning the _____ room after the surgery

    C. Sanitizing and _____ or _____ the instruments used

    D. Restocking _____ as needed

  5. List the items needed when setting up a tray for a typical surgical procedure.

    A. _____

    B. _____

    C. _____

    D. _____

    E. _____

    F. _____

    G. _____

    H. _____

    I. _____

J. _____

K. _____

L. _____

M. _____

N. _____

II. Ambulatory Surgery

1. Ambulatory surgery is performed on a person who is _____ and _____ from a surgical facility on the _____ day.

2. Ambulatory surgery results in cost savings for the _____ and the _____.

3. Each ambulatory facility should develop a consistent _____ procedure to track the patient's _____ after leaving.

4. Outpatient surgery is generally limited to procedures requiring less than _____ minutes to _____.

5. List the categories of surgeries described here.

A. _____—Considered medically necessary but can be performed when the patient wishes

B. _____—Required immediately to save a life or prevent further injury or infection

C. _____—May not be medically necessary, but the patient wishes to have it performed

D. _____—Does not require an overnight stay in a hospital

E. _____—Performed as soon as possible but is not an immediate or acute emergency

III. Principles of Surgical Asepsis

1. Sterile technique results in the killing of all _____ and _____.

2. Surgical asepsis is necessary during any _____ procedure.

3. Requirements of Surgical Asepsis

A. A sterile hand _____ or _____

B. Sterile _____

C. Sterile _____ when handling materials

4. Guidelines for Surgical Asepsis (See Guidelines 41-1 in the textbook.)

A. A sterile item can only touch a(n) _____ item.

B. A sterile item on a sterile field must be within your field of _____ and above your _____.

C. _____ microorganisms contaminate sterile fields.

D. Edges of a sterile field are _____.

E. Sterile _____ must only touch sterile items.

F. Sterile packets may be touched on the _____ with _____ hands.

G. Be honest if you make a(n) _____ or suspect that you have made an error.

5. Surgical Scrubs and Sterile Gloving

A. A surgical scrub removes microorganisms more effectively than regular _____ _____.

B. Hands should be as free from _____ as possible in the event that sterile gloves are _____ during a procedure.

C. If a sterile glove is _____ or if you touch the outside of the glove with your hand, the glove is considered _____ and must be replaced after you perform another _____ scrub.

6. Sterile Packaging

A. Sterile packages (packets) are prepared for use in _____.

B. These packets are _____ with sterilization indicators and dated.

C. Packets are set up on a(n) _____ _____, a small portable table with enough room to hold an instrument tray.

D. After you open a sterile packet, the inside of its wrapper becomes the _____ _____.

E. If the field becomes wet, it is _____, and you must open a new _____.

F. When additional instruments are needed during a procedure, open a sterile packet and _____ the instrument carefully onto the _____ _____.

G. Sterile transfer

i. When placing items onto or moving them within a sterile field, you must put on _____ gloves or use _____ forceps.

ii. Do not _____ _____ the sterile field or turn your back on the field unless it is covered with a(n) _____ _____.

IV. Surgical Instruments

1. Instruments Used in Minor Surgery in an Office

A. Instruments are categorized based on their _____.

B. Instruments are usually made of _____ and treated to be _____ and heat resistant, stain-proof, and _____.

C. _____ instruments may be used for convenience.

2. Cutting Instruments

A. _____ or knives are used to make _____.

B. A scalpel _____ must be inserted into the scalpel handle.

3. Dissecting Instruments

    A. Scissors are used for _____ or to cut _____.

    B. The _____ of scissors vary greatly for performing a variety of

    _____.

    C. Some scissors have _____ tips that can slide under _____ and

    dressings to cut without damaging the _____.

4. Grasping and Clamping Instruments

    A. Forceps are used to grasp _____ or _____.

    B. Forceps often have _____ or _____ edges that prevent tissue from

    slipping out of the forceps.

    C. List the common types of forceps.

        i. _____

        ii. _____

        iii. _____

        iv. _____

        v. _____

        vi. _____

        vii. _____

5. Probing and Dilating Instruments

    A. These instruments are used to enter body cavities for _____ or

    _____ purposes.

    B. List six types of dilating and probing instruments.

        i. _____

        ii. _____

        iii. _____

        iv. _____

        v. _____

        vi. _____

6. Suture Materials and Needles

    A. Suture materials are used to bring together, or _____, a surgical incision or

    wound until _____ takes place.

    B. Absorbable sutures

        i. Absorbable sutures are _____ by tissue enzymes and _____ by

        the body tissues.

        ii. Absorption usually occurs _____ to _____ days after insertion.

iii. Types of absorbable sutures include _____ catgut, _____ catgut, and _____ catgut.

C. Nonabsorbable sutures

   i. Nonabsorbable sutures are used on skin _____ where they can easily be _____ after an incision heals.

D. Suture materials

   i. Suture materials _____ and are selected based on how they are _____.

   ii. List six types of suture materials.

     a. _____

     b. _____

     c. _____

     d. _____

     e. _____

     f. _____

   iii. Suture material is measured by the _____, or _____.

   iv. The _____ material is numbered 0, and the _____ is 000000 (6-0).

E. Suture needles

   i. Suture needles are available in different _____ and are chosen based on _____ they are used.

   ii. List three needle shapes.

     a. _____

     b. _____

     c. _____

F. List three other wound closure materials.

   i. _____

   ii. _____

   iii. _____

G. Guidelines for handling instruments

   i. Surgical instruments are _____ and may be _____.

   ii. Even slight _____ to an instrument can result in _____ at a critical time during surgery.

   iii. Disposable instruments should be disposed of in _____ containers or _____ containers as necessary.

iv. Care for reusable instruments includes the following.

    a. _____ used instruments in an appropriate solution

    b. Gently cleaning them of _____

    c. _____ them if needed

    d. _____ them to sterilize them

V. Surgical Assisting

  1. Nonsterile Assistants

    A. Tasks of a nonsterile assistant

      i. _____ the patient

      ii. Using _____ _____ to bring additional supplies as needed

      iii. Holding the vial of _____ _____ while the surgeon draws up the correct dosage into a syringe

      iv. Applying _____

    B. List four other terms used for a nonsterile assistant.

      i. _____

      ii. _____

      iii. _____

      iv. _____

  2. Actions of a Good Assistant

    A. Anticipating the _____ of the physician

    B. Using care in handing _____ efficiently

    C. Taking care to ensure that _____ does not occur

    D. Accounting for all _____ and _____ used during the procedure

  3. Scrub Assistant

    A. A scrub assistant performs all procedures in _____ _____ clothing, using sterile technique.

    B. Responsibilities of a scrub assistant

      i. Arranging the _____ _____ to meet the operating physician's preferences

      ii. Handing _____

      iii. _____ bodily fluids away from the operative site

      iv. _____ the incision area

      v. Cutting suture _____

    C. Instruments should be passed to the physician firmly and _____ first.

4. Floating Assistant

A. A floating assistant performs _____ duties during a surgical procedure and "floats" between the _____ table, _____, and _____.

B. A major role is to monitor the patient by taking vital signs every ____ to ____ _____.

VI. Preparing the Patient for Minor Surgery

1. Patient Instructions

A. List five formats for providing preoperative and postoperative instructions.

   i. _____

   ii. _____

   iii. _____

   iv. _____

   v. _____

B. Some preoperative patient preparation can take place _____ the patient arrives for the _____.

C. Preoperative instructions may include the following.

   i. An explanation of what _____ _____ is needed and when it is to be done

   ii. _____ and _____ restrictions

   iii. Directions for special bathing/skin _____ preparations or cleansing enemas

   iv. Restrictions on bedtime _____ use

   v. Safe transportation home _____ the procedure

D. Postoperative instructions

   i. Patients should have a clear understanding of what to expect during _____ and how to care for the surgical _____ at home.

   ii. Clear instructions about postoperative medications should be given in _____ as well as _____ to the patient and possibly to _____ _____.

2. Informed Consent

A. The _____ must provide the patient with an honest, thorough explanation of the surgical _____, including the _____ and _____.

B. Written consent is required for the following.

   i. _____ procedures involving a scalpel, scissors, or another device

   ii. Procedures in which a(n) _____ _____ is entered for the purposes of visualization, though no _____ is made

C. The medical assistant can _____ the patient signing the consent form.

3. Positioning and Draping
   A. The patient should remove all _____ and put on a patient _____
      with the ties at the back, unless otherwise instructed.
   B. Have the patient _____ before assisting him/her onto the operating table.
   C. Place the patient in the proper _____ for the procedure.
   D. Ensure the patient's _____ because he/she may have to remain in one position
      for a(n) _____ period of time.
4. Anesthesia
   A. Medical assistants do not _____ anesthetics, but they should be
      _____ with them and their _____.
   B. General anesthesia
      i.   General anesthesia depresses the _____ nervous system to cause
           _____.
      ii. It can be administered through _____ or _____ injection.
      iii. _____ and _____ are usually administered intramuscularly
           before surgery.
   C. Local anesthesia
      i.   Local anesthesia provides a loss of _____ in a particular area of the body
           without overall loss of _____.
      ii. Describe the types of local anesthesia.
           a. Topical and local infiltration—_____.
           b. Nerve block—_____.
           c. Regional, spinal, epidural, or saddle block—_____.
5. Administering Anesthesia
   A. Only _____ or _____ can administer anesthetics.
   B. A medical assistant who draws up the medication must present both the _____
      and the _____ to the physician so that the physician can read the
      _____.
   C. If the physician draws up the anesthetic
      i.   It can be done using a(n) _____ _____ after the physician has
           applied gloves.
      ii. The medical assistant will hold the _____ securely while the physician
           withdraws the _____ without contaminating the needle.
      iii. The physician's _____ gloved hand cannot touch the _____ of
           the vial.

Assisting with Minor Surgery   **489**

6. Preparation of the Patient's Skin

    A. The patient's skin can be cleaned using _____ _____ technique.

    B. Careful cleansing of the skin _____ performing a surgical procedure will reduce the number of _____ on the skin.

    C. The physician may order the surgical site to be _____ because bacteria can reside in _____.

VII. Postoperative Patient Care

  1. Recovery from Anesthesia

    A. The effects of topical and local anesthetics wear off _____.

    B. Patients who are allergic to anesthesia may slip into _____ shock and require _____ treatment.

    C. After surgery, patients must be observed for signs of _____ _____ to the anesthetic, bleeding, and _____ problems.

    D. Vital signs should be monitored immediately after surgery and then every _____ minute(s) for the first _____.

    E. Oral medications for _____, _____, and _____ must be withheld until the patient is fully _____ from anesthesia.

  2. Types of Wounds (List the four types.)

    A. _____

    B. _____

    C. _____

    D. _____

  3. The Healing Process

    A. _____ is the body's protective response to trauma and invasion by _____.

    B. List four signs of inflammation.

      i. _____

      ii. _____

      iii. _____

      iv. _____

    C. Phases of healing

      i. Inflammatory phase (_____ days)—_____ _____ forms to stop bleeding and plug the opening of a wound; _____, or scab, forms to keep out microorganisms.

      ii. Proliferating phase (_____ to _____ days)—_____ threads extend across opening of the wound and pull edges _____; cells multiply to repair the wound.

iii. Maturation phase (_____ days to _____ years)—Tissue cells _____ and
_____ the wound closure and form a scar; the scar eventually
_____ and thins.

4. Wound Complications

    A. List four wound complications.

        i. _____

        ii. _____

        iii. _____

        iv. _____

    B. List four types of wound drainage.

        i. _____

        ii. _____

        iii. _____

        iv. _____

5. Cleansing a Wound

    A. Use a sterile gauze or swab and work from the clean area near the wound _____
    to _____ clean areas.

    B. Wipe in one _____ and then _____ the sterile swab or gauze.

    C. Cleanse a linear wound from _____ to _____ with one
    _____ per sterile gauze or swab.

    D. Use a new sterile gauze or swab for each _____.

    E. To cleanse an open wound, work in _____, beginning in the _____
    and working outward.

    F. Clean at least _____ _____ beyond the edge of the dressing to be
    applied or clean _____ _____ beyond the _____ of the
    wound if a dressing is not being applied.

    G. The size and shape of the dressing needed depend on the _____,
    _____, and amount of _____ from the wound.

    H. Inform the physician if a patient has not received a(n) _____ _____
    within the past 10 years.

6. Sutures

    A. Sutures used to attach tissues beneath the skin are often made of a(n) _____
    material.

    B. _____ sutures are made of nonabsorbable materials.

    C. If sutures remain in the body too long, they can cause skin _____ and
    _____.

D. Suture removal times differ depending on the _____.

E. The medical assistant prepares the patient for suture or staple removal by taking off the

_____.

F. Each edge of the dressing is removed by pulling _____ the suture

_____.

G. In some office _____ and in some _____, medical assistants are

permitted to remove sutures. (Procedure 41-8 in the textbook demonstrates suture removal.)

7. Sterile Dressing

A. A dressing is the application of a(n) _____ _____ over a surgical

site or wound using surgical _____.

8. Bandaging a Wound

A. The physician may instruct you to apply a bandage to _____ the dressing in

_____.

B. Bandages may be _____, _____, or _____ and need not

be sterile.

VIII. Surgical Procedures Performed in the Medical Office

1. List surgical procedures commonly performed the medical office.*

A. _____

B. _____

C. _____

D. _____

E. _____

F. _____

G. _____

H. _____

I. _____

KEY TERMINOLOGY REVIEW

Match each of the following vocabulary terms to the correct definition.

a. biopsy   d. eschar

b. cryosurgery   e. evisceration

c. dehiscence

1. _____ A scab.

2. _____ Microscopic examination of tissue to detect cancerous cells.

---

*These surgical procedures will be further discussed in other activities in this chapter.

3. _____ Separation of wound edges and protrusion of abdominal organs.
4. _____ The use of subfreezing temperatures to destroy tissue.
5. _____ Separation of wound edges.

APPLIED PRACTICE

Follow the directions as instructed for each activity.

Activity 1

Match each surgical procedure with its description.

a. colposcopy   f. cryosurgery
b. electrocautery   g. electrodessication
c. electrofulguration   h. endometrial biopsy
d. endoscopy   i. laser surgery
e. vasectomy

1. _____ Destroys tissue with a spark emitted from the tip of a probe positioned a short distance away from the unwanted tissue.

2. _____ The tying and cutting of the vas deferens, which is a surgical procedure that is now commonly performed in the urologist's office.

3. _____ Performed when an abnormal tissue development is observed by the physician during a routine pelvic examination.

4. _____ Performed to detect inflammatory conditions, if polyps are present, to assess abnormal uterine bleeding as well as the effects of hormone therapy.

5. _____ The use of subfreezing temperatures to destroy tissue, as in the treatment of cervical erosion and chronic cervicitis.

6. _____ Using a beam of light to treat a wide variety of diseases and conditions; it originally was used to treat diseases of the retina.

7. _____ Using high-frequency, alternating electric current to destroy, cut, or remove tissue.

8. _____ Destroying tissue by creating a spark gap when the probe is inserted into unwanted tissue.

9. _____ A procedure that uses an instrument to look into a hollow organ or body cavity such as the larynx, bladder, colon, sigmoid colon, stomach, abdomen, and some joints.

Activity 2

1. Using the information from the following patient chart, correctly identify the instruments that you would prepare for the procedure and briefly explain why the procedure is performed.

> Horsley, Will
> DOB: 10-26-1963
> 04/02/20XX, 12:45 P.M.
> Wt: 175 lbs., T: 98.6°F, P: 104, BP: 118/78
> cc: Pt presents to office complaining of a cut that appears to be inflamed. Upon examination, the area surrounding the cut is red and painful. The physician has requested that the patient be prepped for an I&D. I&D is successfully performed and the patient is discharged on antibiotics.
> Adam Bello, RMA

_____

_____

_____

_____

_____

LEARNING ACTIVITY: MULTIPLE CHOICE

Circle the correct answer to each of the following questions.

1. Which of the following types of drainage exhibits clear, watery drainage, such as the fluid in a blister?

    a. Serous drainage
    b. Sanguineous drainage
    c. Serosanguinous drainage
    d. Purulent drainage

2. Which of the following is an absorbable type of suture?

    a. Silk
    b. Nylon
    c. Chromic catgut
    d. Dacron

3. A wound that has torn edges in an irregular shape is a(n)

    a. puncture.
    b. laceration.
    c. abrasion.
    d. incision.

4. Which of the following is used to grasp foreign bodies?

    a. Tissue forceps
    b. Thumb forceps
    c. Splinter forceps
    d. Needle forceps

5. Laser (regarding surgery) is an acronym for

    a. length amplification by stimulated electricity and radiation.
    b. light application by sustained emission of radiation.
    c. length amplification by sustained emission of radiation.
    d. light amplification by stimulated emission of radiation.

6. Local anesthesia usually takes _____ to become effective.

    a. 20–30 minutes
    b. 40–55 minutes
    c. 5–15 minutes
    d. 1–3 minutes

7. Which of the following is *not* a sign of inflammation?

    a. Decreased drainage
    b. Warmth
    c. Swelling
    d. Pain

8. Sutures on the face are usually removed in
   a. 24–48 hours.
   b. 3–5 days.
   c. 5–7 days.
   d. 7–10 days.

9. Which of the following types of electrosurgery uses a current to incise and excise the tissue?
   a. Electrocoagulation
   b. Electrosection
   c. Electrofulguration
   d. All of the above

10. Which of the following is *not* needed on a tray setup for the removal of a foreign body?
    a. Straight iris scissors
    b. Tissue forceps
    c. Hemostats
    d. Blunt probe

CRITICAL THINKING

Answer the following questions to the best of your ability. Use the textbook as a reference.

1. Patient instructions should be given both orally and in writing. Patients may make many errors if instructions are not clear. Come up with a scenario that illustrates harm that could happen if a patient did not have any written instructions and did not remember the oral instructions provided by the physician or medical assistant.

   _____

   _____

   _____

   _____

2. During a sterile cyst-removal procedure, the physician reaches up to scratch her head briefly. She is wearing a nonsterile surgical cap, and no visible bodily fluids appear to be on her gloves. Has the sterile procedure been compromised? Take some time to think through this scenario and explain your thoughts.

   _____

   _____

   _____

   _____

RESEARCH ACTIVITY

◆

Use your textbook and Internet search engines to research the following topic and write a brief description of what you find. It is important to use reputable websites.

1. Conduct further research on one surgical procedure discussed in the textbook. What are the risks and complications associated with the procedure? How is the procedure performed? What instruments and supplies would be required to perform this procedure?

   _____

   _____

   _____

   _____

   _____

CHAPTER 42
Assisting with Medical Emergencies and Emergency Preparedness

STUDENT STUDY GUIDE

Use the following guide to assist in your learning of the concepts from the chapter.

I. Emergency Resources

  1. Medical Offices

    A. Medical offices provide treatment for conditions that pose no immediate danger to

    _____ or _____.

  2. Freestanding Clinics or Urgent Care Centers

    A. Freestanding clinics or urgent care centers provide treatment for conditions that need to be

    treated _____ but that are not life _____.

  3. Hospital Emergency Departments

    A. Hospital emergency departments provide treatment for most _____, including

    those that are _____ threatening.

  4. Critical Care Centers

    A. Critical care centers treat _____-threatening conditions that require

    _____ critical care.

  5. As a medical assistant, you should be aware of the emergency care _____ available

  in your _____.

  6. Emergency Medical Services

    A. EMS are established to provide _____ emergency care and safe and prompt

    _____ from any location to an appropriate facility.

    B. There are four levels of EMS practitioners.

      i. An emergency medical responder (EMR) can provide immediate _____

      life-saving care while awaiting response from a(n) _____-level EMS

      practitioner.

      ii. An emergency medical technician (EMT) can provide basic _____ medical

      care, administration of a few specific _____, and _____ to a

      hospital or other appropriate facility for definitive care.

  iii. An advanced emergency medical technician (AEMT) can provide basic emergency medical care, some _____ care, administration of a somewhat _____ _____ of medications, and transport.

  iv. A paramedic can provide all the care that an EMT or AEMT can provide plus a broad range of _____ emergency care, a much broader variety of _____, and transport.

 C. Roles played by EMS practitioners

  i. Providing on-the-scene _____ and _____

  ii. Preparing patients with _____, _____ or _____ for transport

  iii. Transporting patients to _____ facilities

  iv. Transferring patients to _____ _____ at receiving facilities

7. Specialized Resources

 A. A medical assistant will occasionally need to consult with specialists in such areas as _____ _____, _____, _____, and _____.

8. Good Samaritan Laws

 A. A health care professional who _____ in an emergency situation in which duty is not owed a victim is generally protected by various _____ laws that hold the medical professional not _____ _____ when rendering first aid.

 B. Health care professionals should be aware of the laws in their own _____ and remember that they must meet the _____ of _____ within their licensure, certification, or training.

II. Guidelines for Providing Emergency Care

1. Medical assistants must stay up to date on the emergency plans of the _____, facility, and _____.

2. Medical assistants should be able to handle emergencies in three settings.

  i. On the _____

  ii. When a(n) _____ occurs near the doctor's office and the patient is brought to the _____

  iii. When the emergency occurs in the _____ setting

3. A physician creates a(n) _____ tree, a map of what action to take in certain circumstances, for a medical assistant to use for _____.

4. Primary Screening and Assessment Steps

 A. Determine the patient's _____, approximate _____, and _____.

B. Determine the patient's need for _____.

C. Obtain the _____ of the event. Past _____ _____ is also important in emergency situations.

D. Gather _____ information.

E. Identify the patient's _____.

F. Take _____ _____.

III. Office Emergency Crash Kit

1. A crash kit, or _____ _____, contains all _____ that may be needed during an emergency and is instantly _____ to anyone in the office.

2. The emergency medical or _____ _____ is kept on or close to the crash cart.

3. Algorithms should be created before a(n) _____ and frequently _____ with staff to ensure that all are trained on how to perform as a team in _____ during an emergency.

4. A crash cart may contain items that are not within the _____ of _____ for a medical assistant.

5. The cart must be _____ after every use and maintained at least _____ a month on a regular basis, with _____ dates checked.

6. Crash cart supplies must include a(n) _____ that names every drug container and every piece of _____ the cart contains.

IV. Medical Emergencies*

1. Cardiopulmonary Resuscitation and Automated External Defibrillation**

A. Respiratory arrest and cardiac arrest may be caused by a(n) _____ airway, electrocution, _____, _____, heart attack, _____, anaphylaxis, drugs, _____, or traumatic _____ or _____ injury.

B. For individuals experiencing loss of _____ with abnormal or no breathing, follow the _____ _____ protocol.

    i. These guidelines vary somewhat according to _____ _____.

C. Defibrillation

    i. Automated external defibrillation is highly effective when provided _____ after or within minutes of _____ _____.

    ii. The AED gives _____ prompts to the rescuer or rescue team that are easy and _____ to follow.

---

*This section has been greatly summarized due to the vast number of procedures discussed.

**Carefully review the procedures in the text related to CPR, rescue breathing, and use of an AED.

2. Obstructed Airway

   A. An obstructed airway prevents the movement of _____ into or out of the respiratory tract.

   B. Certain conditions can cause a blockage from _____ of the upper airway tissue, but _____ _____ cause most obstructions.

   C. There are three types of choking scenarios.

      i. Partial airway obstruction with _____ air exchange

      ii. Partial airway obstruction with _____ air exchange

      iii. _____ airway obstruction

   D. Any time the patient can _____ or _____, air is moving in and out of the airway.

3. Respiratory Distress

   A. Respiratory distress may be a reaction to a long-term _____ disease, or a reaction to a(n) _____ situation, or the result of other disease _____.

   B. _____ control is usually not a factor in respiratory distress.

   C. One of the most serious conditions is a(n) _____ _____ that causes the patient to grasp at the neck and attempt to _____.

   D. List eight other signs and symptoms of respiratory distress.

      i. _____

      ii. _____

      iii. _____

      iv. _____

      v. _____

      vi. _____

      vii. _____

      viii. _____

   E. The physician may ask the medical assistant to administer _____ to the patient.

4. Shortness of Breath

   A. Any individual experiencing shortness of breath needs _____ _____.

   B. A patient experiencing shortness of breath may be _____ for air, looking _____ or cyanotic, and exhibiting nasal _____ and extreme _____.

5. Hyperventilation

   A. Hyperventilation is _____, shallow _____ or rapid,

       _____ breathing.

   B. It results in decreasing _____ _____ in the blood,

       _____ of blood vessels, and _____ blood pressure.

   C. List five signs and symptoms of hyperventilation in addition to faintness.

      i. _____

      ii. _____

      iii. _____

      iv. _____

      v. _____

6. Chronic Obstructive Pulmonary Disease

   A. List the three types of COPD.

      i. _____

      ii. _____

      iii. _____

   B. Air is trapped in the _____, and the patient is unable to expel all the carbon

     dioxide from the _____.

   C. Depending on the situation, the physician may order administration of _____,

     delivery of _____, or transport to a(n) _____ _____

     by EMS.

7. Pulmonary Edema

   A. Pulmonary edema results from _____ accumulation in the lung

     _____ and alveoli.

   B. List seven signs and symptoms of a patient presenting with pulmonary edema.

      i. _____

      ii. _____

      iii. _____

      iv. _____

      v. _____

      vi. _____

      vii. _____

8. Chest Pain

   A. Heart attacks are the leading _____ of _____ for both men and

     women.

B. Pain in the middle to left side of the chest can be described as _____, _____, crushing, _____, or aching.

C. The patient should sit down with feet _____, and the MA should obtain assistance from a(n) _____ to sit with the _____ while the MA informs the _____ of the situation.

D. If oxygen is available, administer it according to office protocol by _____ _____ until the physician or emergency personnel arrive.

E. If the patient has nitroglycerin tablets (from a diagnosis of angina), insert one tablet under the _____.

9. Shock

A. Shock is the collapse of the _____ system and is caused by insufficient cardiac _____.

B. List eight causes of shock.

i. _____

ii. _____

iii. _____

iv. _____

v. _____

vi. _____

vii. _____

viii. _____

C. Anaphylactic shock is a severe _____ _____ to a foreign substance.

i. The physician may order _____ with or without an antihistamine for a patient experiencing anaphylactic shock.

ii. _____ is the most important factor in anaphylactic shock.

iii. In offices where _____ and _____ injections are given on a regular basis, you must be alert to possible _____ and prepared with an emergency drug box for rapid _____.

D. Assisting patients in shock

i. Common signs of shock include pale, _____, or bluish _____; _____, cool skin; _____ pupils; a weak, rapid _____; shallow, rapid _____; and extreme _____.

ii. When a patient exhibits signs of shock, ensure that that patient has an open _____ and proper _____.

iii. Most emergency treatments for shock patients need to be administered by a(n) _____ or _____ personnel.

10. Diabetic Emergencies
   A. _____ is a low blood sugar level, whereas _____ is a high blood sugar level.
   B. A diabetic patient with _____ is at higher risk than one who has hyperglycemia.
      i. The patient may appear intoxicated, have _____, _____ skin, and be anxious or _____.
      ii. Intervention must be _____ and should involve some form of _____ administration.
      iii. Grave danger occurs when blood glucose falls below _____ mg/dL.
11. Bleeding
   A. External bleeding occurs when the _____ is broken.
   B. Internal bleeding occurs with _____ damage and intact _____.
   C. Arterial bleeding is usually copious, _____, and bright _____ and often spurts, echoing the _____.
      i. Apply pressure directly over the _____ and elevate the injured part higher than the _____ to help control bleeding.
   D. _____ blood flows more slowly, is _____ in color, and can usually be controlled by _____ _____.
12. Epistaxis
   A. Nontraumatic epistaxis is a(n) _____ not caused by a(n) _____.
   B. A nosebleed that occurs after a(n) _____ _____ and does not stop should be considered a serious _____.
   C. List circumstances for worry related to persistent nosebleeds.
      i. _____
      ii. _____
      iii. _____
   D. Bleeding from _____ _____ is likely to be more serious than bleeding from just _____ _____.
   E. If _____ is a possible cause, the physician may want 911 to be contacted for transport to the _____ department.
13. Open Wounds
   A. Open wounds are seldom life threatening, unless they penetrate the _____, _____, _____, or _____.
   B. They _____ require irrigation, _____, _____, and antibiotics.

C. List the five types of open wounds discussed in the textbook.

    i. _____

    ii. _____

    iii. _____

    iv. _____

    v. _____

14. Soft Tissue Injuries

A. Soft tissue trauma involves both the _____ and underlying _____.

B. _____, amputations, and _____ are considered soft tissue injuries because underlying _____ as well as skin are involved.

C. _____ are closed soft tissue wounds in which the skin is not broken.

D. For soft-tissue injuries, _____ the body part above the _____ and applying cold are often the only interventions needed.

E. With a more severe injury, the body part should be _____.

15. Wound Care Pointers

A. A dressing is a sterile covering placed directly over a wound to absorb _____ and other body _____, prevent _____, and protect the wound from further _____.

B. A bandage is a strip of _____ _____ used to hold a dressing in place.

C. Simple direct _____ with a dressing will usually stop _____ from a soft tissue injury.

D. Dressing a wound properly helps prevent _____.

    i. Cleanse the wound from the _____ outward, beginning with vigorous irrigation using a(n) _____ solution prescribed by the physician.

    ii. Wipe the edges of the wound in all directions _____ from the wound with _____ gauze.

    iii. Cover with a(n) _____ _____ and fasten the dressing in place.

    iv. Use _____ ointments if directed to do so by the physician.

E. Once bleeding is controlled and the wound dressed, obtain a complete set of _____ _____.

16. Burns

A. The following are some possible causes of burns.

    i. Physical _____

    ii. _____ activity

iii. High _____ current

iv. Heavy exposure to _____

B. The severity of a burn depends on the _____ and _____ of tissue injury.

17. Classification of Burns

A. The _____ of _____ is a useful tool for estimating body surface area.

B. For an adult, each of the following areas represents 9 percent of the body surface.

i. _____

ii. _____

iii. _____

iv. _____

v. _____

vi. _____

vii. _____

viii. _____

C. The _____ region is assigned 1 percent.

D. Percentages are modified for _____ and young children, whose heads are much larger in relationship to the rest of the body.

E. Describe burn severity by depth (refer to Table 42-6 in the textbook).

i. Superficial burn (_____ degree)—_____

_____

ii. Partial thickness (_____ degree)—_____

_____

iii. Full thickness (_____ degree)—_____

_____

iv. Full thickness (_____ degree)—_____

_____

18. Treatment of Burns

A. Treatment for superficial burns involving less than _____ percent of the body surface includes the following.

i. Pain relief by applying _____ _____

ii. Analgesic _____ and _____ if ordered by the physician

B. Partial thickness burns should never be treated with _____ or

_____ because of the risk of breaking blisters and the resulting potential for

_____.

C. Burns of any kind that involve broken skin may need to be _____ by a physician.

D. Full thickness burns of any size warrant treatment at a(n) _____ center or _____ center.

E. Burns should be dressed with _____ _____ dressings.

F. Large surface-area burns should be dressed with dry sterile _____ that are wrapped entirely around the patient's _____.

G. All burn patients should be monitored for signs of _____.

19. Heat- and Cold-Related Emergencies

A. Heat exhaustion

   i. Heat exhaustion is extreme _____ caused by heat that occurs as a result of _____ and _____ depletion from the body.

   ii. Skin is _____, pale, and _____, and body temperature is _____.

   iii. The individual may complain of _____, muscle _____, weakness, dizziness, and _____.

   iv. Apply _____ _____ and give sips of water if the individual is conscious.

B. Hyperthermia

   i. Prolonged _____ to extremely _____ temperatures often results in _____ body temperature.

   ii. It can progress to heat stroke, which occurs when the person fails to _____ and has a body temperature of _____°F or higher.

   iii. If the patient remains exposed to heat, _____ cells begin to die.

   iv. Permanent _____ damage or even _____ may eventually result.

   v. Cool the body down as quickly as possible by _____ cool water over the patient or _____ with a cool, wet cloth.

   vi. Call _____ for transport to an emergency facility.

C. Hypothermia

   i. Hypothermia results from prolonged exposure to _____ or cold _____ and can cause the core temperature to drop below _____°F.

   ii. The patient becomes _____ and eventually unconscious as body functions and organs _____ _____ to the point of complete shutdown.

   iii. Treatment involves removing any cold, wet _____ and wrapping the patient in _____ _____.

iv. The patient should be transported to a treatment facility for assessment by a(n) _____.

20. Seizures*

A. Also called convulsions, seizures are produced by disorganized _____ _____ in the brain.

B. Convulsions can be _____, involving the entire body, or _____ and limited to a specific area of the body.

C. Muscle spasms that come with full-body seizures can restrict _____.

D. Seizure patients may also bite their tongues, causing _____ and _____, which can _____ the airway.

E. Patients may be _____ if a convulsion causes them to fall.

F. A medical assistant can do the following to help a seizing patient.

   i. Prevent _____

   ii. Pay close attention to what the patient is _____ in order to be able to _____ it later

G. Never place anything in the _____ of a seizing patient.

21. Fainting**

A. Fainting, or _____, is sudden loss of _____ sometimes preceded by _____.

B. Patients seldom become _____ or have _____ as a result of simple fainting but may be injured in the course of a fall.

22. Musculoskeletal Injuries

A. Fractures

   i. With a closed or _____ fracture, the bone is broken but does not _____ the skin.

   ii. In an open or _____ fracture, the bone pierces the skin, or the skin is torn open by the bone or by an external force.

   iii. Bone breaks can be _____, _____, or splintered.

   iv. Special precautions must be taken for suspected fractures of the _____ column or _____, and only _____ professionals should stabilize the patient for transport.

   v. Suspected fractures of the _____ and _____ are always severe and dangerous injuries that require _____ and _____ and are best handled by EMS.

---

*Review the procedure in the textbook related to performing first aid for a patient having a seizure.

**Review the procedure in the textbook related to assisting a patient with fainting.

© 2018 Pearson Education, Inc.

B. Splint application

    i. Fractures of _____ bones require immobilization by splinting to prevent joint movement _____ and _____ the fracture.

    ii. After applying a splint, applying a(n) _____ _____ can help with swelling.

23. Sprains, Strains, and Dislocations

A. A(n) _____ occurs when muscles, tendons, or ligaments are torn.

B. A(n) _____, often called a pulled muscle, occurs when a muscle or tendon is overextended by stretching.

C. A(n) _____ occurs when the bone is actually pulled away from the joint, stretching or tearing the ligaments and tendons.

D. The physician assesses the injury and usually orders _____ to eliminate the possibility of _____ and diagnose sprain, strain, or dislocation.

V. Emergency Preparedness

1. Through proper _____, _____, and _____, a medical assistant can play a key role in emergency response.

2. Earthquakes

A. Earthquakes can happen at any _____ and without any _____.

B. FEMA has identified six steps for planning ahead for an earthquake.

    i. Check for _____ around the facility.

    ii. Identify safe places _____ and _____.

    iii. _____ yourself and your coworkers.

    iv. Have _____ _____ on hand.

    v. Develop a(n) _____ _____ plan.

    vi. Help your _____ get ready.

3. Tornadoes

A. Tornadoes are the most _____ storms occurring in nature and can strike with little or no warning.

B. A tornado watch indicates that the _____ conditions are right for a tornado and a tornado is _____.

C. A tornado warning indicates that a tornado has been _____, and all persons are to take shelter _____.

D. Designate a(n) _____ _____ within the office where people can take shelter if a tornado watch occurs during working hours.

    i. The best location is the _____ of a building or the _____ level of a structure.

ii. If a basement is not available, it is advisable to seek shelter in a(n) _____ or an interior _____.

iii. Stay away from _____, _____ and _____ _____.

4. Hurricanes

   A. Most hurricanes allow for some _____ warning, giving the medical office staff time to _____.

   B. Medical office windows may need to be _____; this can be done using permanent _____ _____ or 5/8-inch plywood cut to fit and ready to install.

   C. It is important to listen to the radio or television for _____ and _____ provided by local emergency management personnel.

5. Floods

   A. Floods are considered the most common _____ in the United States.

   B. In the event of a(n) _____ _____, move to higher ground.

   C. If there is time before evacuating, the medical assistant should _____ any electrical equipment and shut off _____ at their main valves.

   D. Be careful not to walk through _____ water.

6. Fires

   A. In just _____ minutes, a fire can become life threatening.

   B. In _____ minutes, a fire can engulf a building.

   C. _____ and _____ from fire are often more dangerous than the flames.

   D. Smoke alarms should be placed on every _____ of the building and in every _____.

   E. Every smoke alarm should be tested and cleaned _____ per _____.

   F. Staff members should _____ escape routes.

   G. _____ _____ should be located throughout the office, and staff should be trained in their use.

   H. Crawl _____ under any smoke on the way to the exit and close _____ as you pass through them to delay the _____ of fire.

7. Terrorism

   A. Explosions

      i. List the questions you should ask the caller if a bomb threat is made.

         a. _____

         b. _____

    c. _____

    d. _____

    e. _____

  ii. Immediately provide all information to the _____.

B. Biological threats

  i. Biological agents can be spread through _____, _____, or

    _____.

  ii. The _____ classifies biological terrorism agents into three categories.

  iii. Category _____ agents are the highest risk.

  iv. List the seven biological agents discussed in the text.

    a. _____

    b. _____

    c. _____

    d. _____

    e. _____

    f. _____

    g. _____

  v. To prepare for a biological attack, the medical facility should have a(n)

    _____ filter installed.

  vi. In the event of a biological attack, the MA should do the following.

    a. Move away from the contaminant _____.

    b. Wash with _____ and _____.

    c. Contact _____.

    d. Listen to the _____ for instructions.

    e. _____ and _____ clothing if contaminated.

C. Nuclear blasts

  i. Take _____ as quickly as possible.

  ii. Remain in a(n) _____ location, listening to the radio for

    _____.

  iii. Lie _____ on the ground with your head _____.

8. Mock Environmental Exposure

A. Organizations within the _____, _____, and _____

may offer mock environmental exposure events.

B. These events provide _____-life _____ and situations that may

arise during times of disaster.

C. List ways an MA can provide assistance.

    i. Aiding in _____ plans

    ii. _____ patients to determine which patients require _____ attention

    iii. Assisting in _____ response for wounded individuals

    iv. Administering _____ and other _____ under the direction of a physician

    v. Facilitating _____ and _____ in the midst of chaos

    vi. Implementing and following through on an environmental _____ _____ plan

9. Community Resources

A. List three examples of community resources related to disasters.

    i. _____

    ii. _____

    iii. _____

B. The Department of Homeland Security has stated that the best way to prepare for a disaster is to get a(n) _____, make a(n) _____, be _____, and get _____.

KEY TERMINOLOGY REVIEW

Match each of the following key terms to the correct definition.

a. anaphylactic shock
b. EMT
c. AEMT

d. hyperglycemia
e. hypothermia

1. _____ A health care professional who can provide basic emergency medical care, administration of a few specific medications, and transport to a hospital or other appropriate facility for definitive care.

2. _____ High blood sugar level.

3. _____ A severe allergic reaction that causes respiratory distress because of swelling of the upper airways.

4. _____ A core temperature below 95°F.

5. _____ A health care professional who can provide basic emergency medical care, some advanced care, administration of a somewhat broader range of medications, and transport.

APPLIED PRACTICE

Read the scenarios and then answer the questions that follow.

Scenario A

Sasha Daniels, CMA (AAMA), is employed at Community Urgent Care. A 47-year-old male patient has been brought to the facility. His right index finger was partially torn from his hand while he was working on a piece of farming machinery. His coworker has driven him to the medical facility.

1. What type of injury has this man sustained?

   _____

   _____

   _____

2. Explain how his injury would be treated.

   _____

   _____

   _____

   _____

Scenario B

Dr. Connors has decided to hold a community seminar titled "Preparing for Natural Disasters." You are her medical assistant, and she has asked you to help her prepare for the seminar by compiling a list of reputable resources to gather helpful information. She also would like for you to choose topics that could be highlighted for discussion throughout the seminar.

1. Which websites would you recommend as reputable resources to gather information for the seminar?

   _____

   _____

   _____

2. What should be considered when choosing topics for the seminar?

   _____

   _____

   _____

LEARNING ACTIVITY: TRUE/FALSE

Indicate whether the following statements are true or false by placing a T or an F on the line that precedes each statement.

_____ 1. An AED can be used on children ages 1 to 8 years old.

_____ 2. An amputation is also known as an avulsion.

_____ 3. A nosebleed that occurs after a head injury and does not stop should be considered a serious emergency until proven otherwise.

_____ 4. In general, perform CPR first for unresponsive children and infants before activating emergency response systems.

_____ 5. Shock, the collapse of the cardiovascular system, is caused by excessive cardiac output.

_____ 6. Blood from arterial bleeding is usually slow and pale red.

_____ 7. Simple direct pressure with a dressing will usually stop bleeding from a soft tissue injury.

_____ 8. Heat exhaustion occurs with a body temperature of 105°F or higher.

_____ 9. The severity of a burn depends on the surface area and depth of tissue injury.

_____ 10. Once a seizure stops, especially a full-body seizure, it is normal for a patient to remain unconscious for as long as 2 hours.

CRITICAL THINKING

Answer the following questions to the best of your ability.

1. Consider the physical and emotional impact an emergency situation has on an individual. For example, assume that you volunteer with the American Red Cross to provide disaster relief to a flooded city that has been evacuated. How might this experience impact you?

   _____

   _____

   _____

   _____

2. Pretend you work as a medical assistant in the front office of a nephrology practice. The practice is located on the third floor of a large building. Suddenly, you hear the building's fire alarm sound, and you can see smoke in the hallway. How would you respond to and handle this emergency situation? (Try not to refer to the textbook and rather recall the information you have already learned regarding responding to a fire.)

   _____

   _____

   _____

   _____

   _____

RESEARCH ACTIVITY

Use Internet search engines to research the following topic and write a brief description of what you find. It is important to use reputable websites.

1. Search for CPR certification agencies in your area. What agencies offer CPR? Do these agencies also offer basic first aid? Are professional-level certifications available? What are the costs associated with various certification levels? Which agency in your area would you recommend to a patient who is interested in becoming CPR certified?

   _____

   _____

   _____

   _____

CHAPTER 43
The Clinical Laboratory

STUDENT STUDY GUIDE

Use the following guide to assist in your learning of the concepts from the chapter.

I. The Role of the Clinical Laboratory in Patient Care

1. Clinical laboratory test results help the patient in the following ways.

    A. _____ for disease

    B. _____ a condition suspected by the physician

    C. _____ _____ a condition

    D. Establishing a(n) _____ level before medication administration

    E. Monitoring _____ of medication or treatment

    F. Assessing the _____ of disease

2. A qualitative test result is typically _____ or _____ for the presence of a specific substance.

3. A quantitative test gives a(n) _____ value.

4. Always determine the _____ _____ associated with the specific laboratory and test before _____ results.

II. Types of Clinical Laboratories

1. Outside Laboratory

    A. An outside laboratory can be either a(n) _____-based or a(n) _____ laboratory.

    B. An outside laboratory handles specimens collected from many types of _____ and performs tests ranging from _____ to very _____.

    C. A medical assistant may be employed in one of these laboratories as a(n) _____ or as a(n) _____ assistant.

2. Reference Laboratory

    A. A reference laboratory may be associated with a(n) _____ hospital or a(n) _____ school, or it may be _____ owned.

    B. A reference laboratory handles tests that are more _____ and often infrequently _____.

3. Physician's Office Laboratory

   A. Some of the _____ that a physician orders are performed right in the _____.

   B. The doctor has the advantage of receiving the results more _____ than if tests are done _____ the office.

   C. Disadvantages of in-house testing are that it may require more _____ and the purchase of _____ _____.

III. The Medical Assistant's Role in the Clinical Laboratory

   1. For the medical assistants working in a laboratory, training in _____ and basic knowledge of _____ _____ is essential.

   2. Record Management

   A. Make sure that the physician's _____ is clearly recorded and the proper _____ _____ are completed.

   B. In-house _____ and _____ must be charted.

   C. Results should be _____ and carefully _____.

   D. A(n) _____ will be transported with specimens that are collected at the physician's office and sent out for testing.

      i. Label the requisition form _____ if the physician wants results immediately for a medical _____.

      ii. Use the laboratory requisition slip designed specifically for the _____ that will receive it.

   E. With POL testing, it is imperative that _____ results be _____ recorded as soon as possible.

      i. A good note states the following.

         a. _____

         b. _____

         c. _____

         d. _____

   3. Paper Versus Electronic Documentation

   A. When paper records are utilized, test results may be _____, couriered, _____, or called in.

      i. If a result is flagged as high _____, always bring it to the _____ attention of the practitioner.

   B. With electronic health records, many offices can _____ with outside labs through the _____.

      i. Test results are _____ accessible, and abnormal results are often _____ or marked for easier identification.

4. Flowcharts, Tables, and Graphs
  A. Flowcharts, tables, and graphs can facilitate the _____ of data and can be shared with patients when educating them on _____ in their health.
  B. Flowcharts, tables, and graphs are often generated by _____ software and allow the physician to make the best plan of care for the patient.
  C. Flow sheets are charts used to evaluate a patient's _____ and response to _____ over time.
    i. With _____ documentation, flow sheets can be generated to _____ the _____ that occur from test to test.

5. Patient Preparation
  A. A fasting specimen means that the patient must not _____ anything other than _____ for a prescribed number of hours _____ collecting the specimen.
  B. _____ (PP), or post cibum (pc), means "after a(n) _____."
    i. A 2-hour PP or pc glucose means that a blood glucose level is drawn exactly _____ hours after completion of the prescribed _____.
  C. The MA should explain special _____ for laboratory tests, which may include the following.
    i. Dietary or _____ restrictions
    ii. _____ limitations
    iii. _____ requirements
    iv. Special _____
  D. Explain to the patient that results may be _____ if directions are not properly followed, and _____ might be required.
  E. Many medical practitioners prefer to speak _____ to the patient about results that are significantly _____.
  F. Other physicians routinely expect _____ _____ to contact patients for them in order to relay new orders or _____.

6. Specimen Management
  A. A specimen is a small _____ taken from the _____.
  B. List five common specimens.
    i. _____
    ii. _____
    iii. _____
    iv. _____
    v. _____

C. It is vital to properly _____ and _____ a specimen to ensure that it truly represents the patient's body functions.

D. Each lab has its own policies regarding which specimen _____ to use and how much to _____.

   i. Some specimens need to be _____, spun, or have _____ added to them.

E. Complications of specimen collection include the following.

   i. Cells may _____ or _____ if there is difficulty drawing blood.

   ii. Accidental _____ or collection in the wrong _____ may occur.

   iii. Exposure to _____ or direct _____ may cause damage.

   iv. If _____ than the required amount of a specimen is collected, testing may not be possible.

F. Avoid collecting a specimen from the wrong patient by using a three-step identification process.

   i. Check the chart to _____ the order.

   ii. During introductions, ask the patient to state his or her _____ _____ and _____ of _____.

   iii. Compare the information the _____ has given with the _____ to verify that this is the right patient.

G. Information needed when labeling a specimen includes two _____ and the date and _____ collected.

7. Quality Assurance (QA)

A. A quality assurance program includes mechanisms for the following.

   i. Evaluating laboratory _____ and _____

   ii. Identifying and correcting _____

   iii. Ensuring _____ and _____ reporting of results and testing by _____ individuals

B. Steps for QA in the laboratory include the following.

   i. Most offices and laboratories have a policies and procedures _____ with a set of routine _____ to follow.

   ii. Checklists generally include the following.

     a. Keeping the lab and patient areas _____

     b. _____ supplies to ensure that the correct _____ are available

     c. Checking _____ instructions and _____ dates for all reagents and test kits

iii. QA includes the following.

   a. Routinely reviewing _____ manuals and testing _____ and following the most recent _____ instructions for correct test performance.

   b. Scheduling or _____ routine equipment maintenance, including _____, to ensure accuracy of results, should always be properly _____.

C. Maintenance

   i. A written record of the maintenance performed must be readily available.

   ii. A record of each piece of equipment with _____ and _____ numbers, date of _____, and manufacturers' _____ should be available when repair is necessary or the laboratory is being _____.

D. Documentation

   i. Documentation of _____ records and _____ logs is important for QA.

   ii. Document daily equipment _____ and _____ testing as well as daily testing with _____ _____ and measurements to assure the _____ of results.

   iii. Monitor and document _____ controls of strips and equipment.

8. Quality Control (QC)

A. Quality control is focused on physical _____ that results are _____.

B. QC is accomplished by routinely performing _____ tests, using one of two predetermined methods.

   i. Calibration devices are specially prepared _____ _____ or _____ that are designed to produce a(n) _____ result.

   ii. _____ _____ are chemicals that produce an expected result.

C. In either case, the _____ should fall within the acceptable _____ listed on the calibration device or control solution bottle.

D. List three causes of abnormal QC results.

   i. _____

   ii. _____

   iii. _____

E. Quality control tests are performed according to manufacturer _____ and _____ policy, often _____.

   i. Results are recorded in a quality control _____.

IV. Laboratory Safety Regulations

    1. _____ enforces the Centers for Disease Control and Prevention's Universal or _____ _____ in health care.

    2. OSHA Regulations

        A. Two programs of standards under the OSHA umbrella impact the clinical laboratory.

            i. _____ hazards

            ii. _____ pathogens

        B. The "general duty clause" means that all _____ must provide a safe work environment, free of _____ that may cause serious _____ or _____.

    3. Clinical Laboratory Improvement Amendments (CLIA)

        A. CLIA was developed by the Centers for _____ & _____ Services in response to widespread concern about the _____ of laboratory tests.

        B. List the three categories of CLIA laboratories.

            i. _____

            ii. _____

            iii. _____

        C. Medical assistants are only qualified to perform _____ testing.

        D. CLIA waived tests frequently come in _____ test kit sets.

        E. Many _____ analyzers are also CLIA waived.

            i. An analyzer is typically a small or _____ machine that processes a specimen with single-use _____ test strips or _____.

        F. A facility is required to have a(n) _____ of _____ from the Centers for Medicare & Medicaid Services so that its employees can _____ perform simple tests to prevent, _____, or _____ a disorder or disease.

        G. To maintain CLIA waived status, facilities must permit _____ _____, as requested.

        H. A medical assistant employed in a facility with a PPM certificate can perform _____-complexity tests with further _____ and under the supervision of a laboratory _____ or physician.

V. Laboratory Equipment

    1. Autoclave

        A. An autoclave is used to _____ equipment or _____ that are used on patients or in certain test procedures.

2. Centrifuge

   A. A centrifuge separates specimens into _____ layers by spinning samples at _____ speed, allowing _____ components to float to the top and _____ components to sink to the bottom.

3. Photometer

   A. A photometer is an instrument that measures _____ _____.

4. Incubator

   A. An incubator is used to maintain a specific _____ to achieve a specific result.

5. Microscope*

   A. Microscopes are frequently used in the medical office to examine _____ sediment, _____ and bacteriological smears, and _____ smears.

   B. List the two sets of lenses on a compound microscope.

      i. _____

      ii. _____

   C. The _____ of a microscope refers to the ability to distinguish clearly between two adjacent but _____ objects.

   D. Using a microscope

      i. The magnification of an object is calculated by multiplying the _____ magnification by the _____ magnification.

      ii. It is important to use the correct _____ for the type of microscopic work to be done.

         a. Low-power objective (10×)—Used to view _____ cells

         b. High dry setting (40×)—Used for _____ RBCs, WBCs, or _____ RBCs

         c. Oil immersion setting (100×)—Used for differential _____ smears or _____ slides

   E. Care of a microscope (Refer to Guidelines 43-1.)

      i. Follow _____ requirements during mandatory _____ maintenance.

      ii. Always use _____ _____ to carry a microscope.

      iii. Clean oculars, objectives, and stage using only _____ paper and _____ cleaner.

      iv. Keep extra _____ _____ on hand.

      v. Document _____ and _____ in a logbook.

_____
*Parts of a microscope will be covered in a separate activity.

vi. Store a microscope with the electrical cord wrapped _____ around the base.

vii. Cover the microscope with a(n) _____ _____ when it is not in use.

KEY TERMINOLOGY REVIEW

Match each of the following key terms to the correct definition.

a. CLIA waived test

b. incubator

c. qualitative test

d. photometer

e. quantitative test

1. _____ A test whose result is typically positive or negative for the presence of a specific substance.

2. _____ A test that is simple enough for a patient to perform at home with basic instructions.

3. _____ An instrument that measures light intensity.

4. _____ A test whose results are usually numerical values.

5. _____ An instrument used to maintain a specific temperature to achieve a specific result.

APPLIED PRACTICE

Follow the directions as instructed for each question.

1. Label the parts of the compound microscope.

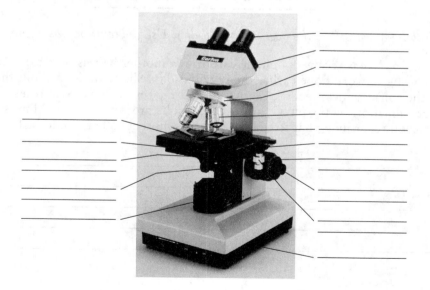

2. Clark LaRiccia has come to the office with complaints of increased thirst, urination, and weight loss, even though he hasn't been trying to lose weight. Dr. Simmons recognizes these as symptoms of diabetes. He wants the patient's blood glucose level tested in the office using a glucometer. Mr. LaRiccia's blood glucose results are very high, at 278 mg/dL. What level of CLIA testing would blood glucose testing (using a glucometer) be considered? Is this a test an MA could perform? Are the results that were obtained by the glucometer considered qualitative or quantitative?

_____

_____

_____

_____

LEARNING ACTIVITY: TRUE/FALSE

Indicate whether the following statements are true or false by placing a T or an F on the line that precedes each statement.

_____ 1. A binocular microscope has one ocular lens.

_____ 2. On a microscope, the diaphragm control moves the slide up and down and back and forth.

_____ 3. On a microscope, the revolving nosepiece holds objectives and rotates for selection.

_____ 4. On a microscope, coarse and fine adjustment knobs are used for focusing.

_____ 5. When you are finished working with a microscope, you must clean the lenses with a soft cloth or paper.

CRITICAL THINKING

Answer the following questions to the best of your ability. Use the textbook as a reference.

1. Clara Jones, RMA, has received a phone call from a mother who is worried about her 8-year-old son, who had bloodwork done earlier the previous day. She is anxious about the results. Upon reviewing the son's medical record, Clara sees that the results have been received but haven't been reviewed or signed off by the physician. All the results are within normal limits. Clara needs to make a decision regarding what to tell the patient's mother. What would be her best course of action?

_____

_____

_____

_____

_____

2. Recall Mr. LaRiccia from the scenario in the Applied Practice activity earlier. The physician explains to the patient that the results of his blood glucose test are indicative of diabetes, and further testing needs to be done. After the physician leaves the room, you begin to review the physician's instructions with the patient regarding blood tests that need to be performed on him. The patient starts to argue with you, saying that no one in his family is diabetic, and he eats healthily. He doesn't believe that the test results completed in the office are accurate, and he doesn't intend to have any further testing completed. What would you say to the patient in this situation?

_____

_____

_____

_____

_____

RESEARCH ACTIVITY

Use Internet search engines to research the following topic and write a brief description of what you find. It is important to use reputable websites.

1. To learn more about the agencies and committees that set and review safety guidelines affecting clinical laboratories, use the Internet to conduct research. Write an essay on your findings and what you learned beyond what is presented in the textbook about these agencies and committees and the guidelines established for laboratories. Be sure to cite your sources.

_____

_____

_____

_____

_____

CHAPTER 44
Microbiology

STUDENT STUDY GUIDE

Use the following guide to assist in your learning of the concepts from the chapter.

I. The Medical Assistant's Role in Microbiology

   1. MAs come in contact with blood and body fluids while _____ and _____ specimens for testing or _____ in patient care.

   2. Preparation of specimens can affect the _____, so it is vital to follow procedures strictly, including _____ and _____ requirements.

   3. Observing _____ _____ is a significant priority to prevent contamination and the spread of _____.

   4. The MA will also assist the _____ and educate the _____ in relation to obtaining specimens.

II. Classification of Microorganisms

   1. Only about _____ to _____ percent of microbes are pathogenic.

   2. Naming Microorganisms

     A. Each organism has two names.

       i. The _____ is always capitalized.

       ii. The _____ is all lowercase.

     B. Understanding the system of nomenclature is necessary when you receive _____ reports over the phone or read a(n) _____ _____.

   3. Retaining Dyes

     A. Many types of microorganisms are classified by their major _____ differences and their reactions to certain _____.

     B. A stain is a(n) _____ used to color microorganisms to make them visible under a(n) _____.

     C. A gram-_____ bacterium retains the violet color of the stain.

     D. A gram-_____ bacterium has the pink color of the counterstain.

4. Use of Oxygen

    A. Bacteria that survive in oxygen-rich environments are called _____.

    B. Bacteria that die in the presence of oxygen are called _____.

    C. Anaerobes that are flexible and can live with some oxygen are called _____

        _____.

    D. Successful _____ requires an understanding of the oxygen requirements of bacteria.

5. Other Identifying Characteristics

    A. Cell _____ and the presence or absence of _____ are also used to classify microorganisms.

    B. Means of _____ are unique to specific categories of microorganisms.

    C. Bacteria are also categorized by their ability to _____ red blood cells in the blood agar.

III. Types of Microorganisms*

  1. Bacteria

    A. Bacteria are small, _____ microorganisms that are capable of rapid _____.

    B. An overgrowth of bacteria can cause a(n) _____ and lead to disease or _____.

    C. Bacteria may be named for their _____ (shape).

    D. *Cocci* (_____ in shape)

      i. *Staphylococci*—Gram-_____, _____ clusters

      ii. *Streptococci*—Round, gram-_____ bacteria arranged in _____

      iii. *Diplococci*—Occur in _____ and can be either gram-_____ or gram-_____

    E. *Bacilli* (_____ shaped)

      i. Gram-negative *Bacilli*—Enterobacteriaceae are a large family found mainly in the _____ tract; however, many of them cause _____ in other body locations.

      ii. Gram-positive *Bacilli*—May be found in _____ or singly and are _____ forming or non–_____ forming.

    F. *Vibrios* are _____-shaped *Bacilli*.

    G. *Spirilla*

      i. These are _____ that are twisted in various shapes.

---

*More specific information about some of the common microorganisms will be covered in later activities in this chapter.

H. Special Categories of Bacteria (List four bacteria that don't fall into the previously mentioned groups.)

    i. _____

    ii. _____

    iii. _____

    iv. _____

2. Viruses

  A. Viruses are the _____ known infectious organisms and can be seen only with the use of a(n) _____ microscope.

  B. A virus is parasitic, depending on _____ cells of other _____ for growth.

  C. Vaccines are available to protect people from diseases such as _____, German _____, measles, hepatitis _____, mumps, and _____.

3. Protozoa

  A. Protozoa are _____-celled parasites that are usually _____ than bacteria.

  B. Most protozoa live in the _____ and receive nourishment from dead or decaying _____ material.

  C. Lack of proper _____ can lead to rapid spread of infections.

4. Fungi

  A. The study of fungi is known as _____.

  B. Fungi include _____ and _____.

  C. *Penicillium* mold was discovered by _____ _____, and its _____ properties changed modern medical treatment.

  D. Most fungi are not _____ and cause few diseases in humans, such as _____ infections.

5. Parasites

  A. Parasites receive _____ from other organisms.

  B. Parasites include _____ (helminths) and _____.

6. Medication-Resistant Microorganisms

  A. Medication resistance occurs when a patient does not complete the full course of _____, and the surviving organism learns to live in the _____ environment.

  B. Medication resistance renders medication _____.

  C. Proper and consistent _____ and _____ hygiene are critically important in decreasing the _____ of these difficult microorganisms.

IV. Diagnosing Infection

1. If an infection can be diagnosed on sight by the _____, further testing will _____ be _____.

2. Diagnosing Open Infected Wounds

   A. The site should be _____, described, and _____.

   B. Charting should include information regarding _____, _____, and level of patient _____.

3. Specimens are _____ and labeled and prepared safely for _____.

4. Specimen Culturing

   A. A specimen is streaked on appropriate _____ _____ in such a way as to allow individual colonies of _____ to develop.

   B. A second culture plate is tested for antibiotic _____.

   C. Culture plates are incubated for _____ hours to allow the microorganisms to _____.

   D. A zone of no growth around a(n) _____ disk indicates that the organism is _____ to that drug, which would be used to treat the patient.

5. Preparation of a(n) _____ _____ may be necessary in cases where the organisms must be kept alive to observe for _____ and morphology.

6. The ultimate goal of all these steps is to select the most _____ _____ that will restore the patient to a(n) _____ condition.

V. Specimen Collection and Processing*

1. Specimens for microbiology must be collected according to _____ established by the _____ department of the _____ performing the testing.

2. Incorrect steps could result in the following.

   A. A(n) _____ or altered specimen

   B. Delayed _____

   C. Postponed or possibly harmful _____

3. Collection Devices

   A. Sterile _____ are frequently used in the collection of specimens.

   B. They are wrapped in a sterile _____ or container to preserve _____.

   C. After a swab is collected, it is placed in a(n) _____ _____ that may or may not contain _____ media.

---

*Carefully review Guidelines 44-1 regarding specimen collection.

4. Culture Tubes and Other Collection Devices

   A. The Culturette^{tm} system is composed of the following.

      i. A disposable clear _____ _____

      ii. A sterile, cotton-tipped _____ _____ inside the tube

      iii. A sealed plastic vial of _____

   B. Some of these units contain two _____ _____—one for

      _____ and one for preparing the _____ _____.

   C. Sterile containers are available for _____, _____,

      _____, and _____ fluid.

5. Specimen Preservation

   A. Specimens should be collected from the area where the microorganisms are most likely to be

      _____ and then stored in _____-proof containers, sealed

      _____.

   B. If a specimen cannot be processed immediately, most specimens can be stored in a(n)

      _____ for up to several hours, except _____ _____

      fluid and _____.

   C. Specimens for *Neisseria gonorrhoeae*

      i. Specimens for *Neisseria gonorrhoeae* must be submitted on appropriate

      _____ plates.

      ii. It is important not to _____ inoculated plates of specimens for *Neisseria*

      gonorrhoeae.

   D. All stool specimens being examined for _____ or _____ require

      preservation in a formalin fixative and PVA or equivalent immediately after collection.

   E. For mycobacterial culture, it is recommended to collect _____ sputum

      specimens for _____-fast smears and culture in patients with clinical and chest

      X-ray findings compatible with _____.

   F. For blood cultures, draw _____ to _____ separate sets within a(n)

      _____-hour period, spaced as far apart as possible (a minimum of _____ minutes between

      sets).

VI. Types of Specimens*

   1. Throat

      A. A(n) _____ will order a throat culture to identify a pathogen when a patient

      presents with signs and symptoms such as _____ _____ infection,

      sore throat, or _____ infection.

---

*This section contains many procedures that should be reviewed carefully with regard to the type of specimen obtained.

B. When performing a throat culture, it is important not to touch the _____ of the

_____ or the _____ with the swab to avoid contaminating it.

C. Nasal swabs are sometimes requested, and care should be taken to label the swabs

"_____" and "_____" to identify from which nostril the specimen

was taken.

2. Sputum

A. The patient must be carefully instructed to cough _____ and _____

the coughed material into a sterile container.

B. This should not be _____ from the mouth.

C. The purpose of obtaining a sputum specimen is to isolate and diagnose diseases such as

streptococcal pneumonia, _____, and _____.

3. Urine

A. A urine specimen for culture must be either a(n) _____ specimen or a

clean-_____ _____ sample.

4. Stool

A. Stool may be tested for the following.

   i. Bacterial, parasitic, or protozoal _____

   ii. The presence of _____ _____

   iii. Excessive amounts of _____

B. Though it can be embarrassing to discuss stool collection, correct _____ is

critical to a(n) _____ result.

5. Stool Culture

A. Collection containers must be _____, and _____ technique must be

used in the collection process.

B. Sterile _____ _____ or applicator sticks can be used to transfer a

small amount of stool to a sterile container for transport to the _____ or office.

C. The sample is transferred to a(n) _____ _____ container and sent to

the lab for testing.

6. Occult Blood

A. A test for occult, or _____, blood may indicate bleeding in the

_____ tract.

B. The patient is given the test units to take _____ to _____ the

specimen.

   i. _____ are provided on each test unit.

   ii. _____ the _____ each time they are given to a patient.

C. Patients should be instructed to refrain from consuming vitamin _____ and red _____ for _____ day(s) before testing because those substances may cause false positives.

7. Stool for Ova and Parasites

   A. The presence of _____ or other forms of a(n) _____ indicate parasitic _____.

   B. Identification of the parasite aids in selecting the correct _____.

   C. If O&P are suspected, _____ specimen collections will be requested.

      i. Specimens are usually obtained in the _____ _____.

   D. The stool specimen samples should be taken from several _____ _____ of the stool.

   E. Collecting pinworm specimens

      i. Transmission is by the _____–_____ route or by ingesting _____ with hand-to-mouth transmission.

      ii. Collection of a specimen should be done first thing in the _____, before a(n) _____ _____ or _____, to detect ova or worms.

      iii. Specimen collection is done by touching the _____ with the sticky side of a piece of _____ and then affixing it to a(n) _____ slide.

8. Wound Specimens

   A. Sterile swabs are used to obtain a specimen from a(n) _____, _____, a(n) _____, or a(n)_____ to test for pathogenic microorganisms.

   B. Several _____ from different _____ may be necessary.

      i. _____ the source of each specimen.

9. Other Types of Specimens

   A. Cerebrospinal fluid (CSF) is always treated as a(n) _____ procedure.

   B. Three tubes are collected under _____ _____ and sent for testing.

   C. Blood and CSF are normally free of any _____.

   D. Commercially available containers containing a(n) _____ media are widely used to grow cultures to test for _____ or _____.

VII. Microbiology Equipment and Procedures

   1. List the microbiology-related equipment found in a typical physician's office laboratory (POL).

      A. _____

      B. _____

C. _____

D. _____

E. _____

F. _____

2. Inoculating Equipment

   A. A(n) _____ is a long instrument with a small loop on the end, designed to pick

      up _____ and transfer them to _____ _____.

   B. After a(n) _____ sterile loop or needle is used, it is discarded in a(n)

      _____ waste container.

   C. A metal loop or needle requires _____ before and after use to ensure sterility.

      i. _____ _____ requiring a natural gas supply or

         _____ incinerators are used.

3. Culture Media

   A. A specimen must be inoculated onto a(n) _____ that will enhance the growth of

      the _____.

   B. Common types of culture media are _____ and _____.

   C. All media should be inspected for _____ before use to ensure the

      _____ of the culturing process.

   D. Media will either _____ or _____ the growth of certain pathogens.

   E. List four ways media are classified.

      i. _____

      ii. _____

      iii. _____

      iv. _____

4. Inoculating Media

   A. _____ of bacteria can be grown only on certain media.

   B. Pathogens are often identified by the manner in which they _____ on a

      particular _____.

   C. The main goal in growing cultures is to separate _____ colonies of organisms

      from colonies of _____ _____.

   D. To isolate colonies, the _____ must be _____ properly.

   E. After inoculation, the lid or top of the _____ _____ is replaced, and

      the agar plate is _____ and placed into an incubator _____

      _____.

F. A secondary culture can be obtained by selecting a(n) _____ _____ from the initial _____ _____ and placing it on another media plate using a sterile loop or needle.

G. Instruments such as Vitek and Autobac use _____ _____ to facilitate organism identification.

5. Direct Examination

    A. Direct smear

        i. A direct smear may be from a(n) _____ of the specimen or from a(n) _____ on a culture plate.

        ii. The swab is _____ carefully across the _____ so all areas of the swab touch the slide.

        iii. The slide is _____ by passing the clear underneath part of the slide through a(n) _____ _____ three to four times or flooding the slide with _____ and letting it dry.

    B. Wet mount preparation

        i. This involves taking a sample either from a(n) _____ or directly from a(n) _____ specimen, placing it on a(n) _____ slide, and adding a drop of sterile normal saline and a(n) _____ _____.

        ii. In the POL, a wet mount for _____ often is performed using potassium hydroxide.

        iii. Preparing a KOH mount involves the following steps.

           a. The specimen is suspended in _____ drop(s) of _____ percent potassium hydroxide, and a(n) _____ _____ is applied.

           b. The specimen sits at room temperature for _____ minute(s) to dissolve the _____.

    C. Staining specimens*

        i. A medical assistant is _____ _____ to perform Gram staining in the medical setting.

        ii. However, it is important to know how to _____ a smear and have general knowledge of the _____ _____ and why it is used.

        iii. Gram staining will differentiate bacteria into two groups: _____ _____ and _____ _____.

        iv. The staining properties, _____, and _____ of the organisms can sometimes be used to identify _____ in specimen samples.

_____
* Review Procedure 44-5 regarding correctly performing Gram staining.

6. Serology Testing

   A. Serology is the study of the _____ and _____ reactions of the body's immune system.

   B. Antigen–antibody reaction is used to test for _____, rheumatoid _____, _____, and _____, among other conditions.

   C. Testing kits standardize testing, ensuring _____, _____, and _____ _____.

      i. It is essential to follow the _____ directions exactly.

7. Strep Testing

   A. The Group A strep screen is a test that is done _____ in POLs.

   B. This test is efficient because it is _____-contained and can be done while the patient _____.

   C. Self-contained test kits include detailed _____ and contain _____, controls, and _____ _____ suggestions.

   D. Other serological test kits are available for _____ mononucleosis, _____ arthritis, and HIV.

KEY TERMINOLOGY REVIEW

Without using any material from your textbook, write a sentence using each selected key term in the correct context as related to the topics presented in the chapter.

1. *enteritis*

   _____

   _____

2. *morphology*

   _____

   _____

3. *normal flora*

   _____

   _____

4. *exudates*

   _____

   _____

5. *steatorrhea*

   _____

   _____

APPLIED PRACTICE

Follow the directions as instructed for each question.

1. List the diseases that can occur from the following pathogens.

Body Location	Pathogen	Disease
Respiratory system	*Streptococcus pyogenes* *Corynebacterium diphtheriae* *Mycobacterium tuberculosis* *Haemophilus influenzae* type B *Streptococcus pneumoniae*	
Central nervous system	*Neisseria meningitides* Polioviruses Rabies virus	
Genitourinary system	Herpes simplex viruses 1 and 2 *Candida albicans* (fungus) *Chlamydia trachomatis* *Escherichia coli*	
Integumentary system	*Staphylococcus aureus* Varicella zoster virus	
Gastrointestinal system	Hepatitis A, B, and C viruses *Salmonella enteritidis* *Escherichia coli*	
Circulatory system and blood, immune system	*Streptococcus pyogenes* *Staphylococcus aureus* *Plasmodium falciparum, P. vivax, P. malariae, P. ovale* Human immunodeficiency virus Epstein-Barr virus *Borrelia burgdorferi*	
Tissue	*Streptococcus pyogenes*	

LEARNING ACTIVITY: FILL IN THE BLANK

Using words from the following list, fill in the blanks to complete the following sentences.

agar
agglutination
cephalosporins
colony
culture medium
facultative anaerobes
feces

hemolysis
laboratory
lawn technique
methicillin-resistant
microorganisms
motility
organelles

ova
oxygen
smear
Streptococci
viable
wet mount

1. The Group A strep screen is an antigen-detection test for group A beta-hemolytic _____ and follows the general procedure for antigen–antibody _____ tests, which produce a clumping of cells.

2. Differences such as cell structure and the presence or absence of _____ are used to classify organisms.

3. The "super bug" _____ *Staphylococcus aureus* (MRSA) produces an enzyme that makes the organism resistant to penicillin and _____, which are normally used for treatment, and renders these antibiotics ineffective.

4. A(n) _____ is a thin layer of _____ spread on a glass slide for identification purposes.

5. One classification of streptococcal organisms is based on the type of _____ the organisms cause on blood _____ plates.

6. Bacteria that are flexible and can live with some _____ are called _____ _____.

7. A(n) _____ is a preparation in a liquid that will preserve the _____ of the microbe.

8. The Mueller–Hinton agar is prepared with the pure culture specimen in overlapping strokes in a technique called the _____ _____ or _____ count.

9. Microorganisms must remain _____ (capable of living) when they reach the _____.

10. The stool, or _____, of the patient can be inspected for the presence of _____ and mature forms of the worm.

CRITICAL THINKING

Answer the following questions to the best of your ability. Use the textbook as a reference.

1. A patient has been instructed to collect stool specimens to be tested for occult blood. He has been asked to refrain from eating red meat or taking vitamin C for 3 days prior to testing for occult blood. Why? What other instructions does this patient need to follow in order to obtain an accurate test result?

_____

_____

_____

_____

2. Mrs. Chen is a 70-year-old who has immigrated to the Unites States from mainland China. She is being seen today with complaints of recent sudden constipation. Mrs. Chen is shy and very hesitant to speak with a male medical assistant about her condition. What can be done to help Mrs. Chen feel more comfortable about discussing her condition?

_____

_____

_____

_____

_____

RESEARCH ACTIVITY

Use Internet search engines to research the following topic and write a brief description of what you find. It is important to use reputable websites.

1. Methicillin-resistant *Staphylococcus aureus* (MRSA) has become a very real threat, not only to health care workers but also to the general population. Visit www.cdc.gov and provide answers to the following questions.

   a. Besides MRSA, what are some other multidrug-resistant organisms (MDROs)?

   _____

   _____

   _____

   _____

   _____

   b. In your opinion, what can be done to prevent the transmission of these organisms?

   _____

   _____

   _____

   _____

CHAPTER 45
Urinalysis

STUDENT STUDY GUIDE

Use the following guide to assist in your learning of the concepts from the chapter.

I. Introduction

  1. The kidneys _____ significant concentrations of certain unwanted _____ from the blood.

  2. The result is _____, which is stored in the bladder until it can be excreted through _____ (urination).

  3. Urinalysis, the testing and evaluating of urine, is performed for the following reasons.

    A. _____

    B. _____

    C. _____

  4. The medical assistant must understand basic _____ and _____, as well as the normal _____ and lab _____ for urine in order to assist in diagnosing diseases and disorders.

II. Asepsis

  1. Asepsis is critical in _____.

  2. Consider all blood and body fluids, including urine, to be potentially _____.

  3. Follow _____ _____, including the following, whenever collecting urine samples or performing urinalysis.

    A. Maintain good _____ principles.

    B. Wear _____ gloves.

    C. Avoid contaminating any equipment with _____.

    D. Use _____ _____ _____ (PPE).

III. Collecting the Specimen

  1. In most cases, urine samples are _____ if testing will not take place within _____ hours.

  2. The patient must be clearly _____ about methods of _____ in easily understood terms.

3. At least _____ mL of urine is usually needed for testing, and appropriate collection

    _____ or _____ must be used.

4. Urine Test Categories

    A. List five types of time-specific tests.

        i. _____

        ii. _____

        iii. _____

        iv. _____

        v. _____

    B. List four types of specialized collection tests.

        i. _____

        ii. _____

        iii. _____

        iv. _____

5. Labeling

    A. List the information that should be included when labeling specimen containers.

        i. _____

        ii. _____

        iii. _____

        iv. _____

    B. Never place labels on specimen _____.

IV. Time-Specific Tests

  1. Random Sample

    A. A random urine sample can be collected at _____ _____ of the day.

    B. The sample is collected in a(n) _____ container and can be collected in the medical office or brought in from the _____ _____.

    C. Random samples are generally used for _____ _____.

  2. Morning Specimen: First Void

    A. A morning specimen is the most _____ urine because it has remained in the bladder _____ or over a(n) _____-hour period of time.

    B. List the reasons a morning specimen is collected.

        i. _____

        ii. _____

        iii. _____

    C. A morning specimen should be brought to the office for testing within _____ to _____ minutes of collection, or the sample should be _____.

3. Timed Specimen

   A. A timed specimen is necessary for _____ analysis.

   B. It may measure amounts of substances such as _____, _____ or _____ in urine.

   C. 24-hour specimen

      i. A 24-hour specimen is used for the following purposes.

         a. Determining the glomerular _____ _____ of the kidneys

         b. Checking specific _____ levels

         c. Checking for other _____ abnormalities

      ii. The patient is given a(n) _____, _____, and properly labeled container to take home.

      iii. Collection begins the next _____, after the _____ void of the morning.

      iv. After the first void, the patient collects every _____ of _____ for 24 hours.

      v. Often _____ are added the container before it is given to the patient.

      vi. Patients should be specifically instructed not to _____ or _____ preservatives.

      vii. The patient should collect the urine in a(n) _____ _____ and then pour it into the 24-hour container.

   D. 2-hour postprandial specimen

      i. This specimen is a single voided specimen collected 2 hours after a(n) _____ has been _____.

      ii. The test detects any _____ that may be spilled into the urine once the blood levels exceed the renal _____.

V. Specialized Collection

  1. Clean-Catch Midstream Specimen

    A. Clean-catch is a method of urine collection that is free of most _____ and other contaminants found in the urethra or around the _____ area.

    B. A patient can collect his/her own specimen without the need for a(n) _____ procedure.

    C. These specimen samples are frequently used to detect urinary tract infections or to perform cytology evaluations to detect _____ _____.

    D. The patient needs clear _____ to obtain a urine specimen that is free of _____.

2. Catheterization Specimen
   A. Catheterization is the process of inserting a(n) _____ tube-like catheter through the _____ and into the _____.
   B. Typically, a(n) _____ will perform this procedure using _____ technique, but a medical assistant may be called to assist and may even _____ the procedure under _____.
   C. There are many sizes, _____, and types of catheters.
       i. Straight catheters are commonly used for specimen collection because they are _____ and easier to _____.
       ii. Foley catheters have inflatable _____ that keep them in place for longer periods of _____.
       iii. A suprapubic catheter enters the bladder through the _____ and may be used when there is _____ obstruction.
   D. Using sterile technique is vital to preventing _____ such as infection.
   E. List the typical contents of a catheter kit or tray.
       i. _____
       ii. _____
       iii. _____
       iv. _____
       v. _____
       vi. _____
       vii. Possibly a(n) _____, prefilled _____, and _____ bag
   F. In some patients, the amount of _____ intake and urine _____ need to be closely monitored and can be _____ by catheterization.
3. Pediatric Specimen
   A. Attaching a(n) _____ pediatric urine _____ _____ is often the method of choice for obtaining a specimen from a pediatric patient.
4. Suprapubic Specimen
   A. To obtain this type of specimen, the physician inserts a(n) _____ into the patient's _____ through the _____ wall, just above the _____ bone, and withdraws the urine sample into a(n) _____.
   B. This procedure is not commonly performed because of its _____ nature.

VI. Routine Urinalysis

1. List the three components of a routine urinalysis.

    A. _____

    B. _____

    C. _____

2. List the five characteristics examined during physical analysis of urine.

    A. _____

    B. _____

    C. _____

    D. _____

    E. _____

3. Chemical analysis is performed by using commercially prepared _____

    _____ that measure the following.

    A. _____

    B. _____

    C. _____

    D. _____

    E. _____

    F. _____

4. _____ blood cells, _____ blood cells, _____, casts, and other

    components may be seen with _____ analysis.

5. Physical Characteristics

    A. Clarity

        i. Note if urine is clear or _____.

       ii. _____ means the urine is cloudy, opaque, or does not allow

          _____ to pass through.

     iii. List seven factors that can cause turbidity.

        a. _____

        b. _____

        c. _____

        d. _____

        e. _____

        f. _____

        g. _____

B. Color

    i. The normal color of urine is _____.

    ii. Urine colors range from _____ yellow to _____.

    iii. Brown or black urine indicates a(n) _____ _____.

    iv. Reddish-brown urine may indicate _____ _____ bleeding or menstruation.

C. Odor

    i. Odor is not recorded unless a(n) _____ aroma is evident.

    ii. A fruity odor may be indicative of uncontrolled _____.

    iii. Putrid or foul odors might indicate _____.

D. Quantity

    i. Quantity is measured for _____-specific tests but not for _____ testing.

    ii. Polyuria may indicate disorders such as _____ or _____ disease.

    iii. Oliguria can be indicative of decreased fluid intake and _____, bleeding, or _____ disease.

    iv. _____ may be the result of renal failure.

E. Specific gravity

    i. Specific gravity compares the density of _____ to the density of _____.

    ii. Normal specific gravity ranges between _____ and _____.

    iii. The higher the specific gravity, the more _____ _____ is in the urine.

    iv. Readings outside the _____ _____ may be the first indication if the _____ are not working properly.

    v. List the two methods used to measure specific gravity.

        a. _____

        b. _____

F. Chemical characteristics

    i. Chemical analysis can be performed by using reagent _____, also called the _____ method.

    ii. Dipsticks are equipped with small _____ treated pads that react with chemicals in the urine to _____ and _____ specific substances.

iii. The _____ changes caused by the chemical reactions can then be compared with a color _____ on the outside of the reagent strip _____.

iv. _____ decide which chemical elements they want to test, based on the patient's status and possible _____.

v. After dipping the reagent strip into the _____, each test should be read at a(n) _____ _____.

vi. Most tests can be read in as little as _____ to _____ seconds after dipping.

G. Reaction pH

i. pH indicates _____ and _____.

ii. Normal kidneys produce urine with pH ranging from _____ to _____.

H. Protein

i. Protein is _____ _____ found in the urine of healthy individuals.

ii. The presence of protein in the urine can indicate _____ _____ from damage to the glomeruli.

I. Glucose

i. Normal urine should not contain glucose since almost all glucose gets _____ back into the blood by the _____.

ii. Glucose spills into the urine when the _____ glucose levels exceed the _____ _____ for glucose, which is approximately _____ to _____ mg/dL of glucose in the bloodstream.

J. Hematuria

i. Blood in the urine is abnormal unless it is contamination from _____.

ii. List the possible problems that the presence of occult blood in urine may indicate.

a. _____

b. _____

c. _____

d. _____

K. Ketones

i. Ketones are byproducts of _____ _____.

ii. They are typically seen only in conditions such as the following.

a. Poorly controlled _____

b. _____

c. _____

d. Ingestion of large quantities of _____

e. High-_____ diets

f. Occasionally after general _____

L. Bilirubin

    i. Bilirubin is _____ _____ found in the urine.

    ii. The presence of bilirubin may be one of the first signs of the following.

        a. _____

        b. _____

        c. _____

        d. _____

M. Urobilinogen

    i. Urobilinogen is a result of _____ destruction, and it is present in _____ _____ under normal conditions.

    ii. High levels of urobilinogen may help detect _____ diseases.

    iii. A(n) _____ or _____ duct obstruction may cause urobilinogen to be absent in the urine.

N. Nitrates

    i. Measurement of nitrites is a method for detection of _____ and may indicate a(n) _____.

    ii. Nitrites are a byproduct of _____ _____ by certain bacteria.

    iii. _____ _____ for the presence of nitrites can happen if the specimen sits at room temperature too long.

O. Leukocytes

    i. Leukocytes are commonly referred to as _____ _____ _____.

    ii. Normally, a(n) _____ leukocytes should be present in urine.

    iii. When performing a urinalysis, the _____ the color on the strip, the _____ the number of WBCs.

6. Automated Urine Chemical Analyzers

    A. These analyzers use light _____ to test the strips, which eliminates the human error associated with _____ _____.

    B. Quality control protocols, including the use of _____ and _____ controls and proper _____, must be followed.

7. Microscopic Examination

    A. Microscopic examination identifies the _____ and approximate _____ of organisms present in a urine specimen.

    B. More often, urine specimens are sent to a(n) _____ _____ for microscopic evaluation.

C. Preparing a urine specimen for microscopic examination

    i. Fresh urine is poured into _____ to prepare for microscopic analysis.

    ii. A(n) _____ rotates the urine tubes at high speeds to separate _____ of different _____.

    iii. The _____ is the solid material remaining at the bottom of the tube after the _____ is carefully poured off.

    iv. A special _____ may be used to provide better _____ to the formed elements present.

D. Reporting and understanding urine microscopic examinations

    i. The slide is moved several times to be able to evaluate different _____ of _____.

    ii. The number of _____ or _____ is counted in each circular field, and an overall _____ is given.

    iii. Microscopic urinalysis is not _____ _____ and, therefore, is not within the medical assistant's _____ of _____ in most states.

    iv. List the elements presented in the textbook that are observed during microscopic examination.

        a. _____

        b. _____

        c. _____

        d. _____

        e. _____

        f. _____

        g. _____

        h. _____

VII. Urine Pregnancy and Ovulation Testing

  1. Blood and urine pregnancy tests are based on the detection of the hormone _____ _____ _____ (hCG).

  2. Levels of hCG can be detectable as early as _____ day(s) after fertilization has taken place.

  3. For the urine dipstick method, the woman urinates into a clean, dry _____ and dips a(n) _____ into the urine sample to detect the presence of hCG.

  4. For a midstream sample, the woman begins voiding into the _____ and then places the absorbent tip of the pregnancy test under the _____ _____ until it is thoroughly wet.

  5. The test should be placed flat on a surface, with the _____ window facing up.

6. Results are shown in the results window as a change in _____, a(n) _____, or a(n) _____.

7. Newer digital pregnancy tests display either the words "_____ _____" or "_____."

8. A more accurate confirmation of pregnancy is often done by _____ _____.

9. List the two categories of CLIA waived pregnancy tests performed in POLs.

    A. _____

    B. _____

10. Most pregnancy tests, including urine home pregnancy tests, have accuracies of _____ to _____ percent.

11. A confirmed diagnosis should always be made by a(n) _____, as certain types of _____ and _____ medications may also cause a test to appear positive.

12. Urine ovulation tests work by detecting the presence of the _____ _____ (LH).

    A. LH surges or peaks _____ to _____ days before ovulation.

VIII. Urine Drug Analysis

1. _____ testing is the most common method for drug analysis.

2. CLIA waived urine drug screening is performed by the _____ _____ in the physician's office laboratory.

3. Drug screening is commonly requested before _____ or state _____.

4. The procedures for collection and testing of urine are very _____ and _____, and the procedures and _____ must be carefully followed.

5. Chain of custody chain assures the following.

    A. The specimen belongs to the individual whose _____ is printed on the specimen container _____.

    B. No post-collection _____ has occurred.

    C. The correct people had _____ of the specimen.

    D. The specimen was _____ and _____ correctly before it was analyzed.

    E. The specimen was _____ in a secure manner.

6. A(n) _____ of _____ _____ is a chronological documentation or paper trail showing the collection, _____, _____, _____, storage, and disposal of the _____.

    A. List what the form identifies.

        i. _____

        ii. _____

    iii. _____

    iv. _____

  B. The chain of custody form is considered a(n) _____ _____ and can invalidate a specimen that has been _____ with or does not have _____ _____ written on it.

7. A medical assistant may be asked to perform a drug test and should ensure that no tampering occurs _____, _____, or after _____.

  A. The primary _____ to tampering with on-site drug testing of specimens is to ensure that collection of the drug test specimen is done under _____ _____.

IX. Quality Control

1. Quality control is a system of ensuring that patients' _____ _____ are accurate and reported in a timely manner.

2. Each testing _____ is sold with a quality control testing _____.

3. All instrumentation associated with urine testing should be _____ and _____ on a regular basis and _____ accordingly.

4. Before any test is used, the _____ _____ of the product should be checked to be sure the product has not _____.

5. It is important to precisely follow the _____ that are supplied by the _____ when using quality control testing material.

6. New employees should be appropriately _____ to perform urine tests, and the training should be _____.

KEY TERMINOLOGY REVIEW

Match each of the following vocabulary terms to the correct definition.

    a. bacturia   d. sediment

    b. hematuria   e. urinalysis

    c. oliguria

1. _____ Blood in the urine.

2. _____ Bacteria in the urine.

3. _____ The solid material that settles at the bottom of a test tube after centrifugation.

4. _____ Testing that provides valuable information about many functions in the body, including kidney function.

5. _____ Decreased amounts of urine production.

APPLIED PRACTICE

Answer the questions related to the scenario below.

Scenario

A clean-catch urine specimen has been provided by Mrs. Gonzalez. The following are the results of the dipstick urinalysis. Fill in the normal value for each, circle those that are abnormal as if you were flagging them for the physician, and then state the possible reasons for the abnormal results.

Tests	Results for Mrs. Gonzalez	Normal Value	Possible Causes for Abnormal Results
Color	orange-red		
Clarity	cloudy		
pH	7.8		
Specific gravity	1.026		
Protein	+ + or positive		
Glucose	0		
Ketones	0		
Bilirubin	0		
Urobilinogen	4		
Blood	+		
Leukocytes	+ + + +		
Nitrite	0		

LEARNING ACTIVITY: FILL IN THE BLANK

Using words from the list below, fill in the blanks to complete the following statements.

acidity	alkalinity
bile duct	foreskin
fruity	labia
organisms	health
physical	positive
random	slows

1. Urine samples provide valuable indicators of the overall _____ of the patient.

2. A(n) _____ sample of urine is the most commonly collected type of urine specimen.

3. When collecting clean-catch specimens, be sure that the female patient understands how to clean the _____ and the male knows how to clean the _____.

4. Refrigeration of a specimen _____ the growth of bacteria and specimen deterioration but does not stop it.

5. The _____ characteristics of urine may be important diagnostic tools for the physician.

6. Individuals testing positive for ketones may have a(n) _____ odor to their urine.

7. The pH of a solution indicates _____ and _____.

8. If urobilinogen is not present in the urine, a(n) _____ obstruction may be present.

9. If a UTI is suspected and the urine tests positive for leukocytes, then a protein test should be _____.

10. Microscopic examination identifies the type and approximate number of _____ present in a urine specimen.

CRITICAL THINKING

Answer the following questions to the best of your ability. Use the textbook as a reference.

1. You are to instruct a 68-year-old female patient in the collection of a 24-hour urine specimen. Explain this, in your own words, as if you were speaking to the patient. Avoid medical terms that the patient may not understand; also avoid treating the patient as if she is a child.

_____

_____

_____

_____

_____

2. Jerry McMathis has been sent to the medical office by his employer for a random drug screening. Mr. McMathis is visibly irritated about the situation. Carlos Vergara, RMA, is preparing to collect the urine specimen for drug screening. According to office policy, Carlos explains to Mr. McMathis that the specimen must be collected in a specimen container that includes a temperature strip to verify specimen temperature. He also tells Mr. McMathis that a bluing tablet has been added to the toilet water, and absolutely no water can be run while he is in the bathroom with the specimen cup. After the specimen has been collected and handed back to Carlos, Mr. McMathis can then flush the toilet and wash his hands. All of this information further irritates Mr. McMathis, and he angrily says to Carlos, "Why do you have to go through all of this just to check my pee? You've got to be kidding me. Don't you trust me?" How should Carlos respond to the patient?

_____

_____

_____

_____

_____

RESEARCH ACTIVITY

Use Internet search engines to research the following topic and write a brief description of what you find. It is important to use reputable websites.

1. Research various types of urine drug screening kits that are available. What types of drugs can be screened using urine? Also, research various policies and procedures related to the chain of custody when collecting and processing urine drug screens. What are the most common policies and procedures related to this type of specimen collection?

   _____

   _____

   _____

   _____

   _____

CHAPTER 46

Phlebotomy and Blood Collection

STUDENT STUDY GUIDE

Use the following guide to assist in your learning of the concepts from the chapter.

I. Introduction

   1. Collection of blood through a tiny incision in the vein is termed _____ or _____.

   2. Blood can also be collected for testing through a simple _____ _____, obtained by pricking the skin.

II. The Medical Assistant's Role

   1. The role of the medical assistant is to properly _____, _____, and perhaps _____ or store the specimen.

   2. Understanding Circulatory Anatomy and Physiology

     A. The heart is a(n) _____ whose job is to keep blood moving.

     B. Blood leaves the heart through blood vessels called _____, which get smaller and smaller farther away from the heart.

     C. Arteries

       i. Arteries have thick _____ _____.

       ii. Arteries carry _____ red blood.

       iii. Arteries actively _____ from the pumping _____ of the heart.

     D. Capillaries act as bridges between the _____ and _____.

       i. Oxygen can pass out of the blood, through the capillary _____, and into the _____.

       ii. Carbon dioxide and other _____ can pass out of the cells, also through the capillary walls, and into the _____.

       iii. Capillary blood is the easiest to collect and is commonly used for _____ of _____ _____.

     E. Veins are vessels that carry blood _____ the heart.

       i. Veins have _____ walls than arteries and do not _____.

       ii. Veins have one-way _____ that prevent backflow.

F. _____ (puncturing a vein) is a common method for obtaining sufficient blood for a variety of _____.

    i. Regulation of _____ _____ is important to remember when performing venipuncture.

    ii. Blood vessels that have shrunk in response to _____ are more difficult to access.

G. Main elements of blood

    i. Plasma, which is the _____ portion, is mostly water.

    ii. Formed elements include _____, _____, and _____.

III. Blood Specimen Collection

  1. List three organizations that have established guidelines for performing specimen collection.

    A. _____

    B. _____

    C. _____

  2. Capillary Puncture

    A. List four CLIA waived tests for which capillary blood is used.

        i. _____

        ii. _____

        iii. _____

        iv. _____

    B. The most common capillary puncture sites for adults is the _____, preferably the fleshy pad of the _____ or _____ finger on the nondominant hand.

    C. The puncture should be a minimum of _____ mm away from the _____.

    D. List six areas to avoid when performing capillary puncture.

        i. _____

        ii. _____

        iii. _____

        iv. _____

        v. _____

        vi. _____

    E. _____ are also a common puncture site for adults.

F. When doing a capillary puncture on an infant, a(n) _____ is usually the best option for obtaining a sample.

    i. The puncture should occur on the _____ and _____ surfaces (sides) of the heel.

    ii. Thoroughly _____ and _____ the heel before the procedure.

    iii. Never place a(n) _____ _____ on patients younger than 2 years.

3. Equipment and Supplies Needed for Capillary Puncture

  A. Lancets

    i. Lancets may be either _____ or _____.

    ii. Many are color-coded according to the _____ _____ they can accomplish.

    iii. After a lancet is used, it should immediately be placed in a(n) _____ _____ to prevent needlesticks.

  B. Capillary blood may be administered directly onto a(n) _____ _____, or it can be collected in a plastic or glass _____.

  C. Microtainer capillary blood collection tubes have a variety of _____, noted by the color-coded _____.

  D. Unopette collection devices can be used for various _____ _____ _____.

4. Venipuncture

  A. The safest and easiest sites to access are located on the _____ _____.

  B. The most popular vein to use is the _____ _____ vein.

  C. The next most popular veins are _____ and _____ veins.

5. The Phlebotomist

  A. A(n) _____ _____ who is trained to perform phlebotomy is considered a phlebotomist and may perform venipuncture in the medical office unless specific _____ _____ say otherwise.

  B. List four places aside from a medical office where venipuncture may take place.

    i. _____

    ii. _____

    iii. _____

    iv. _____

6. Certification in Phlebotomy
   A. Phlebotomy certification is often required at _____, blood _____, and independent _____.
   B. List four benefits of obtaining phlebotomy certification.
      i. _____
      ii. _____
      iii. _____
      iv. _____
   C. Phlebotomy technicians _____ and _____ blood and other body fluid samples for medical laboratory testing.
      i. Credentials for a phlebotomy technician include the _____ _____ _____ (CPT) and _____ _____ _____ (RPT).
      ii. List three nationally accredited phlebotomy credentialing agencies.
         a. _____
         b. _____
         c. _____

7. Venipuncture Methods
   A. The vacuum container method
      i. The vacuum container method is the _____ common method of venipuncture.
      ii. Multiple _____ can be obtained at the same time, requiring fewer _____ for the patient and _____ collection.
      iii. It is important to use a(n) _____ vein because the vacuum can collapse _____ veins.
   B. Sterile syringe and needle method
      i. The amount of _____ that can be collected for testing is limited to the size of the _____ used.
      ii. This method has a higher incidence of _____ or _____ than the vacuum container method.
   C. The butterfly needle method
      i. The _____ _____, or butterfly, method uses a needle that is attached to 6- to 12-inch _____.
      ii. This method is used for _____ _____ that are difficult to draw from with the standard _____ _____ method or syringe and needle method.

iii. The needle used for the butterfly method is a small _____-, _____-, or _____-gauge needle.

iv. The _____ _____ _____ Act has inspired several types of butterfly systems that are designed for both safety and ease of use.

8. List the three types of equipment used for venipuncture.

   A. _____

   B. _____

   C. _____

9. Order of Draw

   A. It is important to fill tubes in the order of draw recommended by the Clinical _____ _____ Institute to prevent _____ of the tubes with skin bacteria or with a(n) _____ from another blood tube.

   B. List the order of draw as presented in Table 46-1 in the textbook.

      i. _____

      ii. _____

      iii. _____

      iv. _____

      v. _____

      vi. _____

      vii. _____

      viii. _____

      ix. _____

      x. _____

   C. Many _____ _____ forms state the tube color to use for each test.

   D. The exact number of tests possible for one tube depends on the size of the container, the type of _____, and the type of _____ being used in the lab.

   E. If more than _____ tests in the same tube are required, it may be wise to draw a(n) _____ tube.

   F. Vacuum blood tubes come in _____-, _____-, _____-, and _____-mL sizes.

   G. Gently invert a tube six to eight times so the _____ and blood mix properly.

10. Blood Cultures

    A. Blood cultures are very _____ tests that look for signs of _____ in the blood.

B. Special _____ are taken while collecting blood for culturing.

    i. The site must be cleaned thoroughly with _____ cleaners, typically

       _____ and then _____, with time for _____ in

       between.

    ii. Cleanse a(n) _____ finger before re-palpation once the site has already

       been cleaned.

11. Patient Preparation

A. The blood tests done in a physician's office typically require _____

   preparation.

B. List three tests for which a patient should fast for 12 to 14 hours beforehand.

    i. _____

    ii. _____

    iii. _____

12. Performing the Blood Draw

A. Phlebotomy _____ can be set up at a height that is easy to access, with

   adjustable _____ _____ that serve to keep the patient both

   comfortable and secure.

B. Blood collection equipment should be kept easily _____ off to the side.

C. List three complications to ask patients about experiencing during previous venipunctures.

    i. _____

    ii. _____

    iii. _____

D. If a patient complains of dizziness, immediately _____ the _____,

   apply _____, and assist in lowering the patient's head between the

   _____.

E. To decrease patient anxiety, it is important to _____ clearly what the process

   involves.

F. If the patient is a child, the participation of the _____ or _____

   may be helpful in calming the patient.

G. List four examples of unexpected events that may occur during venipuncture.

    i. _____

    ii. _____

    iii. _____

    iv. _____

H. It is important to remain _____ and deal with unexpected events
_____.

I. When drawing blood, wear personal protective equipment such as _____ and
a gown or _____ _____.

J. After the blood is collected, it must be carefully _____ to ensure the
_____ of the results.

K. Always check the _____ or book given to you by the _____ for
processing to ensure correct transportation of specimens.

13. Responding to Complications

A. A hematoma is a(n) _____ formed by the collection of _____ at
the puncture site when some of the blood escapes the vein and enters the surrounding
_____.

B. Typically, hematomas can be prevented by having the patient _____
_____ to the insertion site for _____ to _____
minutes after removal of the needle.

14. Patient Refusal

A. One of the fundamental patient _____ is the right to refuse treatment.

B. _____ attempt to collect a specimen from a patient who refuses.

C. Only a(n) _____ _____ order overrides this right.

15. Stress

A. Stress over _____ procedures can cause physical _____ that may
affect people with underlying illness.

B. List two examples of preexisting conditions that can be exacerbated by stress.

   i. _____

   ii. _____

16. Failure to Obtain Blood

A. Failure to obtain blood can be caused by many factors, including the following.

   i. Failure to insert the needle _____ enough

   ii. The needle advancing too far and _____ through both walls of the
   _____.

   iii. The needle resting against the _____ of the vein or a(n)
   _____ within the vein

   iv. The collection tube losing its _____

   v. The veins _____ away

17. Excessive Bleeding

A. Always ask patients before performing venipuncture if they know they have a(n)

_____ _____, are taking anti-_____, or are taking

_____.

    i. If the answer to any of these questions is yes, apply pressure _____ after removing the needle and apply a cohesive _____ dressing after the procedure.

18. Specimen Problems

A. Examples of specimen collection and processing problems include the following.

    i. The wrong _____ is used to draw blood.

    ii. The specimen is not _____ or is incorrectly labeled.

    iii. Blood becomes _____.

    iv. A poor specimen process or _____ _____ occur before or during transportation.

19. Special Needs Patients

A. Avoid the following blood collection sites.

    i. Areas with hematomas, _____, or _____

    ii. An arm with a fistula, _____ _____, or burns

    iii. Sites with _____

    iv. The arm that is on the same side as a(n) _____

B. For a patient with _____ impairment, explain every part of the procedure carefully so as not to _____ traumatize the patient.

KEY TERMINOLOGY REVIEW

Match each of the following terms with the correct definition.

    a. antecubital space   d. platelets

    b. capillaries   e. serum

    c. heparin

1. _____ Plasma without the fibrinogen.

2. _____ A depression in the front of the elbow; it is the most commonly used site for venipuncture.

3. _____ The smallest of the body's blood vessels.

4. _____ A substance that prevents clotting.

5. _____ The smallest cells found in the blood; they are formed in the bone marrow.

APPLIED PRACTICE

Read the scenario and answer the following questions.

Scenario

Julie Turner is working as a clinical medical assistant. A patient, Hector Olanski, comes in for a blood draw. The physician's order reads as follows:

> **COOK FAMILY MEDICINE (188) 555-1111**
>
> Patient: Hector Olanski
>
> DOB: 7-3-1938
> Date: 3-22-20XX
>
> Rx: PTT and CBC
>
> Dx: (1) Heparin monitoring
> (2) Phlebitis of lower extremities
>
> **Dr. Liam Cook**

While gathering supplies, Julie grabs a lavender-topped tube, a red-topped tube, and a light-blue-topped tube.

1. Did Julie collect the correct tubes for Mr. Olanski's blood draw? Why or why not? Explain your answer based on each of the tubes of blood that Julie collected.

   _____

   _____

   _____

2. What would be the correct order of draw?

   _____

   _____

   _____

3. Are there any additives in the tubes that Julie is using for the blood draw? If so, explain which additives are used (based on the color) and the action of each additive.

   _____

   _____

   _____

4. Fill in the label below according to how Julie should label each of Mr. Olanski's tubes of blood.*

_____	_____
(Collection date and time)	(Patient's DOB)
_____	
(Patient's name)	
_____	_____
(Initials)	(Ordering doctor)

*This example of a label may vary based on laboratory or office policy; a patient ID number may also be used if necessary or required.

LEARNING ACTIVITY: TRUE/FALSE

Indicate whether the following statements are true or false by placing a T or an F on the line that precedes each statement.

_____ 1. It is important to shake a tube of blood to ensure that proper mixing occurs between the blood and anticoagulant within the tube.

_____ 2. Occasionally, uncontrollable bleeding can occur when the needle is withdrawn.

_____ 3. Capillary puncture is also called a fingerstick.

_____ 4. Wait until all of the blood tubes have been collected before releasing the tourniquet on the patient's arm.

_____ 5. Plasma is mostly made of formed elements.

CRITICAL THINKING

Answer the following questions to the best of your ability. Utilize the textbook as a reference.

1. A patient needs to have blood drawn for an ESR and a glucose level. The patient is extremely nervous and worried about the pain she will experience with a blood draw and asks if you can "stick her finger" instead. Will that work in this scenario? Why or why not? Explain how you can help the patient with her apprehension.

_____

_____

_____

_____

2. LaShawna has drawn three tubes of blood (gray topped, lavender topped, and dark green topped). She filled the lavender-topped tube first, the gray-topped tube second, and the dark green-topped tube last. Is this the correct order of draw? If not, what could possibly happen because of the mistake?

_____

_____

_____

_____

3. A patient has come in today for a blood draw to have a lipid panel and liver function test performed. She is 78 years old, has fragile skin, and states, "They always have trouble because by veins are so tiny." Which method of phlebotomy would you use on this patient, and why?

_____

_____

_____

_____

_____

RESEARCH ACTIVITY

Use Internet search engines to research the following topic and write a brief description of what you find. It is important to use reputable websites.

1. Visit the Clinical and Laboratory Standards Institute website, at www.clsi.org. Navigate through the website and identify reasons the website would be beneficial for medical assistants working in a clinical or physician's office laboratory.

   _____

   _____

   _____

   _____

   _____

CHAPTER 47
Hematology

STUDENT STUDY GUIDE

Use the following guide to assist in your learning of the concepts from the chapter.

I. The Role of the Medical Assistant

   1. When the physician orders a blood test, the role of the medical assistant is to

    _____ and _____ the specimen.

   2. It is important to know _____ _____ and to understand what test

    results reveal to properly educate the patient and recognize _____ situations.

   3. Blood Specimen Collection

    A. CLIA sets the standards to which all _____ must adhere, including training of

      _____ and testing and transport of _____.

    B. It is part of the role of the medical assistant to _____ between normal and

      abnormal test values and notify the physician of _____ values.

II. Blood Function, Formation, and Components

   1. The main functions of blood are _____ and _____.

   2. Plasma

    A. The _____ component of blood is plasma.

    B. Plasma makes up about _____ percent of the composition of blood.

    C. A key component of plasma is _____, which converts to fibrin, whose

      function is the formation of _____ _____.

    D. Ninety percent of plasma is _____; the other 10 percent is

      _____ substances called _____that dissolve in plasma.

   3. Cellular Components (Formed Elements)

    A. The formation of blood cells is called _____.

    B. All blood cells originate from the hematopoietic _____cell.

    C. Types of cells and their functions include the following.

      i. Red blood cells (_____)—Transport _____ and carbon

      dioxide.

ii. White blood cells (_____)—Provide defense.

    a. Granular leukocytes include _____, _____, and _____.

    b. Nongranular leukocytes include _____ and _____.

iii. Platelets (_____)—Enable clotting.

III. Formed Elements and Associated Tests

  1. Blood tests can be ordered individually or in groups, referred to as _____, _____, or _____.

  2. List the seven tests that make up a complete blood count (CBC).

    A. _____

    B. _____

    C. _____

    D. _____

    E. _____

    F. _____

    G. _____

  3. Red Blood Cells and Red Blood Cell Tests

    A. Red blood cells are formed in the _____ _____ and are routinely replaced every _____ _____.

    B. Hemoglobin is a vital _____ _____ found in red blood cells that has two primary functions: to carry _____ from the _____ to the cells of the body and to carry _____ _____ from throughout the body back to the _____, where it can be expelled with exhalation.

  4. Erythrocyte or Red Blood Cell (RBC) Count

    A. The RBC count is the number of red blood cells per _____ _____ (mm^3) of blood.

    B. The normal RBC range for a male adult is _____ to _____ million/mm^3.

    C. The normal female RBC range is _____ to _____ million/mm^3, although it may slightly decrease during _____.

    D. Anemia is a condition in which the blood has a(n) _____-than-normal level of red blood cells or of _____ within the red blood cells.

    E. Polycythemia is a condition in which the blood has a(n) _____-than-_____ level of red blood cells.

5. Reticulocyte Count

   A. Reticulocytes, or _____ red blood cells, generally mature within _____ hours.

   B. Evaluating the reticulocyte rate helps determine the ability of the _____ _____ to compensate for RBC loss.

   C. Reticulocyte counts are often used to monitor the _____ to treatment for _____.

6. Hemoglobin (Hgb)

   A. Hemoglobin in the blood is responsible for carrying _____ throughout the body.

   B. With higher hemoglobin levels, the body is able to transport more _____, and with lower levels, less oxygen is in _____.

   C. Normal values for adult females are _____ to _____ g/dL and for males are _____ to _____ g/dL.

   D. Hemoglobin can be measured either by a(n) _____ blood analyzer or manually by a(n) _____.

   E. Abnormal levels of hemoglobin can be _____ because they affect the level of oxygen available to the _____.

   F. An Hgb level that is less than 5 g/dL can result in _____ _____ and is considered to be a critical value that must be reported to the _____ at once.

   G. Excessive hemoglobin (over 20 g/dL) can lead to _____ _____ from increased concentration and is considered _____.

7. Hematocrit (Hct)

   A. The _____ (_____) test evaluates the percentage of packed red blood cells in the total volume of blood.

   B. A normal hematocrit is _____ to _____ percent in males and _____ to _____ percent in females.

   C. A low hematocrit may indicate _____ or _____.

   D. An elevated hematocrit may indicate _____ or _____.

   E. The microhematocrit, or "crit," is a hematocrit performed on an extremely _____ quantity of blood collected in a(n) _____ tube.

8. Erythrocyte/RBC Indices

   A. Erythrocyte indices help _____ the type of anemia present by indicating the size of RBCs and the _____ of Hgb.

   B. The _____ _____ _____ measures the average size of RBCs and classifies them according to size.

C. The _____ _____ _____ measures the average amount of hemoglobin in a red blood cell.

D. The _____ _____ _____ _____ measures the amount of hemoglobin relative to the size of the cell.

9. Erythrocyte Sedimentation Rate

   A. The ESR ("sed rate") determines the rate at which RBCs settle at the _____ of a(n) _____.

   B. The sed rate is related to the condition of the RBCs and the amount of _____ in the _____.

   C. When a sed rate test is conducted on a patient, RBCs that fall at a(n) _____-than-normal rate can indicate the possible existence of conditions _____ with increased _____.

   D. Increased values may suggest _____, which can occur from a(n) _____ or a variety of _____.

10. Leukocyte, or White Blood Cell (WBC), Count

    A. A complete WBC count includes the total number of all types of white blood cells in a(n) _____ of blood.

    B. A normal WBC count in adults ranges from approximately _____ to _____ thousand/mm^3.

    C. An elevated level usually indicates _____ because the body is increasing white blood cell production to fight _____.

    D. A low level usually indicates a(n) _____ _____ or autoimmune deficiency, as these conditions typically _____ white cells.

    E. A WBC count can be performed either manually with a(n) _____ or by a(n) _____ blood analyzer.

11. Differential WBC Count

    A. A differential WBC count ("diff") determines the _____ of each type of _____ in a given sample.

    B. This test is most commonly performed by a(n) _____ _____.

    C. The types of leukocytes that are counted in a differential WBC include the following.

       i. Neutrophils—Act as the body's _____ _____ and make up the _____ percentage of white blood cells.

          a. Segmented neutrophils make up _____ to _____ percent of all white blood cells in adults.

          b. Nonsegmented neutrophils make up roughly _____ to _____ percent of all white blood cells.

ii. Eosinophils—Assumed to be produced by the _____

_____.

a. Eosinophils make up less than _____ percent of white blood cell volume.

iii. Basophils—Thought to be produced by the bone marrow; they produce

_____.

a. Basophils are less than _____ percent of white blood cell volume.

iv. Lymphocytes—Produced in the bone _____ and _____

_____.

a. The function of lymphocytes is primarily to produce _____ against

foreign substances such as bacteria, viruses, and _____.

b. Lymphocytes comprise _____ to _____ percent of WBC volume.

v. Monocytes—Formed in bone marrow and stem cells.

a. Monocytes _____ foreign particles or bacteria that the neutrophils

are unable to _____.

b. They assist in cleaning up _____ _____ that may have

been left from an infection.

c. Monocytes make up _____ to _____ percent of the total white blood cell volume.

12. Platelet and Coagulation Studies

A. Platelets are formed in the _____ _____.

B. Platelets live for about _____ days and are continuously _____.

C. The main function of platelets is to assist in the _____ of blood to stop

_____ or assist in _____.

D. Platelet counts

i. There are typically between _____ and _____ platelets/mm^3 in adults.

ii. A condition called _____ occurs when platelet count is over 750,000.

iii. A condition called _____ occurs at a critical level when the platelet

count is less than 50,000.

E. Prothrombin time (PT, protime) International Normalized Ratio (INR)/(PT/INR)

i. Prothrombin time is a(n) _____ test that measures the amount of time it

takes to form a(n) _____.

ii. The International Normalized Ratio (INR) is a(n) _____

_____ that allows specimens performed at different laboratories to have

_____ results.

iii. The protime for an average healthy adult will show clotting at _____ to _____

_____.

F. Partial thromboplastin time (PTT)

    i. A PTT test determines the length of time it takes for a(n) _____

       _____ to form.

    ii. The PTT is commonly used to determine the effectiveness of _____

       therapy such as _____ or _____.

    iii. Normal findings are typically _____ to _____ _____.

IV. Other Blood Tests

  1. List the three tests commonly performed in a lipid panel.

    A. _____

    B. _____

    C. _____

  2. List the four tests included in a liver panel.

    A. _____

    B. _____

    C. _____

    D. _____

  3. Comprehensive Metabolic Panel (CMP)

    A. A CMP is a screening tool that is used to evaluate _____

      _____, check for _____ _____, or monitor the

      progress of current _____ and response to _____.

    B. The CMP includes 14 essential tests in the _____ metabolic panel,

      _____ panel, _____ function tests, and _____.

    C. List the 14 essential tests included in the CMP.*

      i. _____

      ii. _____

      iii. _____

      iv. _____

      v. _____

      vi. _____

      vii. _____

      viii. _____

      ix. _____

      x. _____

      xi. _____

These tests will be discussed in an activity later in this chapter.

xii. _____

xiii. _____

xiv. _____

4. Diabetic Tests

   A. Diabetics monitor their blood sugar with a portable machine called a(n)

     _____.

   B. A(n) _____ _____ (HbgA1C) test measures the long-term

     control of diabetes.

      i. The _____ of glucose in the cells is measured to reveal the patient's

       average plasma concentration of glucose over a(n) _____-month period.

      ii. The typical result for a nondiabetic adult is _____ to _____ percent.

   C. A(n) _____ _____ test is commonly used to detect pregnancy-

     induced diabetes.

      i. Blood is drawn to detect a(n) _____ after fasting.

      ii. The patient is given an oral _____ _____ to drink, and

       blood is redrawn to detect the response after _____ minutes and every

       _____ thereafter for up to _____ hours.

5. Phenylketonuria (PKU)

   A. PKU is a congenital disease caused by a defect in the _____ of the amino acid

     _____.

      i. When it accumulates in the bloodstream and goes undetected and untreated, the result

       is _____ _____.

   B. The PKU test is always performed on _____ to determine the presence of the

     unmetabolized protein phenylalanine.

6. Mono Testing

   A. The mono test is used to help determine whether a patient has _____

     _____.

   B. It is also known as the mononucleosis _____ test.

   C. A mono test is primarily ordered when an adolescent patient has symptoms such as

     _____, headache, _____ glands, and fatigue.

   D. The test may be repeated when it is initially _____ but suspicion of mono

     remains _____.

   E. It is also important to identify _____ _____, whenever present

     because it should be treated promptly with antibiotics.

KEY TERMINOLOGY REVIEW

Match each of the following terms with the correct definition.

a. anemia   d. phenylketonuria
b. erythropoietin   e. polycythemia
c. hematopoiesis

1. _____ A condition in which the blood has a lower-than-normal level of red blood cells or of hemoglobin within the red blood cells.

2. _____ A condition in which the blood has a higher-than-normal level of red blood cells.

3. _____ A congenital disease caused by a defect in the metabolism of an amino acid.

4. _____ The formation of blood cells.

5. _____ A glycoprotein hormone that controls RBC production.

APPLIED PRACTICE

Answer the questions related to the scenario below.

Scenario

Lorraine Spencer is a registered medical assistant. She has been asked to perform a microhematocrit for a female patient with excessive fatigue.

1. What equipment and supplies does Lorraine need to perform this test in the office setting?

_____

_____

_____

2. The patient's result is 30 percent. Is this a normal reading? Explain your answer.

_____

_____

_____

3. Could the results be indicative of any disease process? Explain your answer.

_____

_____

_____

LEARNING ACTIVITY: MATCHING

Match each of the tests below with the correct description.

1. _____ glucose

2. _____ blood urea nitrogen

3. _____ creatinine

4. _____ calcium

5. _____ sodium

6. _____ potassium

7. _____ bicarbonate/carbon dioxide

8. _____ chloride

9. _____ albumin

10. _____ total protein

11. _____ bilirubin

12. _____ alkaline phosphatase

13. _____ aspartate amino transferase

14. _____ alanine amino transferase

a. A liver protein that helps in fluid balance maintenance and assists with movement of small molecules through the blood.

b. A waste product of muscle energy metabolism that is excreted by the kidney. These levels generally rise only when more than half of kidney function has been lost.

c. An enzyme found primarily in the liver. Abnormalities may represent hepatobiliary disease.

d. Helps to maintain activity of the heart and skeletal muscles by influencing the conduction of electrical impulses. Abnormal levels can be dangerous because they are often asymptomatic until very severe changes are present.

e. A group of enzymes found in the liver, gallbladder, intestine, and bones. Testing for it is useful for evaluating bone and liver functions.

f. A simple sugar required by all body cells to produce energy. As levels rise, they become more dangerous, with critical, life-threatening levels above 700 mg/dL while fasting.

g. An enzyme found mostly in heart muscle and the liver. Abnormalities may indicate liver disease or recent heart attack.

h. A substance that controls the distribution of water throughout the body. It also assists in muscle contraction and nerve impulse transmission. Critical values are noted at less than 130 or more than 160 mEq/L.

i. A test that measures the overall state of nutrition in the body, as well as liver or collagen disease.

j. A value that is often tested to evaluate protein intake, the liver's ability to metabolize, and the functioning ability of the kidney. Levels may be abnormally elevated by hormones or a high-protein diet.

k. A substance produced in the liver, spleen, and bone marrow that is also a byproduct of hemoglobin metabolism. A wide variety of disease processes cause increases.

l. Works with other electrolytes to help maintain fluid and acid–base balance and osmotic pressure within the body.

m. Important for neuromuscular activity and blood coagulation; the most dominant mineral present in the human body.

n. Helps balance the levels of acid in the blood, or pH.

CRITICAL THINKING

Answer the following questions to the best of your ability. Use the textbook as a reference.

1. A physician has ordered a renal function panel for Mary Milton. Review some of her results below. Would any of the results need to be flagged for the physician as abnormal values? List the complete names (not just the abbreviations) of all the tests included in a renal function panel.

   BUN 24 mg/dL
   Na 140 mEq/L
   Creatinine 1.8 mg/dL

   _____

   _____

   _____

   _____

   _____

2. Describe how a physician uses blood testing to evaluate and monitor diabetic patients.

   _____

   _____

   _____

   _____

   _____

RESEARCH ACTIVITY

Use Internet search engines to research the following topic and write a brief description of what you find. It is important to use reputable websites.

1. Visit the U.S. Bureau of Labor Statistics website, www.bls.gov, and look up the job of a medical laboratory technician. Describe the responsibilities of a med lab tech, the education requirements, and the projected need for people in this kind of job over the next several years.

   _____

   _____

   _____

   _____

   _____

CHAPTER 48
Radiology and Diagnostic Testing

STUDENT STUDY GUIDE

Use the following guide to assist in your learning of the concepts from the chapter.

I. Introduction

   1. A(n) _____ is a physician who specializes in radiology.

   2. A radiographer is involved in making _____ _____, or X-rays.

   3. Duties of a Radiographer

      A. _____ patients for radiographic procedures

      B. Determining the proper _____, current, and exposure _____ for each X-ray

      C. Adjusting radiographic _____

      D. _____ the film

      E. Assisting the radiologist with _____ _____

   4. Medical assistants might not be able to take X-rays without _____ _____; however, they may refer patients for _____ _____.

II. Radiology

   1. Radiology is the branch of medicine that uses _____ _____, or matter that gives off _____ (radiant energy), and various techniques to visualize the _____ structures of the body for the diagnosis and treatment of disease.

   2. Principles of X-Rays

      A. X-rays were discovered by Wilhelm Konrad _____ in 1895.

      B. When X-rays are emitted from the tube, they form a cone-shaped X-ray _____.

      C. The patient is placed between the _____ producing the X-ray beam and the _____ where the image is recorded.

      D. Bones are _____ and allow fewer X-rays to pass through.

      E. Softer tissues are _____, permitting greater penetration of X-rays.

      F. Radiopaque tissue appears _____ on the film, and radiolucent tissues leave a(n) _____, _____ image.

3. Characteristics of X-rays

   A. X-rays _____ substances of different _____ to varying degrees.

   B. They cause _____ of the substances through which they pass.

   C. They cause _____ of certain substances.

   D. They travel in a(n) _____ _____, so the X-ray beam can be directed at a specific area.

   E. X-rays destroy body cells and can be used to kill _____ cells.

III. Overview of Diagnostic Imaging

  1. Use of Contrast Medium

   A. A contrast medium is a substance that _____ _____ of the tissue or structure being studied.

   B. Contrast media may be _____, _____, or gases.

   C. They are administered _____, by injection, or by _____.

   D. Positive contrast media (which appear _____ on an X-ray) include _____ _____ and _____.

     i. Barium sulfate is frequently used for examination of the _____ tract.

     ii. Iodine is employed for _____ studies, pyelograms, _____, and _____.

   E. Negative contrast media (which appear _____ on an X-ray) include air, _____ _____, and other gases.

     i. These media are used for _____ or _____.

     ii. Negative contrast studies have largely been replaced with the use of _____ _____ _____.

IV. The Medical Assistant's Role in Diagnostic Imaging

  1. The MA's Role

   A. The MA may _____ the procedure ordered by the physician.

   B. The MA may _____ the patient about the procedure.

   C. The MA should explain the _____ needed.

   D. The MA should inform the patient how _____ the entire _____ will take.

   E. The MA must give _____ _____ to the patient and thoroughly review the instructions before the patient leaves the _____.

   F. After additional schooling or certification, an MA can specialize in becoming a(n) _____ _____ X-ray technician.

   G. The credentials that are often obtained include GXMO (_____ X-ray machine _____) and LXMO (_____ X-ray _____ operator).

H. The medical assistant must make every effort to provide a gown that is a(n)

_____ size and _____ the patient to preserve patient

_____.

I. The MA should request that the patient remove all _____ materials such as

jewelry.

J. For some X-rays of the head, mouth, and neck, the patient may have to remove

_____.

2. Positioning

A. It is helpful for the medical assistant to understand that the patient's _____

relative to the source of _____ determines the _____ that are

produced.

B. The position of the patient is critical for a(n) _____ X-ray.

3. Scheduling Guidelines

A. List the four items that must be provided when setting an appointment with an outside

facility.

i. _____

ii. _____

iii. _____

iv. _____

B. Special _____ _____ in preparation for radiographic

procedures often call for a(n) _____-_____ diet on the day before the test.

C. Remind the patient that NPO means "_____ ____ _____."

D. In general, examinations that do not require the use of a(n) _____

_____ are performed _____ examinations with contrast

medium.

E. Some procedures require long _____ _____ between imaging

procedures, and this should be carefully _____ to the patient to schedule

patient time appropriately.

V. Diagnostic Imaging Procedures

1. Radiologic Imaging Procedures Requiring Contrast Media

A. Fluoroscopy is the use of a fluoroscope to see _____ moving images of

internal _____ and _____.

B. Fluoroscopic procedures

i. A gastrointestinal series is a study of the _____ _____

using contrast media to detect abnormalities such as _____, ulcers,

_____, and diverticulosis.

a. An upper GI series is an examination of the _____, stomach, _____, and small intestine that requires the patient to _____ a barium solution.

b. A lower GI series is the administration of a barium _____, which outlines the _____ and _____ on a radiographic picture.

ii. An intravenous pyelogram is a radiologic examination of the _____, _____, and _____.

a. The patient should be screened for _____ sensitivity before this procedure.

iii. Retrograde pyelography involves inserting a(n) _____ into the urinary tract through the _____ and into the ureters.

a. The _____ is sent up the tube into the ureters and kidneys, and X-rays are taken to evaluate the function of the _____, _____, and _____.

iv. A cholecystogram is a radiologic examination of the _____ using a contrast medium, usually _____.

a. This procedure is done to detect abnormalities such as the presence of _____.

v. Myelography is a fluoroscopic procedure of the _____ _____.

a. A lumbar puncture is done to remove some _____ _____ (CSF) and instill contrast medium.

b. This procedure is used to detect compression of the spinal cord or _____ _____.

C. Angiography is X-ray visualization of the internal anatomy of _____ _____ after a radiopaque material has been _____ into the blood vessels.

i. Angiography may be used to study the blood vessels of the brain (_____ _____), the kidneys (_____ _____), and the heart (_____ _____).

D. Arthrography is X-ray visualization of a(n) _____ _____.

i. The procedure involves injecting a(n) _____ _____ followed by contrast medium or air or both into the joint.

ii. A(n) _____ is used to evaluate the function of a joint.

2. Procedures Not Requiring Contrast Media
   A. Mammography is radiologic examination of the soft tissue of the _____ to
      identify benign and _____ neoplasms (tumors).
      i. Some patients may feel discomfort during the procedure, which requires
         _____ of the breast.
   B. Kidneys, _____, and _____ (KUB) radiography is used to
      assess the size, shape, and location of the organs of the _____ tract and to
      detect kidney _____ and diseases of the urinary tract.
3. Tomography
   A. Tomography, which uses radiography to produce _____ views of the body,
      allows the technician to penetrate _____ _____ of the body
      that could not otherwise be visualized.
   B. Computed tomography (CT)
      i. Computed tomography combines radiography with _____
         _____ of tissue density.
      ii. The X-ray camera _____ completely around the patient, and the
          computer accumulates cross-sectional _____ from each rotation of the
          camera.
      iii. CT scan preparation
           a. For some CT procedures, a(n) _____ _____ is used,
              and the patient may be instructed to be _____ for 4 hours before the
              procedure.
           b. Any _____ _____ will interfere with a CT scan, so the
              MA should instruct the patient to remove all metallic objects and ask whether the
              patient has a(n) _____ or metallic _____.
   C. Position emission tomography (PET)
      i. PET is a computerized radiographic method that uses _____ substances
         to examine _____ _____ within the body.
      ii. PET is used to assist in the treatment of _____, _____
          tumors, stroke, Alzheimer's disease, _____ flow, and metabolism of the
          _____ and blood vessels.
4. Magnetic Resonance Imaging (MRI)
   A. MRI uses a powerful _____ _____ to visualize internal tissues,
      organs, and structures.
   B. An MRI scan can give the viewer a(n) _____-dimensional view of tissues or
      organs of the body in total or as _____.

C. The procedure, although painless, can be upsetting to patients who have _____, which is a fear of closed-in spaces.

D. In cases of extreme apprehension, the patient may need to be given a(n) _____ to promote _____.

E. An MRI scan takes from _____ to _____ minutes, depending on the amount of the body to be scanned.

5. Digital Radiography

   A. Digital radiology is the use of standard _____ that is digitized, stored as _____ bits, processed, and then converted into an image on a television or _____ _____ screen.

6. Ultrasound (Sonography)

   A. Ultrasound imaging consists of projecting a beam of _____ _____ into the body.

   B. The waves, at about _____ cycles per second, bounce back as the beam comes into contact with a structure, such as a fetus, which then produces a(n) _____ of the internal structure.

   C. Ultrasound is used to scan organs such as the _____, heart, _____, thyroid, gonads, and _____ _____.

   D. Sound waves cannot penetrate _____.

   E. Ultrasound scanning

      i. A conduction material such as water, a special _____, or _____ is used to conduct the sound waves into the body.

      ii. An ultrasonic _____ (a device that both produces and senses _____ _____) with a conduction head is placed on or near the skin.

      iii. The patient is often able to view the sonogram on the _____ as it occurs.

      iv. The picture can be _____ for the patient's record and, in some cases, a copy of this printout is given to the _____.

7. Bone Densitometry

   A. A bone densitometry test (DXA) uses X-rays to quickly measure the density of bone to detect _____ or _____.

   B. _____ _____ and medications that contain calcium should be discontinued _____ hours before the test.

VI. Radiation Therapy

   1. Radiation therapy is the process of administering a particular dosage of _____ to a specific area on the patient's body for the purpose of killing _____ _____, such as cancers.

2. Radiation actually alters the cells so they cannot _____, and thus they eventually die, leaving no _____ _____ to develop.

3. Radiation Rays

    A. Radioactive substances emit three types of rays: _____, _____, and _____.

        i. Alpha rays are the _____ penetrating rays.

        ii. Beta rays are able to penetrate body tissues a few _____.

        iii. Gamma rays can penetrate most body tissue but are absorbed by _____.

4. Uses of Radiation Therapy

    A. Radiation therapy is implemented for the following types of cancer.

        i. Cancer of the _____, testes, _____, larynx, and _____ cavity

        ii. _____ disease

        iii. _____ tumor (a type of kidney tumor found in children)

        iv. _____ (an eye cancer)

    B. When a cure is not probable, radiation may be used to shrink tumors to alleviate _____, relieve _____, or stop _____.

5. Radiation Techniques

    A. External radiation therapy

        i. External radiation therapy involves administering _____ doses of _____ from a machine positioned at a specific _____ from the site (tumor).

        ii. A computer calculates the dosage required to _____ the largest number of _____ cells while causing the least _____ to surrounding cells.

    B. Internal radiation therapy

        i. Sealed radiation involves the implantation of _____ _____ of radioactive material near the tumor in the body.

        ii. Unsealed radiation involves introducing a liquid form of radioactive substance into the patient by _____, _____, or _____ into a body cavity.

VII. Safety Precautions

    1. The biological effects of radiation exposure vary with the type of _____ and its _____.

    2. A rad, which stands for _____ _____ _____, is the unit used to measure the amount of ionizing radiation absorbed during an X-ray procedure.

3. To measure _____ exposure or other exposure that may involve more than one type of radiation, the unit used is the rem, which stands for _____ _____ in _____.

4. The _____, or personal radiation badge, records the occupational exposure dose, reported in _____.

5. Radiation Exposure

   A. Advances in diagnostic imaging have _____ the radiation dose a patient is exposed to during a(n) _____ _____.

   B. Excessive exposure to radiation causes _____ damage and side effects.

   C. List six symptoms of radiation sickness.

      i. _____

      ii. _____

      iii. _____

      iv. _____

      v. _____

      vi. _____

   D. Cellular effects of radiation

      i. Radiation damages the DNA of cells in both _____ and _____ cells.

      ii. The less specialized a normal cell is, the more it will be _____ by radiation.

      iii. Excessive radiation to embryonic cells causes spontaneous _____, retardation, genetic _____, and increased risk of _____ and other cancers.

6. Personal Safety Precautions

   A. Radiation is discussed in terms of _____ and _____ radiation.

      i. _____ radiation strikes the patient either for therapeutic reasons or for an X-ray procedure.

      ii. Once the primary beam strikes the _____, it can become _____ radiation as it bounces off the patient.

   B. Lead _____, shields, and _____ are provided for personnel coming into close contact with X-ray equipment.

   C. X-ray technicians stand behind a(n) _____-_____ divider.

   D. A dosimeter, or film badge, records the _____ and _____ of radiation exposure.

      i. It is periodically examined to ensure that the health care worker is not _____ to _____ radiation.

E. All radiographic equipment should be checked on a regular basis to ensure that it is in good _____ _____ and to check for radiation _____.

F. Radioactive materials should be stored in _____ containers and handled only with _____, never with bare hands.

7. Patient Safety Precautions

   A. The guiding principle in the use of radiation is "as _____ as _____ _____."

   B. An X-ray may be taken only within _____ days of the last _____ period to avoid taking an X-ray of a female who is unknowingly _____.

   C. Patients should be protected from secondary or scatter radiation by the use of a(n) _____ during radiographic procedures.

      i. The grid is positioned between the _____ _____ and the patient to absorb radiation _____ before it reaches the film.

      ii. Patients should be provided with a lead shield for _____, eyes, _____, and _____ whenever appropriate.

VIII. X-Ray Records: Storage and Ownership

1. X-ray materials for radiologic procedures must be kept in special _____ _____ that protect the film from damage caused by _____, heat, _____ fumes, and _____.

2. X-ray film should be stored on end to prevent _____ _____ from stacking the film.

3. X-ray developer is kept in a(n) _____ location that is _____ free because damage to this fluid can affect the quality of the film.

4. Film should be touched only with _____ _____ and should be hung _____ to avoid damage.

5. All film records are maintained in a(n) _____ or _____ that is kept in the X-ray room.

6. Films that have been processed should be stored in _____ _____ and filed in specially designed film cabinets.

7. Ownership of Film

   A. X-ray film is the property of the _____ _____ or _____ that performed the X-ray.

   B. If the film remains in one location, it can always be accessed for future _____ and _____.

C. Physicians are able to lend their films to _____ _____ for further examination.

D. The patient has to sign a(n) _____ of _____ form for this to take place, but the film must then be returned to the _____ facility.

KEY TERMINOLOGY REVIEW

Match each of the following terms with the correct definition.

a. angiography   d. radiolucent

b. fluoroscopy   e. radiopaque

c. arthrography

1. _____ Procedure using a contrast medium that enables the visualization of real-time moving images of internal structures and organs.

2. _____ X-ray visualization of the internal anatomy of blood vessels.

3. _____ Permits greater penetration of X-rays.

4. _____ X-ray visualization of a joint space.

5. _____ Allows fewer X-rays to pass through.

APPLIED PRACTICE

Use information from the patient's medical record listed below to answer the following questions about the scenario.

Epley, Marguerite V.
11-24-1981

3/18/20XX, 2:15 P.M.

Ht: 5'5" Wt: 115 lbs.   T: 98.6°F   P: 90 bpm   BP: 136/88

cc: Pt. presents to office with rt. lower leg pain, after falling while getting out of her bathtub. Pt. rates the pain as a 6 on a scale of 1 to 10. Rt. lower leg appears to be swollen and without bruising at this time.

Jerry Li, CMA (AAMA), LXMO

Scenario

Dr. Jefferson wants Jerry Li, CMA (AAMA), LXMO, to perform an X-ray of Ms. Epley's lower rt. leg. The order reads as follows:

PT: *Marguerite Epley DOB: 11/24/1981*
Rt. lower leg X-ray. AP and lateral views.
Dx: *R/O Fx (Diagnosis: Rule out fracture)*

1. Dr. Jefferson ordered an AP view. What is an AP view?

   _____

   _____

   _____

2. How do you think Jerry should position the patient for the lateral view?

   _____

   _____

   _____

3. List some of the protective devices that Jerry should use during the X-ray.

   _____

   _____

   _____

LEARNING ACTIVITY: FILL IN THE BLANK

Using words from the list below, fill in the blanks to complete the following sentences.

carbon dioxide	high-frequency
contrast medium	liquid
dietary	rem
dosimeter	pregnant
front to back	Sensitivity
iodine	sonography
negative	ultrasound
stomach	upper GI series
ultraviolet	

1. In preparation for a(n) _____, the patient should not eat or drink after midnight because the _____ must be empty for this procedure.

2. Radiology uses X-rays, radioactive substances, and other forms of radiant energy such as _____ rays.

3. A(n) _____ is a substance that enhances visibility of the tissue or structure being studied.

4. _____ contrast medium is a radiolucent substance that allows X-rays to pass through more easily. Examples include air, _____, and other gases.

5. In the anteroposterior (AP) view, the X-ray beam is directed from _____.

6. Before an X-ray, any female must be asked whether she could be _____.

7. With regard to patient preparation and instructions for an IVP: The patient should be screened for _____ prior to the procedure.

8. _____, or _____, is the use of _____ sound waves to image internal structures.

9. Special _____ restrictions in preparation for radiographic procedures often call for an all-_____ diet on the day before the test.

10. The _____ containing the occupational exposure dose is reported in _____.

CRITICAL THINKING

Answer the following questions to the best of your ability. Use the textbook as a reference.

1. Anna Maria is a 5-year-old who is in need of an X-ray of her upper right leg. She is very apprehensive and scared about the X-ray. When you place the lead shield over her abdomen, you notice a rip and crack in the shield. How would you proceed with this patient?

_____

_____

_____

_____

_____

2. Mr. Abdul has come in for a cholecystogram. As you put the patient into the room, you ask him if he has followed the preparation instructions of taking iodine the day before and then NPO this morning. He states that he took the iodine, but he accidentally ate breakfast prior to the appointment, forgetting the NPO instructions. What would you do?

_____

_____

_____

_____

_____

RESEARCH ACTIVITY

Use Internet search engines to research the following topic and write a brief description of what you find. It is important to use reputable websites.

1. Research your state's laws regarding limited-scope radiography. As a medical assistant with proper training and supervision, would you be allowed to practice limited-scope radiography?

_____

_____

_____

_____

_____

CHAPTER 49
Electrocardiography

STUDENT STUDY GUIDE

Use the following guide to assist in your learning of the concepts from the chapter.

I. Introduction

   1. Electrocardiography is a procedure for recording _____ _____ in the heart.

   2. The record that electrocardiography produces is called a(n) _____ (ECG).

   3. _____ is the abbreviation for electrocardiogram that is most commonly used in the United States, but the abbreviation _____ is also often used.

II. Electrical Cardiac Activity

   1. The electrical charges created by the heart's cardiac _____ _____ can be sensed throughout the body.

   2. When the ECG equipment senses an electrical charge, it is recorded on the readout as either a(n) _____ or a(n) _____ deflection from the horizontal baseline.

   3. The strength, or _____, of the electrical impulse determines the size of the deflection.

   4. Polarity and the Cardiac Cycle

     A. Polarity means having two separate poles, one _____ and one _____.

     B. The sinoatrial node is known as the heart's _____ because it controls myocardial polarity.

     C. When the SA node initiates electrical activity, the atrial cells become _____.

     D. As the cells depolarize, the atria and ventricles _____.

     E. During this stage of _____, the cells become repolarized.

     F. This cycle of electrical impulses—_____ and repolarization, contraction and _____—represents one _____.

   5. PQRST Waves

     A. A normal _____ cardiac cycle is traced on an electrocardiogram as one set of PQRST waves.

       i. The P represents atrial _____.

    ii. The QRS complex represents ventricular _____.

    iii. T represents _____.

  B. A(n) _____ heart rate has more space between the PQRST complexes.

  C. When the heart _____ a(n) _____, there is a long flat line between PQRSTs.

  D. Recordings are made from a variety of perspectives or angles known as

    _____.

  E. Each lead records from a specific _____ of _____.

6. Time and the Cardiac Cycle

  A. Normally, the P-R interval (time from the beginning of _____ to the middle of _____) is between _____ and _____ seconds.

  B. A deviation from these times could represent a(n) _____ in either the electrical system of the heart or in a(n) _____ of the heart that impacts the _____ system.

  C. The process of the QRS complex usually takes less than _____ to _____ second(s).

  D. A medical assistant should not try to _____ an ECG, but understanding what is normal in the _____ _____ is helpful.

7. Calculating Heart Rate

  A. Estimation of heart rate

    i. The 6-second method involves counting the number of P waves across _____ large, _____ squares (30 squares = 6 seconds) and multiplying this number by _____.

    ii. Counting P waves gives the estimated _____ _____ rate.

    iii. Measuring the number of complete QRS complexes across a span of _____ large squares and multiplying by 10 estimates the _____ contraction rate.

  B. Exact calculation of heart rate

    i. An exact calculation of ventricular heart rate is achieved by counting the _____ boxes (the smaller, lighter squares) between two _____ complexes and dividing that number into _____.

    ii. An exact calculation of atrial heart rate is achieved by counting the millimeter boxes between two _____ _____ and dividing that number into _____.

  C. Assessing heart rhythm

    i. There should be a fairly consistent space between _____ to qualify as a(n) _____ rhythm.

III. The Electrocardiogram Machine

1. International standard means that the paper in all machines moves at the same speed of _____ mm/second and, given the same amount of _____ energy, the recording stylus moves the same _____.

2. _____ is a means of verifying that each machine deflects 10 mm in response to 1 mV (millivolt) of electricity in sensitivity.

3. The majority of ECG machines used in the medical office are _____ and have automatic _____.

4. All _____ electrodes are placed on the patient at the beginning of the procedure, and the computer switches from lead to lead in _____ _____.

5. Two main types of ECG machines used in the medical office are _____ channel and _____.

6. A multichannel ECG records all 12 leads _____.

7. Some machines have a built-in _____ feature and print out a statement of the status of the heart.

8. New ECG models allow test results to be _____ transferred directly into the patient's medical _____.

9. It is the medical assistant's responsibility to produce a(n) _____ and _____ tracing for each patient.

10. List the eight features of an ECG machine control panel.

    A. _____

    B. _____

    C. _____

    D. _____

    E. _____

    F. _____

    G. _____

    H. _____

11. Electrocardiogram Paper

    A. Electrocardiogram paper is _____ and _____ sensitive and must be handled carefully.

    B. "Time" markers, referred to as _____-_____ markers, are printed on all ECG paper.

    C. The time markers are small squares with a(n) _____ line and larger squares with a(n) _____ line.

    D. Small squares are _____ mm by _____ mm square and represent _____ mV of voltage in the height and _____ second time in the width.

E. Larger squares are _____ mm by _____ mm square and represent _____ mV of voltage in the height and _____ second time in the width.

IV. Performing Electrocardiography

1. Electrode Placement

   A. The ECG machine records the cardiac cycle through 10 _____ (sensors) placed on the bare skin of the _____ (extremities) and the _____.

   B. The term "lead" often refers to both _____ and _____.

   C. Limb leads are placed over the _____ part of the _____ aspect of both lower legs and either both _____ arms or both _____, avoiding the bony prominences.

   D. _____ leads are placed on the chest.

   E. Identify the locations of the six precordial leads.

      i. V1— _____

      ii. V2— _____

      iii. V3— _____

      iv. V4— _____

      v. V5— _____

      vi. V6— _____

   F. An intercostal space is a space between _____.

   G. The sternal border is the border of the sternum, or _____.

   H. The midclavicular line is an imaginary _____ line that runs through the middle of the _____, or collarbone.

   I. After the electrodes have been applied to the correct anatomical locations, the _____ are attached.

   J. By recording from different _____ of directionality of electrodes, the electrical activity of the heart is seen from different _____.

2. Patient Preparation

   A. Explain the equipment, the _____, and what the patient is expected to do.

   B. The ECG is performed in an exam room, with the patient in the _____ position.

   C. Patients must be bare to the _____.

      i. Offer female patients a(n) _____ to be worn with the opening at the _____.

   D. Instruct patients to remove _____ or stockings and roll long _____ _____ out of the way.

E. Jewelry, particularly _____ jewelry, must be removed so it does not interfere with the _____ _____ of the ECG.

F. Prepare the skin where the _____ will be applied.

G. If men have large amounts of chest hair, it might be necessary to _____ small areas of the chest where _____ will be placed.

3. Special Considerations

A. If a patient has an amputated leg, one electrode should be placed on the _____ leg _____, and the other electrode should be placed _____ _____ from the electrode on the stump.

B. Patients with cognitive disabilities or small children may be unusually _____ of the procedure and may need to be reassured that no electricity is going into the body.

C. _____ _____ near leads may need to be removed.

D. Avoid placing leads on _____ or _____ if possible.

4. Technical Preparation

A. Plug the ECG machine into a properly _____ outlet on a(n) _____ exam room wall.

B. Verify that the machine is _____ and in compliance with the _____ standard.

C. When storing equipment after use, make sure it is _____ and stored according to _____ recommendations.

D. Have extra _____, electrodes, and _____ in stock for future use.

5. Mounting and Uploading

A. When cutting and pasting strips into the chart, cut part of the _____ strip that includes the indicated number of _____.

B. Paste strips into the chart, making sure to align the correct _____ with its _____.

C. If the equipment produces digital results, these can be _____ or electronically _____ into the EMR.

V. Adjustments and Troubleshooting

1. Making Adjustments

A. A satisfactory tracing is one that is _____, readable, and clear; travels across the _____ of the page; and has a baseline that is consistently _____.

B. If the baseline begins to drift upward or downward, use the _____ _____ knob to return it to the _____ of the page.

C. Sometimes it is necessary to adjust the _____ or sensitivity controls.

D. If you have to change the speed or sensitivity, mark the _____ to indicate that it was changed.

2. Artifacts

   A. Deflections, or artifacts, impair accurate _____ of the tracing.

   B. List the four common causes of artifacts.

      i. _____

      ii. _____

      iii. _____

      iv. _____

   C. Most ECG machines today are so technologically advanced that they are able to _____ and _____ artifacts.

3. Evaluating an Electrocardiogram

   A. Interpreting an ECG is beyond a medical assistant's _____ of _____.

   B. A medical assistant must be able to _____ and _____ an ECG to ensure that it is an acceptable tracing.

   C. What is normal?

      i. A normal sinus rhythm means that each heartbeat has _____ distinct waves.

      ii. In a normal rhythm, the beats come at regular _____, indicating that the impulse originates in the _____ _____.

      iii. Most newer ECG machines print out a(n) _____ with _____ identified.

   D. An observant medical assistant will recognize the _____ abnormalities and draw them to the attention of the _____ or will follow office protocol, which often calls for an additional recording of a particular _____.

VI. Special Procedures

1. Additional Tracings

   A. A(n) _____ _____ is run on lead II for 20 seconds at the physician's request or if the medical assistant sees anything that appears abnormal on the tracing.

   B. A(n) _____ _____ is run on lead II for 10 seconds with the patient holding his or her breath.

2. Exercise Tolerance Testing

   A. A(n) _____ test, or treadmill test, involves an evaluation of the heart's response during moderate _____ while a 12-lead ECG is performed.

B. It is performed to determine the likelihood of _____ _____ _____ (CAD).

C. The stress test is continued until _____ percent of the _____ _____ heart rate is achieved or the patient becomes symptomatic.

D. The formula for determining the maximum target heart rate is

_____.

E. Patient preparation

  i. In addition to providing the patient with the scheduled date and time, it is important to provide patient _____ and _____ about the procedure.

  ii. The patient should be instructed to wear comfortable _____ or _____ shoes and _____-fitting clothes on the day of the test.

  iii. Patients should not eat a large meal for at least _____ hours before the test to avoid _____.

  iv. Normal _____ should be taken unless otherwise instructed by the physician.

  v. Inform the patient that baseline _____ _____ and a(n) _____ ECG are recorded first.

  vi. Another ECG is taken with the patient standing and _____.

3. Varieties of Stress Tests

A. Additional types of stress tests may be ordered either based on the _____ of an exercise tolerance test or based on patient _____.

B. Two varieties of stress tests are _____ and _____ scan.

4. Holter Monitor

A. A Holter monitor records _____ activity while the patient is ambulatory for at least a(n) _____-hour period.

B. A small _____ device and a patient _____ are used to detect heart irregularities that are infrequent and not detected on the standard 12-lead cardiogram.

C. While wearing the monitor, patients carry out all routine daily activities except _____ or _____.

D. List six examples of activities a patient would record in a Holter monitor diary.

  i. _____

  ii. _____

  iii. _____

  iv. _____

  v. _____

  vi. _____

E. Patients also indicate in the diary or by pressing a(n) "_____ button" when they experience any cardiac symptoms, such as _____ _____, _____ of breath, or _____.

F. Five special _____ chest electrodes are attached more _____ than in the 12-lead ECG because they must remain in place during all activity.

G. Electrode placement

    i. _____ intercostal space, 2 or 3 inches to the _____ of the sternum

    ii. _____ intercostal space, 2 or 3 inches to the _____ of the sternum

    iii. _____ intercostal space at the _____ sternum margin

    iv. _____ intercostal space at the _____ anterior axillary line

    v. _____ intercostal space at the left anterior _____ line

5. Cardiac Event Monitor

A. Patients who have _____ cardiac events might be asked to wear a monitor for up to _____ days to ensure that any events can be captured.

B. Electrodes are worn much as they would be for a(n) _____ monitor.

C. The patient presses a button on the monitor when perceiving a cardiac event such as a(n) _____ or _____ heartbeat or dizziness or feeling _____.

6. Mobile Cardiac Telemetry (MCT)

A. Mobile cardiac telemetry allows a device to send data _____ to a facility that is staffed 24 hours per day.

B. The data are interpreted by a qualified, _____-trained registered _____.

C. There are a wide variety of telemetry monitors—with _____, _____, and _____ leads.

D. Leads are placed according to _____ _____.

7. Pacemakers

A. Pacemakers are electronic devices that help the heart maintain _____ _____.

B. Pacemakers may be _____ or _____ installed in the patient.

C. The type of permanent pacemaker implanted depends on the patient's _____ and the type of _____ problem involved.

D. An atrial-paced pacemaker shows a spike with the _____ wave.

E. Pacemakers that spike with the _____ wave are ventricular paced.

KEY TERMINOLOGY REVIEW

Match each of the following vocabulary terms to the correct definition.

    a. artifacts   d. stress test

    b. ischemic   e. thallium

    c. perfusion

1. _____ Any irregular or erratic markings on an EKG.
2. _____ A radioisotope that emits gamma rays and is used in nuclear medicine.
3. _____ Blood flow to the myocardium.
4. _____ Heart muscle that is receiving less than the normal amount of blood flow.
5. _____ Involves an evaluation of the heart's response during moderate exercise while a 12-lead ECG is performed.

APPLIED PRACTICE

Follow the directions as instructed for each question.

1. Identify the type of artifact shown in each of the following figures.

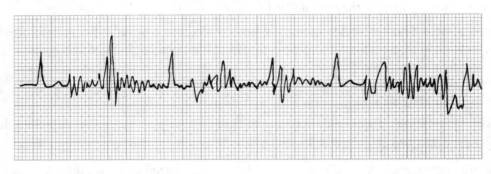

a. _____

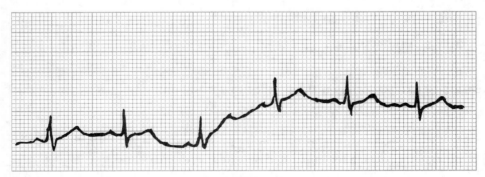

b. _____

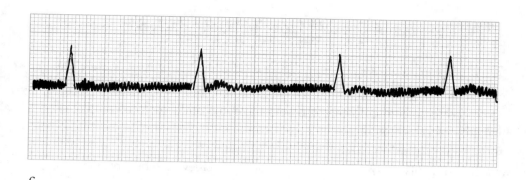

c. _____

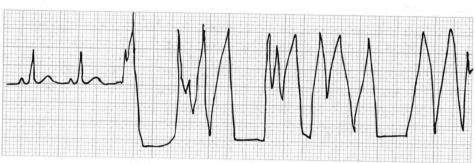

d. _____

2. Using the figure provided, identify the placement of electrode chest leads V1–V6.

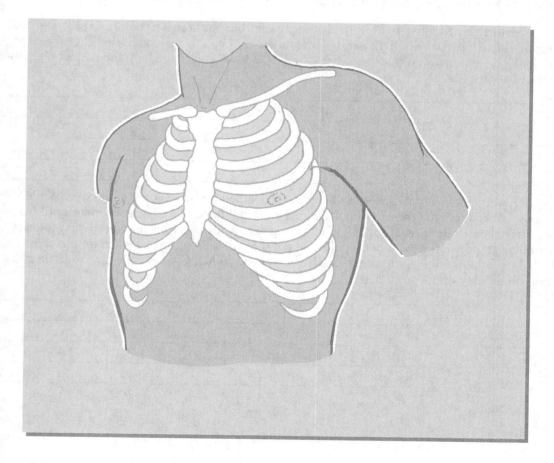

LEARNING ACTIVITY: TRUE/FALSE

Indicate whether the following statements are true or false by placing a T or an F on the line that precedes each statement.

_____ 1. The abbreviations ECG and EKG have different meanings and cannot be used interchangeably.

_____ 2. Electrocardiography introduces electricity into the heart.

_____ 3. Limb leads should be placed over bony prominences to achieve the best results.

_____ 4. Atrial and ventricular depolarization and repolarization, contraction and relaxation, represents one heartbeat.

_____ 5. When completed, a 12-lead EKG produces a two-dimensional record of cardiac impulses.

_____ 6. Normally, the P–R interval is between 0.12 and 0.20 seconds.

_____ 7. A P–R interval that is too long may indicate a conduction delay in the AV node.

_____ 8. A somatic tremor is caused by a tense muscle or a muscle contraction.

_____ 9. A rhythm strip is run on lead II for 60 seconds at the physician's request.

_____ 10. Pharmacological stress testing involves no exercise.

CRITICAL THINKING

Answer the following questions to the best of your ability. Use the textbook as a reference.

1. You need to perform an ECG on an elderly female patient, but she seems to be nervous or fearful. What are some signs the patient might exhibit that might lead you to the conclusion that she is fearful of the ECG? How would that fear affect the ECG? How could you help the patient feel more at ease about the procedure?

_____

_____

_____

_____

2. Henry Clymer is a 49-year-old patient who has been scheduled for an exercise stress test. While explaining the procedure, you mention that the physician will have Mr. Clymer exercise until his maximum target heart rate is reached. Mr. Clymer wants to know how his maximum target heart rate is figured out and what it is. What would you tell the patient regarding his maximum target heart rate? What additional information should be provided to Mr. Clymer in regard to patient preparation on the day of his procedure?

_____

_____

_____

_____

RESEARCH ACTIVITY

Use Internet search engines to research the following topic and write a brief description of what you find. It is important to use reputable websites.

1. Over the past 10 or more years, advancements have been made in addressing heart disease. Conduct research online to find out about some of the procedures and treatments that have been discovered recently. Write an essay on your findings. Be sure to cite your sources.

_____

_____

_____

_____

_____

CHAPTER 50
Pulmonary Function

STUDENT STUDY GUIDE

Use the following guide to assist in your learning of the concepts from the chapter.

I. The Role of the Medical Assistant in Pulmonology

    1. Medical assistants may perform several different tests to assess respiratory

        _____, assist in the _____ of patients with suspected

        obstructive or restrictive pulmonary disease, and assess the _____ of drug and

        other pulmonary therapies.

    2. The medical assistant must be knowledgeable about the _____ and

        _____ of the respiratory system and should be prepared to assist in or perform

        specialized _____ in this field.

II. Pulmonary Disorders

    1. _____ lung diseases include conditions that make it hard to exhale all the

        _____ from the lungs.

    2. Patients with _____ lung diseases have difficulty fully _____

        their lungs with air.

    3. Define the following common symptoms related to pulmonary conditions.

        A. Dyspnea—_____

        B. Coughing—_____

        C. Wheezing—_____

        D. Cyanosis— _____

        E. Rales— _____

        F. Stridor— _____

        G. Rhonchus— _____

        H. Hemoptysis—_____

III. Pulmonary Function Tests (PFTs)

    1. PFTs assess lung _____ and _____ and are often performed

        when a patient complains of shortness of breath, especially after _____

        exertion.

2. PFTs are also commonly performed to monitor lung function if a patient has been diagnosed with asthma, chronic _____, _____, or cystic fibrosis.

3. An awareness of the long-term effects of _____ and exposure to occupational or environmental _____ has increased the number of PFTs performed.

4. PFTs might be a component of a patient's annual _____ _____ to provide a(n) _____ measurement of the patient's lung function.

5. PFTs may also be a component of some pre-_____ physicals.

6. List six different types of PFTs.

   A. _____

   B. _____

   C. _____

   D. _____

   E. _____

   F. _____

7. The most common tests and procedures performed by the medical assistant are _____, _____ _____ meter instruction, and pulse _____.

8. Spirometry

   A. Spirometry is a noninvasive test that determines the ability of the lungs to effectively _____ and measures how _____.

   B. Spirometry is used to diagnose airflow _____ in patients with respiratory symptoms and can also be used to monitor disease _____ and improvements with _____.

   C. All spirometers consist of a(n) _____ and _____ connected to a(n) _____ device.

   D. During the spirometry test, the patient is asked to inhale as _____ as possible and then to exhale as _____ and as _____ as possible while measurements are being taken.

   E. At least _____ acceptable spirometry tests must be obtained to ensure the _____ of the measurements.

9. Spirometry Volumes and Capacities

   A. _____ rates are measurements of different _____ of air moving in and out during breathing.

      i. Forced vital capacity (FVC) measures the volume of air a patient can _____ with force after inhaling as _____ as possible.

ii. Forced expiratory volume (FEV) is the volume of air that can be

_____ exhaled in one _____.

iii. FEV^1 is forced expiratory volume after 1 _____.

iv. FEV^1 is a good indicator for patients with _____.

B. _____ _____ _____ measure lung

volumes and are indicators of patients' ability to expand their lungs.

C. List four types of pulmonary volumes measured.

   i. _____

   ii. _____

   iii. _____

   iv. _____

D. Define pulmonary capacities that are calculated based on pulmonary volumes.

   i. Total lung capacity (TLC)— _____

   _____

   ii. Vital capacity (VC)— _____

   _____

   iii. Inspiratory capacity (IC)— _____

   _____

   iv. Functional residual capacity (FRC)— _____

   _____

10. The Medical Assistant's Role in Spirometry Testing

    A. The medical assistant will most commonly perform spirometry testing as it relates to

    measuring the patient's _____ _____

    _____ (FVC).

    B. The patient must be prepared for the spirometry procedure, which requires proper

    _____ and _____ to obtain accurate results.

    C. The medical assistant should act as both _____ and _____

    to encourage the patient to give the best performance.

11. Patient Preparation and Testing Procedures*

    A. The patient should be instructed to refrain from _____ and from eating a

    large meal for _____ to _____ hours before the test.

    B. The patient should not use bronchodilators or _____ for _____ hour(s)

    before the test.

    C. When the patient arrives on the day of the test, _____ the test again, review

    the _____ involved, and answer any _____.

*Carefully review the steps to perform a spirometry test to measure FVC found in Procedure 50-1.

D. Reasons a test should not be performed include the patient being sick with the

_____ or a(n) _____ or having active

_____.

12. Peak Flow Meters*

   A. A peak flow meter is often used for patients who have _____ to monitor

   their _____ respiratory function and condition.

   B. The peak expiratory flow rate measures the _____ rate at which the patient

   exhales after taking a(n) _____ breath.

   C. The medical assistant may be responsible for teaching the _____ and

   _____ members how to use a peak flow meter.

   D. It is also important to instruct the patient to keep a(n) _____ of the flow

   rates to see if _____ is helping or if the disease is getting worse.

   E. The information from the diary will help the _____ determine the most

   effective medication and _____ regimen.

13. Arterial Blood Gasses

   A. Testing arterial blood gases is one of the most accurate methods of measuring the amount of

   _____ and _____ _____ in the blood, as

   well as the _____.

   B. Blood gas levels are helpful in evaluating breathing conditions such as

   _____ and _____.

   C. They also provide information on the effectiveness of _____

   _____ and other therapies.

   D. Arterial blood gases are usually drawn by _____ _____ or

   IV (intravenous) technicians.

IV. Pulmonary Treatments

   1. Treatments for obstructive lung disease may include drugs that reduce _____

   or relax _____ _____ to improve air flow.

   2. Treatments for restrictive lung diseases may include _____ and other drugs

   that suppress the body's _____ system.

   3. Nebulizers**

   A. A nebulizer is a handheld device that delivers medication directly to deep areas in the

   _____ through a fine _____ mist that is inhaled.

   B. A small amount of liquid medication is placed in a(n) _____ and mixed

   with sterile _____ or water.

---

*Carefully review the steps related to instructing a patient on the use of a peak flow meter in Procedure 50-2.
**Carefully review the steps related to administering a nebulizer treatment in Procedure 50-3.

Pulmonary Function **599**

C. The aerosol of the medication, delivered into the patient's respiratory tract through the _____ or a(n) _____, is absorbed directly into the lungs.

D. The preferred delivery method is with a(n) _____.

E. The _____ may be preferred for children or when the patient is unable to use a(n) _____.

F. Nebulizing treatments are often administered in the _____ _____ by the medical assistant but can be done by the patient at _____.

4. Inhalers

A. An inhaler is a handheld _____ or _____ attached to a mouthpiece that delivers a measured amount of medication into the respiratory tract to _____ the airways.

B. List the three basic types of inhalers.

  i. _____

  ii. _____

  iii. _____

C. Patient education is very important because MDIs are frequently _____, resulting in _____ treatment.

D. Some inhalers may have a spacer, sometimes called a(n) _____, which is used to improve the _____ and _____ of the medication.

E. A dry powder inhaler (DPI) usually comes in the shape of a(n) _____.

F. A dry powder inhaler does not have any mechanism that _____ the particles toward the _____.

G. Dry powder inhalers are rarely given to patients experiencing a(n) _____, a flare-up, or _____ symptoms.

H. A soft mist inhaler (SMI) is a newer type of inhaler that delivers a premeasured amount of _____ in a slow-moving _____.

5. Oxygen Treatments and Delivery Systems

A. Oxygen may be provided as _____ or long-term therapy for adults and children with chronic lung _____.

B. Patients on oxygen therapy are managed by a(n) _____ and a respiratory therapist.

C. List three oxygen delivery sources.

  i. _____

  ii. _____

  iii. _____

D. Compressed-oxygen cylinders are under extreme _____, so they must be kept _____ and handled carefully.

E. An oxygen concentrator extracts air from the room air, removes _____, and, thus, is able to deliver a higher _____ of oxygen to the patient than would be obtained by breathing room air.

F. In the liquid system, oxygen is converted to a liquid by _____-_____ oxygen in its gas form.

G. Liquid oxygen cannot be stored for more than a(n) _____ _____ because it will evaporate.

H. The most common devices for administering oxygen are a nasal _____, a simple mask with or without a(n) _____ bag, and a transtracheal or tracheostomy _____.

KEY TERMINOLOGY REVIEW

Match each of the following vocabulary terms with the correct definition.

a. tidal volume (V_T)
b. forced vital capacity (FVC)
c. peak expiratory flow rate (PEFR)
d. residual volume (RV)
e. vital capacity (VC)

1. _____ Measures the volume of air a patient can exhale with force after inhaling as deeply as possible.

2. _____ The fastest rate at which the patient exhales after taking a maximum breath.

3. _____ The amount of air that can be exhaled following forced inspiration, including maximum expiration.

4. _____ The volume of air left in the lungs at the end of an exhalation.

5. _____ The amount of air inhaled or exhaled during normal, relaxed breathing.

APPLIED PRACTICE

Read the scenario and answer the questions that follow.

Scenario

Clark Charleston smoked for 35 years. At the age of 54 he quit smoking, but he was diagnosed with emphysema a few years later. He frequently requires the use of supplemental oxygen, which he has supplied via a compressed-oxygen cylinder.

1. Is emphysema considered an obstructive or restrictive lung disease? What is the difference between the two types of lung disease categories?

   _____

   _____

   _____

   _____

2. Mr. Charleston often complains of shortness of breath and hearing hoarse, whistling sounds when he breathes. He also has noticed blood in his sputum. What are the medical terms for these respiratory symptoms?

   _____

   _____

   _____

   _____

3. What are some precautions Mr. Charleston must take into consideration in regard to the compressed-oxygen cylinder that supplies his supplemental oxygen?

   _____

   _____

   _____

   _____

LEARNING ACTIVITY: TRUE/FALSE

Indicate whether the following statements are true or false by placing a T or an F on the line that precedes each statement.

1. _____ Cystic fibrosis is an example of a restrictive pulmonary disease.
2. _____ Rales are crackles heard while listening to the chest.
3. _____ The most common pulmonary function tests and procedures performed by the medical assistant are spirometry, peak flow meter tests, and pulse oximetry.
4. _____ Smokers are at increased risk for bladder cancer.
5. _____ Flow rates are the measurements of different volumes of air moving in and out during breathing.
6. _____ Total lung capacity and functional residual capacity decrease in COPD.
7. _____ When performing PFTs, it is not necessary to obtain the patient's height and weight.
8. _____ Keeping a record of peak flow helps the physician develop an effective treatment plan.
9. _____ The medical assistant should encourage the patient to cough at the end of a nebulizer treatment.
10. _____ The most common method of oxygen delivery is with oxygen pressured cylinders.

CRITICAL THINKING

Answer the following questions to the best of your ability. Use the textbook as a reference.

1. Janine works as a medical assistant for a pulmonology practice. She has been smoking for 15 years. She makes it a point to only smoke behind the medical practice so that patients won't see her smoking. How do you feel about Janine's decision?

   _____

   _____

   _____

   _____

   _____

2. Dustin O'Donnel has recently been hired by an asbestos removal company. He has an appointment for a pre-employment physical, which includes a PFT. During his appointment, Tonya, the medical assistant, begins to explain the PFT procedure. Dustin becomes agitated. He tells Tonya that the company is targeting him because he is a smoker. He explains that he feels the only reason they want him to have this test is so that they can charge him more in health insurance premiums as a punishment for being a smoker. If you were Tonya, how would you respond?

   _____

   _____

   _____

   _____

   _____

RESEARCH ACTIVITY

Use Internet search engines to research the following topic and write a brief description of what you find. It is important to use reputable websites.

1. Visit www.lungusa.org. What information do you think will be most useful with regard to patient education? As you navigate throughout the site, identify information you think will be most helpful to you as you begin a career in the health care field.

   _____

   _____

   _____

   _____

CHAPTER 51
Physical Therapy and Rehabilitation

STUDENT STUDY GUIDE

Use the following guide to assist in your learning of the concepts from the chapter.

I. The Therapeutic Team

1. Rehabilitation is the process of bringing a patient back as close as possible to his or her normal _____ _____ after injury or _____.

2. Restorative care is care provided to _____ and maintain _____ and independence.

3. Members of a Therapeutic Team (List eight team members.)

   A. _____

   B. _____

   C. _____

   D. _____

   E. _____

   F. _____

   G. _____

   H. _____

II. Rehabilitation

1. Rehabilitation is the process of assisting a patient to regain a(n) _____ of _____ and the highest level of function possible after a(n) _____, a(n) _____, or a condition.

2. The rehabilitation process is a(n) _____ approach.

   A. Holistic medicine focuses on the whole patient and addresses the _____, _____, and _____ needs of a patient as well as the physical treatment.

3. The first element of rehabilitation is short-term and long-term _____ setting, based on the _____'s orders and the patient's willingness to _____.

   A. Short-term goals include objectives such as learning _____ _____ and performing exercises to increase _____ of _____.

   B. Long-term goals aim at achieving _____ and a feeling of _____.

III. Patient Assessment
  1. A physiatrist completes the following patient assessments.
      A. Inspect and palpate _____ and _____ to evaluate muscle strength and _____.
      B. Evaluate range of _____.
      C. Evaluate _____ for clues to specific problems.
      D. Evaluate _____ for asymmetry.
  2. Types of Spinal Curvature (List three types.)
      A. _____
      B. _____
      C. _____
  3. Treatment of any abnormal curvature may include physical therapy _____, surgery, a body _____, or a brace, depending on the specific _____ and its severity.
  4. For the patient's safety, a(n) _____ belt may be used.
      A. This is a safety device that can be used to hold up a weak patient while _____, standing, or _____.
  5. To assess the patient's ability to use stairs, the physician may ask the medical assistant to assist the patient on and off a(n) _____ _____.

IV. Conditions Requiring Physical Therapy
  1. Conditions That Can Result in Loss of Function (List five conditions.)
      A. _____
      B. _____
      C. _____
      D. _____
      E. _____
  2. Patients requiring physical therapy may be inpatients, _____, _____, home residents, _____ health patients, and those in special facilities such as _____ hospitals.

V. Physical Therapy Methods
  1. Exercise Therapy
      A. _____, the decrease or wasting away of muscle tissue, occurs rapidly in a(n) _____ patient.
      B. _____ may result, increasing the original disability.

C. Effective exercise programs can help increase or establish lost _____ _____, improve _____, relieve _____, correct poor _____ and body alignment, and increase _____.

D. List four types of recommended exercises.

  i. _____

  ii. _____

  iii. _____

  iv. _____

2. Range of Motion (ROM)

A. ROM exercises can help maintain muscle tone and _____.

B. ROM is measured with a special type of protractor called a(n) _____.

C. List three types of ROM exercises, matching each to the description.

  i. _____—The patient is able to move all limbs through the entire ROM unassisted.

  ii. _____—The patient must have someone else move his or her limbs through the ROM exercises because he or she is unable to do it.

  iii. _____—The patient participates to a limited extent in ROM exercises but requires assistance.

3. Application of Heat*

A. Heat and cold are used to treat conditions resulting from _____ and _____.

B. _____ damage may result if hot and cold applications are not monitored closely.

C. Heat application

  i. The application of heat to a body part causes _____ of blood vessels and allows more blood to _____ to injured tissues.

  ii. This increased circulation assists in providing the body with _____ and _____ necessary for repair and healing.

  iii. Heat can help relieve pain and _____ spasms and also soften hard crusts of _____ produced by damaged body tissues.

  iv. Two forms of heat therapy are _____ heat and _____ heat.

4. Application of Cold**

A. The application of cold to the body results in the _____ of blood vessels, which helps prevent or reduce _____.

---

*Carefully review the steps in the procedures related to the application of heat and cold therapies.
**Carefully review the steps in the procedures related to the application of heat and cold therapies.

B. Benefits of cold application may include the reduction of _____ and control of _____ because blood circulation has slowed.

C. Cold application consists of cold _____, soaks, _____ packs, and hypothermia _____.

D. Cold _____ packs can be used as an alternative to ice packs.

E. _____ _____ applications, such as cold compresses, may be used to treat pain and fever.

5. Ultraviolet Radiation

A. Ultraviolet rays stimulate the growth of new _____ cells and are capable of killing _____.

B. Rays are used therapeutically for the treatment of disorders such as _____, acne, and _____ sores.

C. Both the timing of the _____ and the _____ of the ultraviolet lamp from the patient must be carefully controlled.

D. Treatment is ordered by the _____, such as a 20-_____ lamp treatment placed at least _____ inches from the patient and directed only on the area to be treated.

E. Eye protection, in the form of _____ _____, should be worn by both the patient and medical assistant to protect the eyes from ultraviolet ray exposure.

6. Diathermy

A. Diathermy is the therapeutic use of a high-_____ current that induces an electrical field within a portion of the body.

B. Diathermy is useful in treating muscular disorders as well as _____, arthritis, and _____.

7. Ultrasound Therapy

A. Ultrasound waves vibrate at the rate of 1 _____ times per second, which cannot be heard by the human ear but produce mechanical and _____ effects.

B. Ultrasound is used effectively to treat _____, relax muscle _____, stimulate _____ in patients with vascular disorders, relax tendons and ligaments, and break up calcium _____ and scars.

C. Ultrasound is administered via a machine with an applicator _____ attachment that can be placed directly on the _____.

D. A conducting medium, such as a special _____ or _____ oil, must be placed on the skin to conduct the ultrasound into the body.

VI. Adaptive Equipment and Devices

   1. Examples of adaptive equipment include wheelchairs, _____, canes, and

      _____.

   2. Mobility aids or mobility- _____ devices are designed to enable the patient to

      _____.

   3. Crutches*

      A. List the three most common types of crutches.

         i. _____

         ii. _____

         iii. _____

      B. Steps for measuring crutches

         i. Have the patient wear _____ shoes and stand _____.

         ii. Place the crutch tips 4 to 6 inches to the _____ and 4 to 6 inches in

            _____ of each foot.

         iii. Adjust the crutch, using the bolts and nuts at the _____ of the crutch, so

            that the axillary crutch bars are _____ finger widths below the

            _____.

         iv. Adjust the _____ so the patient can flex his or her elbows at a(n) _____-degree

            angle when the crutch is in place and the patient's hands are on the hand bars.

      C. Crutch-Walking Gaits

         i. The type of crutch gait or walk that the patient will use depends on the amount of

            _____ bearing the patient's leg or legs will support, _____

            coordination, age, and overall _____ condition.

         ii. The four-point gait is a(n) _____ and steady gait that is used when a

            patient can bear weight on _____ legs.

         iii. The three-point gait is used when one leg is _____ than the other or when

            there is _____ _____ bearing on one leg.

         iv. The two-point gait is faster moving than the _____-point gait and is used

            by a patient who can bear _____ weight on both feet and maintain good

            _____.

         v. Swing gaits are used by patients with severe leg _____.

           a. Two types of swing gaits are _____ and _____.

   4. Canes

      A. Canes are used by patients who have _____ or _____ weakness

         on one side or need assistance with _____.

---

*Carefully review the steps in Procedure 51-7 for teaching or reinforcing instructions on the correct use of crutches.

B. A cane should have a(n) _____ _____ on the end to prevent slipping.

C. A(n) _____ _____ determines the most suitable cane for a patient.

D. To determine the correct cane height, the patient should stand tall so that the handgrip of the cane is level with the _____ _____ and the elbow is flexed at an angle of _____ to _____ degrees.

5. Walkers*

A. Walkers are assistive devices made of _____ that provide a base of support for patients who need help with balance and _____.

B. A stationary walker requires strong _____ _____ development.

C. A walker with wheels can be used by patients who have good _____ and _____.

6. Wheelchairs**

A. Wheelchairs are hand _____ or _____ driven.

B. Wheelchair transfer

  i. Help move a patient with hemiplegia or general weakness from a wheelchair by _____ the patient so he/she can use the _____ leg to assist you.

7. Braces

A. List the uses of a brace.

  i. _____

  ii. _____

  iii. _____

B. Braces may be made out of _____, _____, or _____ and are customized to the patient's needs and anatomy.

C. Any orthotic positioned over a bony point must be _____ to avoid skin breakdown.

8. Casts

A. Casts are made of _____, plastic, or _____ and are used to hold a bone in place after reduction of a fracture.

9. Cast Care

A. Casts are generally applied using a wet _____-type material around a(n) _____ liner and cotton padding over the limb.

---

*Carefully review the steps in Procedure 51-9, which outlines how to teach a patient to use a walker.

**Carefully review the steps in Procedure 51-10, which outlines how to successfully transfer a patient from a wheelchair to a chair or an examination table.

B. The patient should be instructed to call the physician if problems such as the following occur.

    i. Restricted _____

    ii. Pain as a result of the cast _____ the skin

    iii. Excessive _____ under the cast

    iv. Numbness or tingling of the _____ or _____

    v. _____ toes or fingers

    vi. _____ of the limb around the edge of the cast

    vii. Discoloration _____ through the cast

    viii. _____ fitting cast

    ix. Foul _____ coming from the cast

10. Traction

    A. Traction is a method of _____ or _____ in two directions.

    B. List three uses of traction.

      i. _____

      ii. _____

      iii. _____

11. Prosthesis

    A. A prosthesis is an artificial _____ for a missing body part.

    B. The decision to select a specific type of fitting rests with the _____ and must include an assessment of the patient's overall _____, age, and willingness to learn to use the _____ _____.

    C. Prosthetic devices are _____ _____ for the patient, and _____ may be necessary to ensure a comfortable fit for the patient.

VII. Diagnostic Testing

  1. Diagnostic testing may be used to evaluate the following.

    A. Muscle _____

    B. Muscle _____

    C. _____ of joints

    D. _____ function

    E. _____ and sensory function

  2. Electromyography (EMG)

    A. EMG consists of using an electromyograph to test the _____ _____ of muscles.

    B. It is most often performed when a patient complains of muscle _____ or _____.

C. The EMG consists of inserting a fine-gauge _____ electrode through the skin and into a muscle and then sending a small amount of _____ _____ into the muscle.

D. Abnormal results are found in conditions such as _____ _____ _____ (ALS), muscular _____, and peripheral _____ damage.

3. Electrical Stimulation

A. Electrical stimulation with low-_____ current is helpful to stimulate _____ that supply muscles.

B. An electrical current is applied using disposable _____ _____.

C. This type of stimulation is used to avoid _____ of muscle tissue.

4. Evoked Potential Studies

A. Evoked potential studies examine _____ within the brain to external stimuli such as _____, _____, and _____.

B. Two types of evoked potential studies are _____ _____ _____ _____ (BAER) and _____ _____ _____ _____ (SEP).

VIII. Complementary and Alternative Treatments

1. Alternative medicine is a non-mainstream practice that is used instead of _____ _____.

2. Non-mainstream practice that is used in addition to conventional medicine is called _____ _____.

3. Chiropractic

A. Chiropractic is an approach to health care that uses _____ _____ to relieve pain.

B. Doctors of chiropractic usually also promote healthy _____, beneficial lifestyle changes, and _____.

4. Massage

A. Massage is kneading or applying pressure with the hands to a part of the patient's body to promote _____ _____, improve blood _____, and reduce _____.

B. List common terminology associated with massage.

   i. _____

   ii. _____

   iii. _____

   iv. _____

C. Traditional, or _____, massage includes stimulating blood _____ through the soft tissues.

D. Deep tissue massage is used to release chronic patterns of _____ or pain.

E. Trigger point massage concentrates finger pressure directly to individual _____ to release trigger points or _____ in the muscles.

5. Reiki

A. Reiki involves channeling the body's _____ and _____ through gentle touch and massage.

B. It is a Japanese technique to reduce _____ and promote _____ and healing.

6. Acupuncture and Acupressure

A. The medical theory behind the ancient _____ science and art of acupressure is that special acupoints lie along _____, or channels, in the body.

B. The meridians begin at the _____, connect to the _____, and then connect to a(n) _____ associated with a certain meridian.

C. Acupuncture differs from acupressure in that it involves inserting very thin _____ through the _____ at key points.

D. It is believed that inserting these needles rebalances the _____ of _____.

7. Tai Chi

A. Tai chi has become a popular means of _____ reduction.

B. Tai chi involves gentle flowing _____ that promote _____ and _____ health.

KEY TERMINOLOGY REVIEW

Without using your textbook, write a sentence using each of the selected key terms in the correct context as discussed in material covered in the chapter.

1. *ambulation*

_____

2. *cryotherapy*

_____

3. *gait belt*

_____

4. *petrissage*

_____

5. *complementary medicine*

_____

APPLIED PRACTICE

Read the scenario and answer the questions that follow.

> ## Scenario
>
> It is a busy Monday morning, and you are working as a clinical medical assistant at an orthopedic office. Rachel Dade, an administrative MA, has just informed you that an emergency appointment was just scheduled for Li Chen, a teenager who injured his lower leg while participating in a soccer game during physical education class. While he is currently en route to the office, his parents have arrived and are insisting that he be treated using traditional Chinese medicine.

1. Explain how you would address their wishes and traditions.

   _____

   _____

   _____

2. After discussion, the physician and Li Chen's parents agree to incorporate acupuncture and acupressure into Li's overall treatment plan, which also includes physical therapy and medication for pain control. Why are acupuncture and acupressure good choices in this scenario?

   _____

   _____

   _____

3. Considering the treatment plan, would the incorporation of acupressure and acupuncture be considered alternative or complementary medicine? Explain your answer.

   _____

   _____

   _____

LEARNING ACTIVITY: TRUE/FALSE

Indicate whether the following statements are true or false by placing a T or an F on the line that precedes each statement.

_____ 1. Holistic medicine focuses on the whole patient and addresses the social, emotional, and spiritual needs of the patient as well as the physical treatment.

_____ 2. The two-point gait is considered the safest of all gaits.

_____ 3. Arthritis is inflammation of a joint that usually occurs with pain and swelling.

_____ 4. Diathermy is useful in treating muscular disorders, tendonitis, arthritis, and bursitis.

_____ 5. All patients should be able to operate their own wheelchair.

_____ 6. Cryotherapy is the use of cold for therapeutic purposes.

_____ 7. Prolonged use of a brace may weaken muscles.

_____ 8. Casts are made of plaster, plastic, fiberglass, and metal.

_____ 9. Kyphosis is an abnormal inward curvature of the lumbar spine.

_____ 10. There are four types of crutches: axillary, Lofstrand or forearm, Canadian or elbow, and bipedal crutches.

CRITICAL THINKING

Answer the following questions to the best of your ability. Use the textbook as a reference.

1. A patient calls 5 days after her broken arm was placed in a cast. She says she "feels disgusting" because she isn't allowed to take a shower. She admits she lost her cast care instructions, but she knows that her cast isn't supposed to get wet. How would you handle this telephone call?

   _____

   _____

   _____

   _____

2. Harriette Langdon is 85 years old and lives with her son and his family. She recently had hip surgery and requires physical therapy to improve her range of motion. She needs assistance with her ROM exercises because she is unable to move her hip and leg with her own strength. She doesn't want to burden her son by requiring extra help, but the physical therapist warns her that muscle atrophy could occur. Ms. Langdon doesn't understand what atrophy means and why ROM exercises would be helpful. How could you explain this to her? What type of ROM exercise would Ms. Langdon require due to her physical limitations?

   _____

   _____

   _____

   _____

RESEARCH ACTIVITY

Use Internet search engines to research the following topic and write a brief description of what you find. It is important to use reputable websites.

1. Research new materials and advances being made in prosthetics. What information do you find most interesting, and why?

   _____

   _____

   _____

   _____

CHAPTER 52
Math for Pharmacology

STUDENT STUDY GUIDE

Use the following guide to assist in your learning of the concepts from the chapter.

I. Mathematics Review

  1. Addition and Subtraction

    A. Addition and subtraction are used in everyday tasks in the medical office, including drug _____, _____ tracking, and _____ collection.

  2. Multiplication and Division

    A. It is very important to have a strong knowledge of the basic multiplication ("_____") tables when working in the medical office.

  3. Fractions

    A. A fraction consists of a(n) _____ (the top number), a(n) _____ (the bottom number), and a(n) _____ _____ that separates the two.

    B. Fractions are used when indicating _____ and _____.

    C. A mixed number is made up of both a(n) _____ number and a(n) _____.

  4. Decimals

    A. Anything less than the number _____ is often written as a decimal.

    B. To convert a fraction to a decimal, simply divide the _____ by the _____.

    C. Decimal place values

      i. It is necessary to correctly identify the decimal point and _____ _____ of a number.

      ii. When speaking or verbalizing decimal values, state the decimal placeholder (_____, _____, or _____) where the _____ digit falls.

5. Equivalents
   A. Equivalents are _____ and have the same _____.
   B. The ratio 1:2, the percentage _____ percent, and the decimal _____ all have the same fraction value of ½.

6. Leading Zero and Trailing Zero
   A. When writing a decimal number less than 1, you must apply the _____ _____ _____.
      i. A zero must be written _____ the decimal point, such as 0.5 mg.
   B. The trailing zero rule states that it is never appropriate to include a zero _____ a(n) _____ number.
      i. For example, write _____ rather than 5.0.

II. Weights and Measures
   1. Three systems of weights and measures are used to calculate medication dosages: the _____ system, the _____ system, and the _____ system.
   2. _____ measurements are often used by medical assistants and other health care professionals in _____ patients because patients are generally more _____ with them.
   3. Apothecary System
      A. The apothecary system is considered to be the _____ system of measurement.
      B. List the dry units of measurement in the apothecary system.
         i. _____ (gr)
         ii. _____ (dr)
         iii. _____ (oz)
         iv. _____ (lb)
      C. List the fluid units of measurement in the apothecary system.
         i. _____ (m)
         ii. _____ (fl dr)
         iii. _____ (fl oz)
         iv. _____ (pt)
         v. _____ (qt)
         vi. _____ (gal)
      D. Apothecary notation rules
         i. The unit or abbreviation comes _____ the amount.

    ii. Use _____ _____ numerals to express whole

       numbers 1 through 10, 15, 20, and 30.

       a. Use _____ numerals for all other quantities.

    iii. Use _____ to designate amounts less than 1.

    iv. The symbol _____ is used to designate the fraction ½.

4. Household System

  A. The household system is used as frequently as the _____ system in the
    United States.

  B. List the liquid measurements in the household system.

    i. _____

    ii. _____

    iii. _____

    iv. _____

    v. _____

    vi. _____

    vii. _____

  C. Dry weights can include the _____ and _____.

  D. To help patients understand medication dosages, the medical assistant may frequently need
    to convert _____ and _____ measurements to the
    _____ system.

5. Metric System

  A. The metric system is commonly used for dosage calculations and _____.

  B. Identify the prefix that corresponds with each metric value.

    i. _____ = 1,000 of a unit

    ii. _____ = 100 of a unit

    iii. _____ = 10 of a unit

    iv. _____ unit of 1

    v. _____ = 0.1 (one-tenth) of a unit

    vi. _____ = 0.01 (one-hundredth) of a unit

    vii. _____ = 0.001 (one-thousandth) of a unit

    viii. _____ = 0.000001 (one-millionth) of a unit

  C. Metric conversions are simply accomplished by multiplying or dividing by _____.

    i. Multiplying by 1,000 is the same as moving the decimal point _____
      places to the _____.

    ii. Dividing by 1,000 is the same as moving the decimal point _____
      places to the _____.

D. The common metric units of measure are the _____ (volume), the _____ (weight), and the _____ (length).

E. In the metric system, the dosage is written as a(n) _____ number first, with the unit of _____ following.

6. Rules for Conversion

A. When converting from one system to another, it is important to remember that the equivalents may be only _____, especially when using _____ _____.

III. Drug Calculations

1. Stock medications, which are stored by medical offices for use by their office, are sometimes packaged in a different _____ than the physician's _____.

2. It is important to understand basic drug _____ to ensure that the _____ dose of medication is given.

3. Factors that impact drug dosage calculations include the patient's _____, _____, and current state of _____.

4. The first step in the drug calculation is to confirm that the system of weights and measures in the _____ is the same as in the container of _____ _____.

5. Ratio Method*

A. A ratio establishes a relationship between _____ _____: the amount of drug _____ to the amount on _____.

B. When two ratios are equal, it is a(n) _____.

C. If three of the four numbers for the _____ _____ in a proportion are known, you can solve for the fourth number by using _____ principles.

D. The symbol _____ is used for the unknown quantity.

E. Provide two examples of ratio method equations that solve for x.

    i. _____

    ii. _____

6. Formula Method**

A. It is possible to calculate dosages using a very simple _____.

---

*Carefully review the sample problems provided in the textbook to master this method.

**Carefully review the sample problems provided in the textbook to master this method.

B. In the formula below, D represents the _____ _____,
H represents the _____ on _____, and Q represents
the _____ of the dose on hand.

$$\frac{D}{H} \times Q$$

IV. Calculating Pediatric Dosages*

1. It is imperative that the calculations be _____ when administering
medications to a(n) _____.

2. Often, the _____ takes responsibility for this task, but the medical assistant
may be asked to assist or to _____ the dosage.

3. Clark's Rule

A. Clark's rule is based on the _____ of the child.

B. This is the _____ _____ calculation of drug dosage
for children.

C. Write the formula for Clark's rule.

_____

_____

4. Fried's Law

A. Fried's law is applied to children under the age of _____ _____.

B. Fried's assumption is that a 12½-year-old child could take a(n) _____
dose, and a(n) _____ of that is taken to figure dosages for a young child.

C. Write the formula for Fried's law.

_____

_____

5. Young's Rule

A. Young's rule is used for children who are _____ 1 year of age.

B. Write the formula for Young's rule.

_____

_____

6. West's Nomogram

A. West's nomogram is the preferred method of dosage calculation for

_____ and _____ care patients and

_____ children.

---

*Carefully review all the sample problems provided in the textbook that relate to calculating pediatric dosages.

B. It takes into consideration the child's body surface area (BSA), which is based on a calculation of the child's _____ and _____ and is expressed as _____ (meters squared).

C. To calculate the child's BSA, a(n) _____ _____ is drawn on the nomogram chart from the patient's _____ in inches or centimeters across the columns to the patient's _____ in kilograms or pounds.

D. The straight line will intersect on the _____ column.

E. Write the formula for West's nomogram.

_____

_____

F. 1.73 square meters is the standard _____ _____.

7. Body Weight Method

A. The body weight method uses calculations based on the patient's weight in

_____.

B. This method requires converting a patient's weight into kilograms.

   i. 1 kg = _____ lb.

   ii. Divide the number of _____ by 2.2 to determine weight in kilograms.

C. To calculate dosage based on body weight, calculate the safe drug dose in _____ (as recommended by a reputable drug reference) and then multiply that amount by the child's _____ in _____.

KEY TERMINOLOGY REVIEW

Complete the following sentences using the correct key terms found at the beginning of the chapter.

1. The bottom number in a fraction is called the _____.

2. The _____ is considered the oldest system of measurement.

3. A(n) _____ is a comparison between two numbers.

4. When writing a decimal number less than the number 1, you must apply the

_____.

5. _____ is the preferred method for calculating pediatric dosages, particularly for oncology and critical care patients and underweight children.

APPLIED PRACTICE

Complete the following exercises.

1. Basic math review: Do not use a calculator.
   a. Addition
      1. 18 + 49 = _____
      2. 142 + 730 = _____
      3. 1,799 + 283 = _____
      4. 7,839 + 943 + 41 = _____
      5. 28,845 + 83 = _____
   b. Subtraction
      1. 75 − 52 = _____
      2. 429 − 81 = _____
      3. 1,648 − 379 = _____
      4. 612 − 419 = _____
      5. 3,527 − 274 = _____
   c. Multiplication
      1. 9 × 3 = _____
      2. 32 × 5 = _____
      3. 815 × 4 = _____
      4. 711 × 30 = _____
      5. 3,780 × 210 = _____
   d. Division
      1. 150/15 = _____
      2. 1,152/12 = _____
      3. 450/60 = _____
      4. 327/6 = _____
      5. 825/50 = _____

2. Dosage calculations

   a. The physician orders digoxin 0.125 mg to be given to a patient. On hand is a vial of digoxin marked 250 mcg/mL. How much should the medical assistant administer?

   _____

   _____

   b. The physician orders 500 mg of metformin to be given to a patient. On hand is a bottle of metformin that reads 1,000 mg/tablet. How much should the medical assistant administer?

   _____

   _____

   c. The physician orders 125 mg of a medication. On hand is a bottle of the same medication that reads 500 mg/5 mL. How much should the medical assistant administer?

   _____

   _____

   d. The medication that the physician ordered reads 20 mg/kg/day. Your patient weighs 220 lb. The physician wants the patient to take the medication BID in equal doses. How much will the patient be given for each dose?

   _____

   _____

e. The physician orders 40 mg of furosemide to be given to a patient. On hand is a bottle of furosemide that reads 20 mg/tablet. How much should the medical assistant administer?

_____

_____

LEARNING ACTIVITY: MULTIPLE CHOICE

Circle the correct answer to each of the following questions.

1. If the doctor orders 4 mg of a certain medication, and the vial states that there are 2 mg in 1 cc, how many ccs would you give to deliver 4 mg?

   a. 2 cc
   b. 4 cc
   c. 6 cc
   d. $^1/_2$ cc

2. If the doctor orders 1 dram of medication to be given and the vial states that there is 1 mg in 1 cc, you must

   a. give 1 cc.
   b. ask the doctor how to determine the number of ccs.
   c. ask the pharmacy.
   d. convert from the apothecary system to the metric system and then calculate the dosage.

3. When adding and subtracting fractions, which of the following is correct?

   a. You do not always need to have a common denominator.
   b. To obtain the common denominator, you must multiply the entire fraction by the correct multiplier.
   c. Subtract the numerators; the denominator remains the same.
   d. All of the above

4. When converting an improper fraction to a mixed number, which of the following is correct?

   a. Divide the numerator by the denominator.
   b. The remainder, if any, is placed over the denominator to form the fractional component of the mixed number.
   c. Reduce the fractional component to its simplest form.
   d. All of the above

5. To accurately write an apothecary notation, which of the following rules should be applied?

   a. The unit or abbreviation comes after the amount.
   b. Use lowercase Roman numerals to express whole numbers 1 through 10, 15, 20, and 30.
   c. Use fractions to designate amounts greater than 1.
   d. The symbol ss is used to designate the fraction ¾.

6. Metric conversions are simply accomplished by multiplying or dividing by _____

   a. 100.
   b. 500.
   c. 1,000.
   d. None of the above

7. The apothecary measurement of 5 gr is equivalent to _____ in the metric system.
   a. 65 mg, or 0.065 g
   b. 325 mg, or 0.33 g
   c. 650 mg, or 0.67 g
   d. 4 mL

8. The apothecary measurement of 8 oz is equivalent to _____ in the metric system.
   a. 160 mL
   b. 240 mL
   c. 500 mL
   d. 15 mL

9. The measurement of 60 gtts (drops) is equivalent to the common household measurement
   a. 1 teaspoon (tsp).
   b. 1 tablespoon (T).
   c. 1 oz.
   d. 2 oz.

10. Which of the following factors should be considered when calculating the correct dose of a drug?
    a. Patient's age
    b. Patient's weight
    c. Patient's current health
    d. All of the above

CRITICAL THINKING

Answer the following questions to the best of your ability. Use the textbook as a reference.

1. You have received a physician's order to administer 1 mg of a medication to a patient. It is a medication that is injected into the muscle. As soon as you have given the medication, you realize you measured 1 mL instead of calculating 1 mg. What would you do?

   _____

   _____

   _____

   _____

2. An established patient has come in to ask for a new prescription for a medication that she has taken for many years because she is out of refills. The physician is not in the office today, but after checking the medical record and noting that it is the patient's usual medication, the medical assistant (MA) calls in a new prescription to the pharmacy and makes a note to have the doctor write the order in the chart when she returns. Is this an appropriate action for the MA? Explain you answer.

   _____

   _____

   _____

   _____

RESEARCH ACTIVITY

Use Internet search engines to research the following topic and write a brief description of what you find. It is important to use reputable websites.

1. Visit www.rxlist.com. Navigate through the site and determine how the information on this site could be best used by patients. How could a medical assistant working in health care benefit from this website?

   _____

   _____

   _____

   _____

   _____

CHAPTER 53
Pharmacology

STUDENT STUDY GUIDE

Use the following guide to assist in your learning of the concepts from the chapter.

I. Introduction

  1. Pharmacology is the study of medications and drugs, including their _____, intentions for _____, and _____.

  2. Some drugs come from natural sources, including _____, _____, and _____, and others are _____ created.

  3. Reasons Drugs Are Prescribed (List three reasons.)

    A. _____

    B. _____

    C. _____

  4. The Medical Assistant's Role in Pharmacology

    A. _____ medication

    B. Keeping accurate medication _____

    C. Providing patients with _____ pertaining to the medications they are _____

II. Drug Names

  1. Generic Name

    A. The generic name is typically written in _____ letters and is the _____ name for the drug.

    B. List the ways, according to the FDA, that a generic drug compares to a brand name drug.

      i. _____

      ii. _____

      iii. _____

      iv. _____

      v. _____

      vi. _____

      vii. _____

2. Brand Name
   A. The brand is typically written with the _____ letter capitalized.
   B. The brand name is also called the _____ name.
   C. A company holds a patent on a brand name drug for _____ years.
   D. _____ _____ cannot be sold while a company holds a patent on the brand name.
   E. If a physician wants the patient to receive only a brand name drug, the physician must write "_____ ____ _____" on the prescription.
3. Chemical Name
   A. The chemical name of a drug is the _____ _____ used by manufacturers and pharmacists.
   B. Pharmacists are specially trained and _____ professionals who specialize in the _____ and _____ of drugs.

III. Regulations and Standards
   1. The Food and Drug Administration (FDA) ensures that human drugs are _____ and _____ and that these products are honestly, _____, and informatively represented to the _____.
   2. The Drug Enforcement Administration (DEA) is responsible for _____ _____ enforcement.
   3. All physicians are required to register with the DEA to _____, _____, or _____ controlled substances.

IV. References
   1. Commonly Used Drug Reference Books (List three books.)
      A. _____
      B. _____
      C. _____
   2. Physicians' Desk Reference (PDR)
      A. The PDR is the most commonly _____ resource.
      B. It is updated _____, and the information is provided by drug _____.
      C. Describe the information found in each of the colored sections of the PDR.
         i. White— _____
            _____
         ii. Pink— _____
            _____

iii. Blue— _____

_____

iv. Gray/multicolored— _____

_____

v. White— _____

_____

vi. Green— _____

_____

3. Electronic Resources

  A. Many _____ _____ _____ (EHR) platforms
    have electronic versions of the reference books.

  B. This is _____ and saves _____ for health care providers and
    helps improve patient care.

4. Online Resources

  A. Many online medical _____ _____ are available.

  B. _____ and _____ are two Internet resources that are
    considered to be reliable.

V. Drugs

  1. Prescription Drugs

    A. A prescription is a written explanation to a pharmacist specifying the _____
      of the medication, the _____, the _____, and the times of
      _____.

    B. Besides physicians, other professionals who have special licenses to prescribe medications
      include _____ _____ and advanced _____
      _____.

    C. A label on a prescription container must read "Caution: Federal law _____
      _____ without _____."

      i. It is _____ to give someone a(n) _____ medication that
        was not prescribed for that person, even when the intention is to _____
        the person.

  2. Nonprescription Drugs

    A. Nonprescription drugs are also called _____-____-_____
      (OTC) drugs.

    B. Examples of OTC drugs include medications such as _____,
      _____ medications, and _____ ointments.

    C. OTC drugs are regulated by the _____.

D. Some OTC drugs may react _____ with a(n) _____ drug the patient is taking.

E. The medical assistant should be sure to review and _____ OTC medications and prescription medications the patient is taking at _____ office visit.

F. Remind patients that they need to list supplements such as _____ and _____ that they might not think of as drugs.

3. Side Effects of Drugs

A. The intended effects on a patient's medical condition are known as _____ _____.

B. _____ effects are called side effects, and they are generally accepted because the _____ of taking the medication _____ the unwanted effects.

C. _____ effects require that the patient discontinue the medication because the _____ effects outweigh the _____.

D. List nine examples of unexpected side effects.

    i. _____

    ii. _____

    iii. _____

    iv. _____

    v. _____

    vi. _____

    vii. _____

    viii. _____

    ix. _____

E. Adverse effects can be _____, which means they may cause death.

    i. For example, _____ shock is a life-threatening adverse reaction.

4. Patient Reactions to Medications

A. Patient's age

    i. _____ and _____ patients are more susceptible to the effects of medications than others and usually require _____ doses.

B. Patient's weight

    i. There is a direct correlation between the patient's weight and the optimum _____ level.

    ii. The typical medication dosage is based on the weight of a(n) _____-pound adult.

    iii. Dosages may increase if the patient weighs _____ or may decrease if the patient weighs _____.

C. Method of administration

    i. The method of administration affects the _____ at which the body _____ the medication.

D. Allergies

    i. Generally, the _____ an allergic reaction develops, the more _____ and dangerous it is.

    ii. Patients who have been prescribed new medications should be provided education regarding the _____ _____ and _____ of allergic reactions to medications.

    iii. If a reaction is _____, a patient should be instructed to _____ the medication and call the medical office immediately.

    iv. If a reaction is _____, a patient should call _____ for immediate transport to the nearest _____ department.

5. Drug Tolerance and Intolerance

A. Drug tolerance

    i. Drug tolerance is a(n) _____ in the _____ of a drug as the body gets used to having the drug in the system.

    ii. When tolerance develops, it takes a(n) _____ dose of the drug to achieve the _____ result.

B. Habituation

    i. Habituation is _____ or _____ dependence on a drug.

C. Drug intolerance

    i. Drug intolerance or drug sensitivity is a lower _____ to the normal pharmacologic _____ of a drug.

    ii. Vomiting, _____, and _____ cramping can be indications of intolerance.

    iii. Patients who experience intolerance to medication should alert the _____, who may then adjust the _____ or change the _____ as needed.

6. Inventory and Record Keeping

A. In the medical office, medications that are kept on hand can range from _____ provided by _____ companies to medications _____ _____ within the office.

B. Offices and facilities store both _____ medications and _____ drugs.

C. All medication inventory is maintained in a logbook that contains the following.

    i. The _____ of each medication stored

    ii. The _____ of each medication

    iii. The _____ on hand for each dosage

    iv. The _____ dates

D. A separate section in the logbook is used to indicate when a(n) _____ is dispensed to a(n) _____.

E. Many _____ health record platforms allow for medications that are _____ to be _____ into the patient's record.

F. Once a(n) _____ it is important to review the inventory to ensure that a sufficient _____ of each drug is available and that no medication has _____.

G. _____ staff members should document the destruction of _____ substances.

H. The local _____ office should be contacted regarding practices for _____ _____ amounts of controlled substances.

I. Medication errors should be documented according to _____ _____, which usually includes immediately reporting to a(n) _____ and filling out a(n) _____ report.

7. Controlled Substances

A. The Controlled Substances Act (CSA), enacted in _____, states that certain drugs are classified as controlled substances because they have a potential for _____ or _____.

B. The _____ strictly enforces the control of these medications.

C. The psychoactive drugs regulated by the CSA include _____, hallucinogens, _____, and stimulants.

D. Controlled substances are divided into five categories (schedules) based on their potentially _____ level of _____.

E. Controlled substances are generally kept under _____ lock and key in a(n) _____, secured cabinet.

F. The following information is included in a controlled substance log.

    i. The _____ in stock

    ii. Who _____ the controlled substance

    iii. How _____ was given

    iv. How much was _____

    v. The date and name of the _____ receiving the drug

G. The controlled substance log must be kept on file for at least _____

_____ and must be available for _____ by the Drug
Enforcement Administration (DEA).

H. Physicians are required to register with the DEA to _____,

_____, or _____ controlled substances.

VI. Drug Abuse

1. Drug abuse is defined as the use of a drug _____ or wrongly.

2. Drug dependency is relying on or using a medication for _____

_____.

3. Individuals who become physically _____ are those who continuously use a
substance to function or to avoid _____ _____.

4. Identifying Drug Abuse

A. Be alert when patients are requesting medication refills or new prescriptions

_____ than _____, particularly if the medication request is

for a(n) _____ _____ drug.

B. Take the following steps if drug abuse is suspected.

   i. Notify the _____ immediately of the suspicion.

   ii. Check local _____ to see if the patient is obtaining medications from

_____ pharmacies.

   iii. Tell patients who are frequently calling for refills that another refill will require a(n)

_____ _____.

C. List three items it is important to safeguard that could be stolen and misused for drug
abuse.

   i. _____

   ii. _____

   iii. _____

VII. Routes and Methods of Drug Administration

1. Common Routes of Drug Administration (List seven common routes.)

A. _____

B. _____

C. _____

D. _____

E. _____

F. _____

G. _____

2. Be sure the patient understands the directions for correct medication _____

   because the right _____ must be followed for the medication to be

   _____.

3. Frequently Administered Drugs

   A. List six frequently administered types of drugs.

       i. _____

       ii. _____

       iii. _____

       iv. _____

       v. _____

       vi. _____

   B. Two websites that are useful resources providing information about the drugs prescribed

   and sold the most in the United States are _____ and _____.

VIII. Medications and Pregnancy

   1. Very few drugs are considered _____ for use during pregnancy.

   2. Pregnant women should consult their _____ before taking any medication,

   including over-the-counter medications and _____ _____.

   3. Pregnancy classifications range from _____ to _____.

   4. Class A drugs are the safest for pregnant women; Class _____ drugs have been shown to cause

   health risks, _____, or both to the unborn _____.

   5. Drug Use and the Breast-feeding Mother

   A. Several medications are _____, which means that the medications are so

   _____ for the infant that the mother must _____ breast-

   feeding while she is taking them or must forgo taking them at all.

   B. List six medications that are contraindicated for breast-feeding mothers.

       i. _____

       ii. _____

       iii. _____

       iv. _____

       v. _____

       vi. _____

IX. Reading and Writing a Prescription

   1. Main Parts of a Prescription (List seven parts.)

   A. _____

   B. _____

C. _____

D. _____

E. _____

F. _____

G. _____

2. When a pharmacist fills a prescription, the patient _____ are placed on the label as instructed by the _____.

3. Special instructions and _____ for taking the medication are also included that can help ensure that the _____ is as _____ as possible.

4. The pharmacist also includes a package insert with each medication that contains information regarding possible _____ effects, _____ effects, and _____.

5. Only _____ are permitted to sign prescriptions. However, a medical assistant in some cases may _____ the prescription form, which the physician then checks for _____ and signs.

6. E-prescriptions

A. E-prescriptions are growing in _____ and becoming the norm, preferred by both physicians and patients.

B. E-prescriptions are _____ generated and sent via _____ and _____ computer connections.

C. Not only do e-prescriptions provide _____ for the patient, they also eliminate the _____ factors involved with the interpretation of _____ prescriptions.

7. Computerized Physician Order Entry (CPOE)

A. Computerized electronic records allow _____ and entries, including _____, to be directly entered into the patient's health record.

B. These computerized entries _____ the number of medical errors and improve the _____ and _____ of the delivery of health care.

C. CPOE falls under the Electronic Health Record (EHR) _____ _____.

D. _____ medical assistants are allowed to enter orders into the electronic health record.

E. A credentialed medical assistant must obtain his or her credential from a(n) _____ credentialing _____.

X. Abbreviations Used in Pharmacology

1. Because of the risk of _____ resulting from _____ information, many physicians choose not to use abbreviations in _____ writing and chart _____.

2. The use of abbreviations in EHRs is _____ because everything is typed out.

3. It is still important to understand abbreviations, which may appear in the _____ or _____ and _____ plans for patients.

4. The _____ _____ has issued a "Do Not Use" list that includes all abbreviations that are not acceptable for use because of the high _____ of error or _____.

KEY TERMINOLOGY REVIEW

Match each of the following terms with the correct definition.

a. Drug Enforcement Administration (DEA)
b. habituation
c. over the counter (OTC)
d. proprietary name
e. Food and Drug Administration (FDA)

1. _____ Nonprescription drugs.
2. _____ Dependence on a drug.
3. _____ The name given to a drug by a specific manufacturer.
4. _____ The agency which ensures that human drugs are safe and effective.
5. _____ The agency of the federal government responsible for enforcing drug control.

APPLIED PRACTICE

Complete the following exercise.

1. On the right-hand side of the following table, explain the use for each drug listed.

Name	Use
Adrenergic	
Adrenergic blocking agent	
Analgesic	

(Continued)

Name	Use
Anesthetic	
Antacid	
Antianxiety	
Antiarrhythmic	
Antibiotic	
Anticoagulant	
Anticonvulsant	
Antidepressant	
Antidiabetic	
Antidiarrheal	
Antidote	
Antiemetic	
Antifungal	
Antihelminthic	
Antihistamine	
Antihypertensive	
Anti-inflammatory	
Antineoplastic	
Antipruritic	
Antipyretic	
Antiseptic	
Antitussive	
Astringent	
Bronchodilator	
Cardiogenic	
Cathartic	

(Continued)

Name	Use
Contraceptive	
Decongestant	
Diuretic	
Emetic	
Expectorant	
Hemostatic	
Hypnotic	
Hypoglycemic	
Immunosuppressant	
Laxative	
Miotic	
Muscle relaxant	
Mydriatic	
Narcotic	
Purgative	
Psychedelic	
Sedative	
Stimulant	
Tranquilizer	
Vaccine	
Vasodilator	
Vasopressor	
Vitamin	

LEARNING ACTIVITY: MULTIPLE CHOICE

Circle the correct answer to each of the following questions.

1. Which of the following is *not* a Schedule II drug?

   a. Heroin
   b. Morphine
   c. Opium
   d. Secobarbitol

2. A shallow injection just within the top layer of skin is a(n) _____ injection.

   a. intramuscular
   b. Z-track
   c. subcutaneous
   d. intradermal

3. What is the medication abbreviation for twice a day?

   a. BID
   b. TID
   c. prn
   d. q2h

4. The drug acetaminophen is also known as

   a. Motrin.
   b. Tylenol.
   c. iso-butyl-propanoicphenolic acid.
   d. aspirin.

5. The PDR is divided into six sections. What does the first white section contain?

   a. An alphabetical listing of the generic and brand names of each product
   b. An alphabetical listing by category or classification of generic and brand names
   c. Current information regarding drugs grouped by therapeutic purposes
   d. The manufacturer's index with company names, addresses, phone numbers, emergency contacts, and lists of products

6. Which organization regulates OTC medications?

   a. AMA
   b. FDA
   c. CSA
   d. DEA

7. Schedule III drugs have

   a. the highest potential for addiction and abuse.
   b. moderate to low potential for addiction and abuse.
   c. lower potential for addiction and abuse.
   d. the lowest potential for addiction and abuse.

8. Common controlled substances include which of the following?

   a. Anabolic steroids
   b. Butabarbital
   c. Chloral hydrate
   d. All of the above

9. How often should a medical assistant review the inventory to ensure that a sufficient supply of all drugs is available and that no medication has expired?

   a. Once a day
   b. Once a week
   c. Once a month
   d. Once a quarter

10. Which of the following is the abbreviation meaning "before meals"?

    a. aa
    b. ac
    c. bf
    d. pc

CRITICAL THINKING

Answer the following questions to the best of your ability. Use the textbook as a reference.

1. A patient has finished seeing the doctor, and on her way out, she asks the medical assistant for a sample of Motrin, which is an OTC medication. The MA gives her two packages without asking the doctor and fails to document it. The MA felt that because Motrin is an OTC medication, giving it without an order would be appropriate. Is this appropriate? Explain your answer.

   _____

   _____

   _____

   _____

   _____

2. It is important for patients to understand the instructions when taking medications. If a patient has a difficult time understanding the English language, it is important to overcome this communication barrier. List the various methods you might use to overcome this barrier.

   _____

   _____

   _____

   _____

RESEARCH ACTIVITY

Use Internet search engines to research the following topic and write a brief description of what you find. It is important to use reputable websites.

1. Visit the FDA website at www.fda.gov. Navigate through the site to learn more about this organization and the information provided. Identify information that would be most helpful for you, a medical assistant, when performing various functions of your job.

   _____

   _____

   _____

   _____

   _____

CHAPTER 54
Administering Medications

STUDENT STUDY GUIDE

Use the following guide to assist in your learning of the concepts from the chapter.

I. Medication Administration

  1. Routes of Medication Administration (List six routes.)

     A. _____

     B. _____

     C. _____

     D. _____

     E. _____

     F. _____

  2. The "Three Befores" of Checking Medication (List them.)

     A. _____

     B. _____

     C. _____

  3. The "Ten Rights" of Medication Administration (List them.)

     A. _____

     B. _____

     C. _____

     D. _____

     E. _____

     F. _____

     G. _____

     H. _____

     I. _____

     J. _____

  4. Oral Medication Administration

     A. Oral medications are _____, enter the tissues of the

        _____ system, and are then _____ absorbed into

        the circulatory system and carried to the _____ of the body.

B. Oral medications can be _____, syrups, or other _____.

C. It is important to educate the patient on the proper _____ of these medications.

D. Instruct patients to keep the measuring cup _____ when pouring liquid medication to be sure to get an accurate dose and to assess it at _____ level on a flat surface.

E. _____ medications are held under the tongue, where they diffuse through the tissues and into the _____ for distribution to the body.

F. _____ medications are placed between the patient's _____ and _____ area for absorption through the tissues into the bloodstream.

5. Inhaled Medication Administration

A. Inhaled medications are dispensed into the _____ tract.

B. The advantage to this route is that the medication is absorbed _____ from the _____ system into the bloodstream.

C. Sometimes the physician will order that the inhalation medication be administered by a(n) _____, which delivers the medication more _____ into the respiratory system than a(n) _____.

6. Topical Medication Administration

A. List three topical medication forms used for skin conditions.

    i. _____

    ii. _____

    iii. _____

B. List six topical medications applied to mucous membranes.

    i. _____

    ii. _____

    iii. _____

    iv. _____

    v. _____

    vi. _____

C. When administering any form of topical medication to a patient, it is important to _____ _____ so medication isn't absorbed through your own skin.

D. Some topical medications and medication patches are _____ to _____ locations to avoid skin irritation.

E. List four medications that are effectively administered with transdermal patches.

    i. _____

    ii. _____

    iii. _____

    iv. _____

II. Equipment for Administration by Injection

  1. Syringes

    A. Identify the seven parts of a syringe.

      i. _____—The bore of the hollow needle. The size of the lumen determines the gauge of the needle, and the higher the gauge, the smaller the lumen.

      ii. _____—The length of the hollow needle.

      iii. _____—Connects the shaft to the hub.

      iv. _____—Connects the needle to the syringe.

      v. _____—Holds the liquid in the syringe.

      vi. _____—Prevents the needle from rolling on flat surfaces.

      vii. _____—When pressed, expels medication from the syringe. When pulled, gathers medication into the syringe.

    B. The smallest syringe is a(n) _____ syringe, and the measurements are calibrated in hundredths of a(n) _____.

    C. With an insulin syringe, units marked on the _____ are the amounts the physician may order for _____ administration.

    D. Larger syringes are calibrated in _____-, _____-, _____-, and _____-mL sizes and larger, up to _____ mL.

  2. Needles

    A. Needles are categorized according to _____ and length.

    B. The _____ the size of the needle (lumen), the _____ the gauge.

    C. Intramuscular injections are usually given with _____- or _____-gauge needles, usually _____ inch(es) to _____ inch(es) long.

    D. Subcutaneous injections are given with _____- to _____-gauge needles.

    E. Intradermal injections are given with _____- to _____-gauge needles.

    F. To prevent needlesticks, always use _____ needles and syringes.

    G. It is important to ensure that the _____ is in place any time you are changing the _____ on a syringe.

    H. All needles and syringes should be placed in a(n) _____ _____ container, needle _____, immediately after they are used.

3. Medications for Injection

   A. Injectable medications are available in various _____.

   B. _____-dose and multidose vials are available.

   C. An ampule is a small, _____ glass bottles that contains a(n) _____ dose of medication.

   D. Powders to be reconstituted are injected after reconstituting the powders with diluents, such as _____ _____.

   E. With unit dose packaging, medications are packaged in _____ containers that deliver dosages one at a time by a(n) _____ route, as ordered by the prescriber.

   F. Prefilled _____ _____ systems are prefilled, single-dose cartridges that fit into a special cartridge holder.

III. Safety Procedures: OSHA Standards

   1. OSHA has established specific _____ regarding the disposal of contaminated needles and syringes.

   2. OSHA's Bloodborne Pathogens Standard has provisions for follow-up procedures for health care workers who are exposed to _____ from contaminated needles.

   3. If you are accidentally stuck with a contaminated needle, immediately _____ the wound and then notify the _____ and _____ _____ manager.

   4. The employer is responsible for providing free _____ _____ and _____ for exposure to contaminated sharps or needles while at work.

   5. By law, all medical offices must have a(n) _____-proof, rigid, _____ container labeled with an international biohazard _____ for the disposal of sharps.

   6. Any time a medical assistant has the potential to come in contact with _____ body fluids, _____ _____ must be observed and followed.

IV. Intramuscular Injections

   1. Intramuscular (IM) injections administer medication directly into _____ tissue.

   2. They are always given at a(n) _____-degree angle.

   3. Deltoid Muscle

     A. The deltoid muscle is located on the _____ _____ surface of the upper arm.

     B. This site works well for _____-volume injections.

     C. A(n) _____-gauge, _____-inch needle is used to give injections in the arm.

D. For individuals with small arms, a(n) _____-gauge, _____-inch needle is more appropriate.

E. Up to _____ mL can be injected in a large adult's deltoid muscle.

4. Vastus Lateralis Muscle

A. The vastus lateralis muscle is located on the _____ portion of the upper _____ and is part of the quadriceps.

B. This muscle is well developed in _____ and recommended by the American _____ of _____ as the preferred injection site for infants and _____.

C. Typically, it is one handbreadth below the greater _____ and extends to one handbreadth above the _____.

5. Dorsogluteal Muscle

A. The dorsogluteal muscle, located on the upper outer quadrant of the _____, may be used for _____-volume, deep IM injections or for _____ viscous (thick) medications.

B. If the dorsogluteal site is used for an injection, landmarks must be observed to avoid _____ to the _____ nerve.

C. Up to _____ mL can be injected into this site.

6. Ventrogluteal Muscle

A. The ventrogluteal muscle is considered a safer injection site than the _____ site because there are no major _____ or _____ vessels in this muscle.

B. This site is considered safe for _____, _____, and adults.

C. Up to _____ mL can be injected safely into a large adult ventrogluteal muscle.

7. Z-track Method

A. The Z-track method is used when a medication is _____ to the subcutaneous tissues or when the medication may _____ the skin.

B. When giving a medication using the Z-track method, pull the _____ to the side before inserting the needle.

   i. Then _____ the medication, _____ the skin, and remove the _____, and the medication will not be able to _____ back to the skin's surface.

V. Subcutaneous Injections

1. A subcutaneous injection is given just _____ the skin, in the _____ (adipose) tissue.

2. This method is used for small doses of _____ medications such as _____, insulin, and _____.

3. Common Injection Sites for Subcutaneous Injections (List four sites.)

A. _____

B. _____

C. _____

D. _____

4. A subcutaneous injection is given at a(n) _____-degree angle to the skin surface, unless the injection is heparin or insulin, in which case a(n) _____-degree angle is used.

5. For patients who self-inject, the site of injection must be _____ so as not to form _____ tissue by repeatedly injecting the same sites.

VI. Intradermal Injections

1. Intradermal (ID) injection is commonly used for _____ skin testing, in which a minute amount of material is injected within the _____ _____ of skin to determine a patient's sensitivity.

2. A tuberculin skin test is done intradermally to determine whether a patient has ever been exposed to _____.

3. The _____ _____ _____ (PPD) skin test uses a measured amount of TB antigens via an injection that is administered under the top layer of skin on the patient's _____.

4. TB Skin Test Results

A. A(n) _____ _____ is a positive reaction to the test.

B. The size of the firm bump (not the red area) should be measured _____ to _____ days after the test to determine the result.

C. Interpreting the results of the TB skin test is _____ within the _____ of practice for a medical assistant and should _____ be done.

VII. Intravenous Therapy (IV)

1. IV therapy involves injecting medications or therapeutic solutions directly into the _____ for immediate _____ and use by the body.

2. Medical assistants must consult their _____ _____ _____ before attempting any IV procedure.

3. Medical Office Settings and Outpatient IV Therapy

A. List three reasons medical office and outpatient settings are becoming more acceptable for IV therapy.

i. _____

ii. _____

iii. _____

4. Three indications for administering IV therapy include administering _____ and _____ _____, replacing _____ _____ and correcting _____ imbalances, and aiding in the administration of _____ _____.

5. Medications Commonly Administered Intravenously (List five.)

   A. _____

   B. _____

   C. _____

   D. _____

   E. _____

6. Administration of _____ _____ is not within the scope of practice of a medical assistant.

7. Special Requirements for IV Therapy*

   A. IV administration requires special knowledge and _____ because it involves direct access to the _____.

   B. The _____ and the _____ site must be assessed regularly during the infusion for signs of adverse reactions.

   C. Any combination of _____, swelling, _____, bleeding, and loss of _____ at the site of the infusion must be immediately reported to the physician.

8. The MA's Role in Intravenous Therapy

   A. In addition to setting up the IV _____, the MA should be available to provide the patient with _____ during the procedure.

   B. If present during the procedure, the MA should be able to recognize some of the possible _____ _____ that intravenous therapy can cause.

   C. _____ occurs when the tip of the IV catheter withdraws from the vein or pokes through the vein into surrounding _____.

   D. List six possible reactions that may occur during IV therapy.

      i. _____

      ii. _____

      iii. _____

      iv. _____

      v. _____

      vi. _____

*If your state allows medical assistants to participate in components related to IV therapy, carefully review related information to acquaint yourself with IV therapy, including preparing an IV tray and observing IV therapy.

9. After an IV procedure, it may be the MA's responsibility to make sure the area is cleaned up and that the _____ and _____ have been properly placed where they belong.

VIII. Immunizations

1. Immunizations, or _____, are given to humans to decrease their susceptibility to disease.

2. Antibodies defend against _____ or _____ substances.

3. This defensive process of the body occurs when an individual contracts a(n) _____.

4. During the illness, the body begins to develop _____ to fight off the disease.

5. After an individual has recovered from an illness, he/she is less likely to contract the _____ _____ again.

6. When this occurs, the individual is said to have developed _____ or a resistance, to the disease.

7. Immunity can be either _____ or acquired.

8. Artificially acquired active immunity to a certain disease develops in response to receiving a vaccination with _____ (dead) or _____ (weakened) organisms of that disease.

9. Sometimes, an immunization or a vaccine can cause an individual to experience some mild _____ of the disease or to develop _____ at the site of injection.

10. Childhood and Adolescent Immunizations

   A. List three organizations that are associated with issuing the annual recommended childhood and adolescent immunization schedule.

      i. _____

      ii. _____

      iii. _____

   B. The _____ provides vaccine information sheets (VIS) that are to be given to parents or guardians _____ the _____ of a vaccine to a child.

   C. List 11 common childhood vaccinations.

      i. _____

      ii. _____

      iii. _____

      iv. _____

      v. _____

vi. _____

vii. _____

viii. _____

ix. _____

x. _____

xi. _____

11. Adult and Other Immunizations

A. In addition to the _____ vaccination, adults 65 years of age and older should receive the _____ _____ _____ vaccine (PPV) and the _____ _____ (Zostavax).

B. Adults and children who travel abroad must also obtain, _____ _____, additional _____, immunizations, and _____ medications recommended by the _____.

KEY TERMINOLOGY REVIEW

Complete the following sentences using the correct key terms found at the beginning of the chapter.

1. The _____ site is most commonly used for large-volume, deep IM injections or for irritating viscous (thick) medications.

2. _____ are placed between the patient's cheek and gums area for absorption through the tissues into the bloodstream.

3. Meningitis is a result of _____, which affects about 12,000 children a year.

4. _____, also known as chickenpox, is one of the most common childhood diseases.

5. An alcohol pad or cotton pad must be used to hold the vial to prevent glass cuts when opening a(n) _____.

APPLIED PRACTICE

Complete the following exercises.

1. On the figure below, label each part of the syringe.

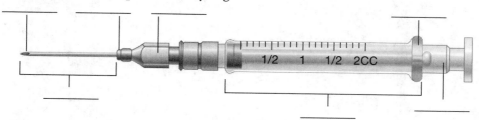

2. To demonstrate your knowledge of the angle of insertion for intramuscular, subcutaneous, and intradermal injections, indicate on the figure provided which angles represent each type of injection. In addition, provide the names of each of the layers of the skin.

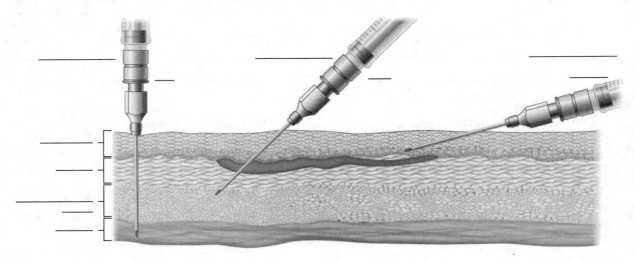

3. Demonstrate your knowledge of intramuscular injection sites by labeling the image below.

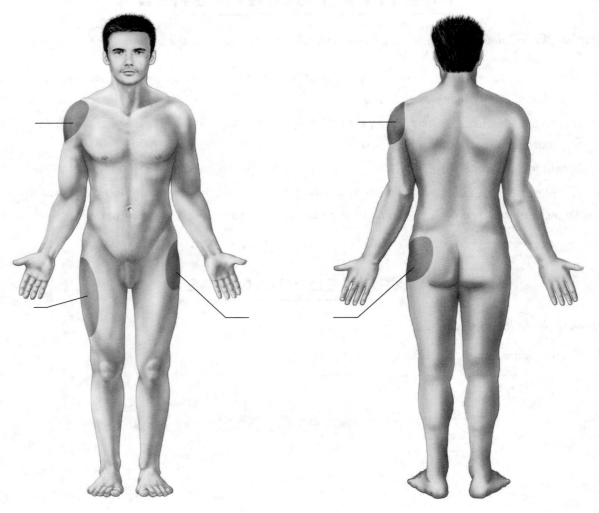

LEARNING ACTIVITY: TRUE/FALSE

Indicate whether the following statements are true or false by placing a T or an F on the line that precedes each statement.

_____ 1. Artificially acquired active immunity develops in response to receiving vaccinations that contain active organisms.

_____ 2. The deltoid muscle is located on the lower outer surface of the upper arm.

_____ 3. Transmission of diphtheria occurs through direct and indirect contact.

_____ 4. Hepatitis B, a form of viral hepatitis, is highly contagious and can be fatal.

_____ 5. There are three forms of the polio vaccine.

_____ 6. Intramuscular injections are usually given with 27- or 28-gauge needles.

_____ 7. Many liquid medications are prescribed for pediatric patients because of the ease of administration.

_____ 8. The MMR vaccination is given in three doses.

_____ 9. Subcutaneous injects are usually administered at a 45-degree angle.

_____ 10. When giving a medication using the Z-track method, you need to pull the skin upward prior to inserting the needle.

CRITICAL THINKING

Answer the following questions to the best of your ability. Use the textbook as a reference.

1. Elenora Kiesel is a 35-year-old woman of normal body weight and size. The doctor has ordered tetanus vaccination to be administered intramuscularly. The vaccine does not have a thick viscosity, and 0.5 mL will need to be drawn up in the syringe. Based on this information, what size needle/syringe would be used? Identify the angle of injection and which muscle would be an ideal injection site for this vaccine. Explain your choice.

_____

_____

_____

_____

_____

2. Although injecting a very small of amount of bubbles or air into the muscle or the subcutaneous tissue would not be harmful, *the medical assistant must never let this happen.* Explain why it is not acceptable to have even tiny bubbles within the medication inside the syringe.

_____

_____

_____

_____

_____

RESEARCH ACTIVITY

Use Internet search engines to research the following topic and report what you find. It is important to use reputable websites.

1. Some parents believe that it is not necessary to immunize their children. To learn more about this issue, conduct research online and then write an essay on your findings. Conclude with a synopsis of what you believe about the necessity of immunizations for children. Be sure to cite your sources.

   _____

   _____

   _____

   _____

   _____

CHAPTER 55
Patient Education

STUDENT STUDY GUIDE

Use the following guide to assist in your learning of the concepts from the chapter.

I. The Patient Coach

  1. Ways a Patient Coach Can Help a Patient (List four.)

    A. _____

    B. _____

    C. _____

    D. _____

  2. Any information that could be perceived as patient education must first be _____ by a(n) _____ or other _____ health care provider.

  3. Health Maintenance

    A. Health maintenance focuses on the idea of a patient's overall _____.

    B. Proper coaching from a medical assistant can empower a patient to make positive life changes.

    C. An increasing number of applications (apps) focus on _____ and _____.

    D. For additional motivation, app users are often able to post their successes and _____ directly on social _____ sites.

  4. Disease Prevention

    A. It is important to focus on _____ measures that can reduce the risk of illness and disease.

    B. Many illnesses are related to _____ behaviors.

    C. List examples of basic hygiene procedures that play a role in disease prevention.

      i. _____

      ii. _____

      iii. _____

      iv. _____

    D. Patients must be able to identify personal _____ factors for disease.

5. Treatment Plan Compliance

   A. Patient compliance is the patient's ability to follow through on all suggestions and _____ as given by the _____.

   B. In order for a patient to be _____ with a treatment plan, the patient must understand all the _____ of the plan and why the plan is _____ for health and wellness.

6. Impact of Finances on Patient Education

   A. The patient may want to comply with a treatment plan but may be inhibited in doing so because of _____ of _____.

   B. A wise and efficient medical assistant will create a list of _____ _____ that can help patients who need _____ assistance and provide the information to patients in a discreet and _____ manner.

7. Handling Noncompliance

   A. Noncompliance is _____ following the _____ orders.

   B. Health care costs _____ with noncompliance because disease processes progress and _____, leading to other health complications.

   C. Lack of compliance may be indicated by failure to take _____ as ordered, return for _____ appointments, practice _____ changes, or follow a(n) _____ program.

   D. _____ have the least problem with noncompliance as long as their _____ are compliant and assist them.

   E. A medical assistant can reinforce learning and reduce noncompliance by working out a(n) _____ plan that includes regular _____ of progress.

II. Understanding and Developing Patient Education

   1. The patient education process begins with _____, or evaluation of the patient's needs.

   2. The next step is to _____ or determine how to begin the task of teaching.

   3. _____ the plan involves teaching the patient specifically what to do.

   4. Documenting the teaching done by _____ it in the patient's health record helps ensure _____ of care.

   5. The final component is evaluating the _____ of the teaching plan.

   6. How Adults Learn

      A. Adult learning is a(n) _____ process.

      B. Adult learners most desire practical _____ of learning.

      C. Adults often prefer a(n) _____-learning atmosphere because of the _____ support a group setting offers.

D. Motivational incentives for adult learners include better _____, improved _____, pride of _____, self-_____, and praise from others.

7. Teaching Methods

   A. Choose teaching methods based on _____ and preferences of the _____.

   B. Use a combination of teaching methods and techniques to enhance patients' learning _____ while maintaining their _____.

8. Learning Environments

   A. Patients are inclined to be more open to learning and honest about situations if they have a sense of _____.

   B. If it is necessary to teach a patient how to use equipment, the equipment should be available for _____.

   C. The learning environment is also cultivated by _____ and communication.

   D. The following are some roadblocks to effective communication.

      i. Ordering, _____, and directing the patient to learn through force or _____ tones

      ii. Warning or _____ remarks

      iii. Moralizing or _____

      iv. _____

      v. _____

      vi. Name calling, _____, and labeling

      vii. _____

      viii. _____

      ix. _____ inappropriate treatment plans

      x. Speaking loudly to a(n) _____ person

      xi. _____-inappropriate speech

9. Teaching Resources

   A. When creating a plan for patient education, consider using _____ players, compact _____, videos, or _____.

   B. Pharmaceutical and manufacturer _____ can be valuable resources.

   C. Free videos regarding _____ _____ can be found on the Internet.

   D. It is always important to make sure that the source providing a video is _____ and _____.

10. Electronic Health Records and Patient Education

    A. Many offices that use electronic health records send out _____ patient education information via _____.

    B. An office that use electronic health records is able to query its records and obtain _____-specific information that can be e-mailed.

    C. Sending such e-mails requires _____ from the patient but it is an efficient and _____-effective means to deliver patient education.

III. Patient Coaching and Education: Meeting Patient Needs

  1. Patient education must be adapted to fit not only the _____ style but also the special _____ of the patient.

  2. Teaching Children

    A. Patient education should be modified to the appropriate _____ stage to reach each child.

    B. Children may need to see a treatment or procedure performed on a(n) _____ before tolerating it well.

    C. Many children like to _____ equipment that will be used on them.

    D. Older children also will have numerous _____ about their treatments and should receive adequate _____ in response.

    E. Regarding educating children about their own health issues, it is important to direct the education to both the _____ and the _____.

  3. Hearing-Impaired Patients*

    A. Patients who have hearing impairments frequently _____ _____.

    B. Face a hearing-impaired patient and speak _____ but be sure not to speak so slowly that it is _____ to the patient.

    C. Do not stand with your back to a(n) _____ or _____ source when speaking to a hearing-impaired patient because such positioning will cast _____ over your mouth.

  4. Visually Impaired Patients

    A. For visually impaired patients, consider making _____-recorded instructions of _____ that is usually written.

    B. This might be done using the patient's own _____ device.

    C. Be sure to clear _____ from the office and _____ that might impede a visually impaired patient.

---

*Carefully review Procedure 55-2, which details effective patient education for hearing-impaired patients.

D. Ask a visually impaired patient if he/she would like a(n) _____ arm while navigating the examination room.

5. Developmental Delays, Mental Challenges, Illiteracy, and Language Barriers

   A. Patients who have developmental delays or are mentally challenged may have trouble understanding _____ or multiple-_____ patient education and instruction.

   B. When directing instructions toward the caregiver, do not _____ the patient or act as if he or she isn't in the _____.

   C. Make appropriate references and _____ _____ with both the patient and the caregiver, showing that you _____ and appreciate them both.

   D. Be alert to behaviors that might indicate someone has difficulty with _____ and writing.

   E. Always provide the patient with _____ _____ and highlight or underline especially important information.

   F. It is very likely that a patient has a(n) _____ _____ or friend who is able to read to and _____ the patient.

   G. Advanced notice and preparations can be made for a non–_____-speaking patient at the time the patient's _____ is scheduled.

   H. When such an appointment is being scheduled, ask if a(n) _____ will accompany the patient to the appointment or if the _____ _____ will need to provide an interpreter.

   I. If a relative is acting as an interpreter, it is necessary to obtain the patient's _____ permission to discuss _____ information with the interpreting relative.

   J. If a large _____ of patients in the office speak a certain language other than English, it may help to construct _____ in that language.

6. Teaching Older Adults

   A. An older adult's intellectual capacity usually does not _____; it merely _____.

   B. An older person is able to learn quickly if the learning requires _____ acquired in the _____.

   C. Teaching methods that are useful with an older adult range from using handouts with _____ _____ to using video and audio _____.

   D. Slowed processing time

      i. Older patients need more time to think through and _____ new information.

     ii. It is helpful for you to break down information into _____

         _____.

     iii. It is also helpful to give _____ _____ so the patient can

         process the instructions more slowly later.

E. Decreased short-term memory

     i. An older adult patient often will have an easier time remembering what happened in

         the _____ but may have difficulty remembering _____

         _____ information.

     ii. Work with an older patient to devise methods to reinforce _____ or

         prod the _____.

     iii. New information should be linked to a well-known _____

         _____ when possible.

F. Decreased mobility and dexterity

     i. Some elderly patients are not _____ able to do the same things they

         could when they were _____.

     ii. It is helpful to be aware of _____ equipment and _____

         devices that are available for elderly patients.

G. Increased anxiety about new situations

     i. Many circumstances cause _____ for an elderly patient.

     ii. A newly diagnosed medical condition will likely cause a(n) _____ in

         patient anxiety levels.

     iii. As an advocate, an MA can help patients by encouraging and building their

         _____ levels.

     iv. Practice positive _____ and provide _____ when patients

         display an understanding of a new concept.

7. Culture and Patient Education

A. The best way to find out about a patient's culture is to _____ the

   _____.

B. Make every attempt to _____ the wishes of the patient while not taking

   personal _____ if someone else will make the patient feel more comfortable.

C. _____ _____ can be key allies in assisting the patient with

   learning and with reinforcing your teaching.

D. Always ask the patient if religious _____ could interfere with the ability to

   _____ with a treatment or if special considerations need to be made to

   comply with religious and _____ beliefs before or following a(n)

   _____.

IV. Community Resources

1. Community resources are programs and services that are available to improve the
_____ of life of an individual by providing help, _____, and
_____.

2. Medical assistants should be familiar with _____ available within their
community that can _____ and _____ the lives of their patients.

3. Referrals to Community Resources

A. Physicians and their staff are given personal access not only to the patient's
_____ health but also information related to their personal
_____.

B. Physicians may ask medical assistants to refer patients directly to _____
_____ that can help meet patient needs.

C. When medical assistants work as _____ _____, they help
patients streamline services available to meet their health care needs and improve
_____ in the ever-changing and sometimes confusing world of
_____.

KEY TERMINOLOGY REVIEW

Complete each sentence by selecting the correct key term from the textbook. A few of the sentences use more than one key term.

1. The education process begins with _____, or _____ of the patient's needs.

2. _____ refers to the patient's ability to follow through on all suggestions and orders as given by the physician.

3. _____ a plan involves actually teaching the patient what to do.

4. Some procedures that require small-muscle _____, such as flossing the teeth and opening medication bottles, are almost impossible for elderly persons with arthritis.

5. _____ are programs and services that are available to improve the quality of life of an individual by providing information and assistance.

APPLIED PRACTICE

Explain how you would handle the following scenario.

Scenario

Pearson Endocrinology Associates has chosen to begin weekly, group-centered patient education sessions for children who have been newly diagnosed with type 1 diabetes. Dominick, a CMA (AAMA) in charge of helping lead the education sessions, has been given the task of creating a shopping list of items that will help the children with the patient education process. What types of items might Dominick want to include on his shopping list?

_____

_____

_____

_____

_____

LEARNING ACTIVITY: TRUE/FALSE

Indicate whether the following statements are true or false by placing a T or an F on the line that precedes each statement.

1. _____ Patient education should be modified to the appropriate developmental stage to reach each child.

2. _____ Intellectual capacity diminishes with advanced age.

3. _____ Sarcasm is considered a roadblock to effective patient learning.

4. _____ Adult learning is an active process.

5. _____ Religious beliefs do not have an impact on health care.

6. _____ Wellness is the ongoing process of practicing a healthy lifestyle.

7. _____ A lack of finances might impact patient compliance with treatment plans.

8. _____ Medical assistants often decide which patient education will be provided to patients.

9. _____ Patients who do not speak English are always required to pay for their own interpreter to accompany them to medical appointments.

10. _____ An older adult patient often will have a harder time remembering what happened in the past but may easily recall newly acquired information.

CRITICAL THINKING

Answer the following questions to the best of your ability. Use the textbook as a reference.

1. You are a medical assistant at an OB/GYN office. The physician has recently put you in charge of creating a list of resources and materials to be used in a patient education library. What patient education topics would you include in an OB/GYN resource library? List at least three topics and explain why you chose them.

   _____

   _____

   _____

   _____

   _____

2. The physician has asked you to lead a discussion group that focuses on educating patients about health maintenance. What discussion points would you include for this patient education session?

   _____

   _____

   _____

   _____

   _____

RESEARCH ACTIVITY

Use Internet search engines to research the following topic and write a brief description of what you find. It is important to use reputable websites.

1. Search the Internet for reputable resources related to patient education about diabetes. List three reputable websites that could be beneficial to a newly diagnosed diabetic patient. Explain why you chose each website.

   _____

   _____

   _____

   _____

   _____

CHAPTER 56
Nutrition

STUDENT STUDY GUIDE

Use the following guide to assist in your learning of the concepts from the chapter.

I. Nutrition Professionals

   1. A well-nourished person is better able to ward off _____, remain _____, and perhaps even live _____.

   2. Nutrition professionals are able to help individuals develop healthy _____ _____ to improve and prolong their _____ of life.

   3. Registered Dietitians and Nutritionists

     A. A registered dietitian provides patients with information about nutrition and creates _____ _____ that will help treat and prevent _____.

     B. The services registered dietitians offer are considered medical _____ _____.

     C. _____ laws vary regarding who is allowed to be designated as a "nutritionist," but a nutritionist may or may not be a(n) _____ health care provider.

     D. All registered dietitians could be considered _____, but not all nutritionists are _____ _____.

   4. The Medical Assistant's Role in Nutrition

     A. List the duties a medical assistant may perform related to nutrition and patient care.

       i. _____

         _____

       ii. _____

         _____

       iii. _____

         _____

       iv. _____

         _____

II. A Review: Digestion and Metabolism

  1. Digestion

    A. Digestion is the body's process of converting food into _____ substances that can be absorbed into the bloodstream and used by body _____ and _____.

    B. The digestive process is accomplished by breaking down, _____, dissolving, and chemically _____ the food we consume into _____ compounds.

    C. The digestive process that takes place in the stomach reaches a peak about _____ hours after a(n) _____.

    D. When a person who has eaten too _____, still feels _____, and goes on eating after he or she has actually eaten _____, excess food and calories are consumed.

  2. Metabolism

    A. Metabolism is the sum of all _____ and _____ changes that take place inside the cells of the human body.

    B. List four enzymes that are required to maintain metabolism.

      i. _____

      ii. _____

      iii. _____

      iv. _____

    C. Approximately _____ percent of the energy created by cell metabolism is used by the body to carry on its _____ _____.

    D. The remaining _____ percent of the energy produced by metabolism becomes _____.

III. Nutrients

  1. Nutrients are the _____ and _____ chemical substances found in foods that supply the body with the elements necessary for metabolism.

  2. More than _____ nutrients are required for the human body to function properly. These nutrients must be consumed in the diet on a(n) _____ basis.

  3. Carbohydrates

    A. Carbohydrates are the _____ _____ of energy from the foods we consume.

    B. Carbohydrates are the sugars and _____ that are found mainly in _____.

    C. Sugars are either _____ or complex.

D. Starches are _____, which are reduced to _____ during the digestive process and transported into the blood.

E. Complex carbohydrates are considered _____ foods for a healthy diet because they are generally _____ in fat, _____ in fiber, and a good source of _____ and minerals.

4. Fiber

A. Fiber is a type of carbohydrate that is _____.

B. It helps move food through the digestive system _____.

C. List six common sources of fiber.

    i. _____

    ii. _____

    iii. _____

    iv. _____

    v. _____

    vi. _____

5. Proteins

A. Proteins are called the "_____ _____" of the body because they form the base of every living _____.

B. Complete proteins include proteins from animal sources, including _____, eggs, _____, milk, and _____, as well as _____ and quinoa.

C. Incomplete proteins, which cannot supply the body with all the essential _____ _____, include vegetable proteins, such as _____, beans, _____, and wheat.

D. Proteins are necessary for producing _____, promoting _____ and repair of _____, and providing the framework for _____, _____, and blood.

6. Fats

A. Fats, also called _____, are fatty acids.

B. Two critical fatty acids, _____ and _____, are "essential" to the diet.

C. Fat is important for proper growth, _____, and maintenance of good _____ but should be eaten in _____.

D. Infants and toddlers have the _____ energy needs per unit of body _____.

E. Saturated fat

    i. Saturated fat has many _____ effects on the body, including raising the level of blood _____.

    ii. It is recommended that no more than _____ percent of the daily _____ intake come from saturated fat.

F. Unsaturated fat

    i. Unsaturated fat is further classified as either _____ fat or _____ fat.

    ii. Monounsaturated fat has the ability to lower _____ levels and low-_____ _____.

G. Trans fat

    i. Trans fat is formed when manufacturers add _____ to _____ oil.

    ii. Saturated fat and trans fat _____ LDL cholesterol levels in the blood.

    iii. In _____, the FDA introduced a proposed _____ on artificial trans fat in processed foods.

    iv. The ban of artificial trans fat is based on the hope that, by _____ trans fats completely, more lives will be _____ through the prevention of heart attacks and _____ disease.

7. Water

  A. The human body can survive for several _____ without food but cannot live more than a few _____ without water.

  B. Water comprises between _____ and _____ percent of average human body weight.

  C. List six functions of water in the body (refer to Box 56-1).

    i. _____

    ii. _____

    iii. _____

    iv. _____

    v. _____

    vi. _____

  D. The recommended amount of daily water intake is _____ to _____ 8-ounce glasses.

  E. Water intake is balanced by fluid output through the _____, lungs, _____, and feces.

8. Vitamins

  A. Vitamins are _____ substances that are essential for metabolism, _____, and _____ of the body.

B. The two main classifications of vitamins are _____ soluble and

_____ soluble.

    i. Fat-soluble vitamins include ___, ____, ____, and K.

    ii. Water-soluble vitamins include _____ and _____.

C. Vitamins can be destroyed in foods through improper _____ and prolonged

_____.

D. Recommended dietary allowances are the recommended _____ intake

levels that meet the _____ requirements of most _____

individuals.

9. Minerals

  A. Minerals are _____ elements that are of neither _____ nor

plant origin.

  B. List seven _____, or major minerals.

    i. _____

    ii. _____

    iii. _____

    iv. _____

    v. _____

    vi. _____

    vii. _____

  C. List 11 _____, or trace minerals.

    i. _____

    ii. _____

    iii. _____

    iv. _____

    v. _____

    vi. _____

    vii. _____

    viii. _____

    ix. _____

    x. _____

    xi. _____

D. Minerals are necessary for physiological processes such as _____

contraction and _____ action.

10. Dietary Supplements

    A. Dietary supplements come in various forms, including _____,
_____ caps, liquids, and _____.

    B. List ingredients found in dietary supplements.

        i. _____

        ii. _____

        iii. _____

        iv. _____

        v. _____

    C. Dietary supplements should never be used to _____ food.

11. Cholesterol

    A. Cholesterol is a(n) _____ material that is normally found in the body.

    B. It is produced naturally by the _____ and other body cells.

    C. Cholesterol moves into and out of the body cells within compounds called

    _____.

        i. High-density lipoproteins are considered _____ cholesterol.

        ii. Low-density lipoproteins are considered _____ cholesterol.

    D. It is believed that the _____ the HDL level in the blood, the lower the risk
for _____ disease.

    E. It is important to examine _____ labels for the amounts of both cholesterol
and _____ fat.

IV. A Healthy Diet and Lifestyle

    1. List four examples of healthy eating choices.

        A. _____

        B. _____

        C. _____

        D. _____

    2. MyPlate

        A. In 2012, the USDA retired the traditional food _____ with a concept called
MyPlate.

        B. MyPlate shows a plate and glass divided to show recommended relative

        _____ of the five major _____ _____.

        C. Suggestions from the USDA also include the following.

            i. Half of your plate should be filled with _____ and

            _____.

ii. Half or more of your grains should be _____ _____ foods.

iii. When making dairy choices, switch to _____ or ____ percent low-fat milk and low-fat or fat-free _____ and cheeses.

iv. Choose lean cuts of _____ and _____.

v. Avoid drinks that contain additional _____; stick with water or 100 percent natural _____ juice.

D. A program called _____ allows individuals to track, analyze, and plan their diet and _____-_____ levels.

3. Understanding Caloric Intake

A. A calorie measures the amount of _____ produced by the foods we eat.

B. Daily calorie requirements of individuals vary based on factors including gender, _____, _____, and _____ level.

C. When more calories are taken in than are used by the body, they are stored as _____.

D. When fewer calories are taken in than are needed, the body begins to use the _____ _____.

4. Determining the Number of Calories in Food

A. 1 g of protein has ____ calories.

B. 1 g of carbohydrate has ____ calories.

C. 1 g of fat has ____ calories.

5. Measuring Body Fat

A. Ideal weight varies with _____, gender, body _____, and _____ charts.

B. Another consideration is a person's percentage of _____.

C. The skin fold measurement of body fat involves using special _____ _____ to measure the thickness of _____ folds.

6. Body Mass Index (BMI)

A. A patient's BMI is calculated using the formula BMI = Weight in _____ / Height in _____ squared.

   i. A patient's height is measured in _____ (1 m = ____ ft or ____ in.).

   ii. A patient's weight is measured in _____ (1 kg = ____ lb).

B. A helpful feature of electronic health records (EHRs) is automatic BMI _____.

C. A BMI between 19 and 25 is considered a(n) _____ weight; 25 to 30 is considered _____; over 30 is considered _____.

7. Exercise

   A. Exercise and other physical activity should be included as part of the patient's

    _____ _____.

   B. Activity helps to _____ the fat in the diet so that it does not become

    _____ in the body.

   C. It is important to match exercise with the interests, _____, and

    _____ of the patient.

8. Limiting Alcohol

   A. Alcohol is not a food product but contains _____ and lowers the rate at

    which calories are _____.

   B. Excessive alcohol intake is associated with problems such as alcoholism or alcohol

    _____, _____ accidents, and family and work

    _____.

   C. Pregnant women are advised to _____ alcohol during pregnancy because of

    its potential to cause birth defects such as _____ _____

    _____.

V. Special Dietary Needs and Modifications

  1. A diet modified for health reasons is called a(n) _____ diet.

  2. In many cases, the physician will refer the patient to a(n) _____

   _____ who can discuss all aspects of a therapeutic diet.

  3. All the principles of adult _____ must be considered when

   _____ patients about dietary changes.

  4. Restrictive/Food-Sensitive Diets

    A. A patient may have a food _____ or may not be able to physically

     _____ certain ingredients in food.

    B. A patient may experience symptoms ranging from mild _____ upset and

     _____ rashes to more severe allergic reactions that can cause swelling of the

     _____ and respiratory distress.

    C. Gluten-free diets

      i. Gluten is a protein found in _____, _____,

      _____ and grains that is most often derived from wheat.

     ii. This protein works as a(n) _____ to help keep food together.

    iii. Symptoms of gluten intolerance _____ _____, as

      does the level of symptom _____.

    iv. Patients with gluten sensitivity should only eat foods that are labeled

      _____ _____.

D. Lactose-free diets

   i. Dairy products such as _____, cheese, _____, and ice cream contain a sugar known as lactose.

   ii. Lactose intolerance is due to the body's inability to properly break down and _____ the sugar, which results in _____ upset.

   iii. Some patients choose to eliminate _____ products from their diet, while others choose to use dairy _____.

5. Dietary Considerations for Cancer Patients

  A. Higher-_____ and higher-_____ foods can help a cancer patient maintain weight, which is often lost as a side effect of both the _____ and _____ treatments.

  B. Cancer patients are encouraged to eat diets that are rich in fresh _____ and _____ and healthy _____ grains.

  C. Increased protein intake helps facilitate _____ and promote the regeneration of _____.

  D. Increased fluid intake is also encouraged to help prevent _____ and promote _____.

6. Weight-Control Diets

  A. High-protein diets

   i. Protein can help control _____ and maintain lean muscle mass, which helps with burning _____ _____.

   ii. Diets are considered to be high protein when _____ percent of the daily calories come from _____-rich sources.

  B. Calorie-count diet

   i. A 1,200-calorie diet that includes a balance of the _____ food groups and low-_____ foods will result in weight loss.

   ii. Patients are encouraged to keep a food _____ and record everything they _____ each day.

7. Low-Fat/Low-Cholesterol Diets

  A. A low-fat diet is aimed at keeping the fat content between _____ and _____ grams of fat per day.

  B. A low-fat diet has been found to reduce the risk of _____, breast, and _____ cancer; _____ disease; and _____.

  C. List foods that are recommended on a low-fat/low-cholesterol diet.

   i. _____

   ii. _____

iii. _____

iv. _____

v. _____

D. List foods that are not allowed on a low-fat/low-cholesterol diet.

i. _____

ii. _____

iii. _____

iv. _____

8. Low-Sodium Diets

A. Diets that restrict salt are prescribed for patients with _____ and heart or _____ disease.

B. Salt restriction is also recommended for patients on _____ _____ diets because an excess of salt in the diet promotes _____ retention.

C. Mild sodium-restricted diet

i. A mild sodium-restricted diet allows _____ to _____ mg of sodium per day.

ii. It allows ½ teaspoon of _____ _____ and limited amount of _____ containing salt.

D. Moderate sodium-restricted diet

i. A moderate sodium-restricted diet allows _____ to _____ mg of sodium per day.

ii. All processed and _____ foods containing salt are _____.

iii. No added salt is allowed in food _____.

E. Severe sodium-restricted diet

i. A severe sodium-restricted diet allows _____ mg of sodium per day.

ii. With this type of diet, a patient should eliminate all table salt use, _____ salt, and include only _____-_____ products in the diet.

9. Diabetic Diet

A. List five factors that are considered for therapeutic diabetic diets.

i. _____

ii. _____

iii. _____

iv. _____

v. _____

B. A food _____ system is often used for diabetic patients.

    i. One _____ of food within a group is considered an

      "_____."

    ii. Foods within the same group can be exchanged because they have the same effect on

      the patient's _____ _____ level.

C. _____ counting is also a common dietary tool for patients with diabetes.

D. Carbohydrate counting is based on two concepts.

    i. Of all the nutrients, carbohydrates have the most _____ on blood

      sugar.

    ii. Whether simple or complex, _____ _____ of a

      carbohydrate, will raise the blood sugar the _____ amount.

10. Diets for Gastrointestinal Issues

A. Bland diet

    i. A bland diet is devoid of any foods that contain substances irritating to the

      gastrointestinal tract, such as _____ or _____.

    ii. A bland diet eliminates specific foods that are _____ forming, contain

      _____ or spices, are _____, are highly

      _____, or are high in _____.

    iii. List foods included in a bland diet.

      a. _____

      b. _____

      c. _____

      d. _____

      e. _____

B. BRAT diet

    i. Foods on the BRAT diet are easily _____ and do not cause further

      gastrointestinal upset.

    ii. List the foods on the BRAT diet.

      a. _____

      b. _____

      c. _____

      d. _____

C. Low-fiber diet

    i. Low-fiber diets are used to bind _____ and help with

      _____ issues.

ii. List foods that are allowed on a low-fiber diet.

a. _____

b. _____

c. _____

d. _____

e. _____

f. _____

iii. List foods that are not allowed on a low-fiber diet.

a. _____

b. _____

c. _____

D. High-fiber diet

i. A high-fiber diet is used to treat _____ with existing problems such as _____ _____ disease and _____ as well as to prevent _____ disease and aid in weight loss.

ii. List examples of food that are good sources of fiber.

a. _____

b. _____

c. _____

11. Dietary Modifications Required for Procedures

A. List foods that are allowed on a clear liquid diet.

i. _____

ii. _____

iii. _____

iv. _____

v. _____

vi. _____

vii. _____

B. List foods that are allowed on a full liquid diet.

i. _____

ii. _____

iii. _____

iv. _____

v. _____

vi. _____

C. List foods that are allowed on a soft-mechanical diet.

    i. _____

    ii. _____

    iii. _____

    iv. _____

    v. _____

    vi. _____

KEY TERMINOLOGY REVIEW

Match each of the following terms with the correct definition.

a. calorie

b. lactose

c. lipids

d. minerals

e. Recommended Dietary Allowances (RDAs)

1. _____ Recommendations for the amount of protein, vitamins, and minerals that Americans should try to eat for good nutrition (developed by the Food and Nutrition Board of the National Academy of Sciences).

2. _____ Fatty acids that can be chemically classified as saturated or unsaturated.

3. _____ Inorganic elements that are of neither animal nor plant origin.

4. _____ A measurement of a unit of heat that provides energy.

5. _____ The combination of glucose and galactose that is found in animal milk.

APPLIED PRACTICE

1. Using your textbook as a reference, identify your favorite food sources for each of the nutrient categories listed below.

Nutrient Class	Food Sources
CARBOHYDRATES	
PROTEINS	
FATS	

(continued)

Nutrient Class	Food Sources
MINERALS	
Calcium	
Iron	
Iodine	
VITAMINS	
A	
B1 (Thiamine)	
B2 (Riboflavin)	
B3 (Niacin)	
B12	
C (Ascorbic acid)	
D	
WATER	

LEARNING ACTIVITY: TRUE/FALSE

Indicate whether the following statements are true or false by placing a T or an F on the line that precedes each statement.

_____ 1. Energy released from the metabolism of proteins, fats, and carbohydrates is measured in units of kilograms.

_____ 2. The key to a balanced diet is to eat a variety of foods in appropriate proportions.

_____ 3. Reducing the intake of protein can reduce the risk of certain types of cancer.

_____ 4. A common diet immediately after an operation is a clear liquid diet.

_____ 5. Children are placed on the BRAT diet when they have emotional outbursts.

_____ 6. Creamed and strained soups are allowed on a clear liquid diet.

_____ 7. Honey is an example of a complex carbohydrate.

_____ 8. Carbohydrates are the body's primary source of energy and are found primarily in breads, cereals, pasta products, rice, fruit, and potatoes.

_____ 9. Vitamins are not sources of energy, but they are required for good health.

_____ 10. Minerals make up 10 percent of the total body.

CRITICAL THINKING

Answer the following questions to the best of your ability. Use the textbook as a reference.

1. Mrs. Ortiz is of Hispanic descent. She prides herself in making delicious, authentic Mexican meals for her family and friends. Recently, Mrs. Ortiz was diagnosed with diabetes, and the physician wants her to begin a carbohydrate counting diet. Mrs. Ortiz is very concerned because many of her family's favorite meals are high in carbohydrates. She is discouraged and frustrated about this dietary change. How would you respond to the patient's concerns?

   _____

   _____

   _____

   _____

2. You are working with Millie Stewart, preparing her for annual physical examination. She tells you that she has tried every kind of diet, and many have worked well. She explains that she is able to lose weight rapidly, but the weight always comes back. Ms. Stewart says that she has decided to accept the fact that she is 20 pounds overweight, and she is not going to diet anymore; she is going to enjoy her food and her life. How would you respond to her?

   _____

   _____

   _____

   _____

RESEARCH ACTIVITY

Use Internet search engines to research the following topic and write a brief description of what you find. It is important to use reputable websites.

1. Visit www.choosemyplate.gov. Using the information that you find on the website, develop a diet plan for yourself or for one of your family members.

_____

_____

_____

_____

_____

CHAPTER 57
Mental Health

STUDENT STUDY GUIDE

Use the following guide to assist in your learning of the concepts from the chapter.

I. Psychology

    1. Psychology is the science of _____ and the human _____ process.

    2. A psychologist is trained in the methods of psychological _____, _____, and research.

    3. A psychiatrist is a(n) _____ doctor who has chosen to specialize in psychiatry and can _____ medications.

    4. Behavior that interferes with a person's activities of daily living is often considered _____.

    5. Abnormal psychology is the branch of psychology that focuses on abnormal _____, psychopathy, and disruptions of _____ and _____.

II. Psychological Disorders

    1. Causes of Psychological Disorders (List five causes.)

        A. _____

        B. _____

        C. _____

        D. _____

        E. _____

    2. Mental disorders are defined as any behavior or emotional state that causes an individual great _____ or _____, is self-defeating or self-_____, or disrupts the person's day-to-day _____.

    3. The guide for terminology and classifications related to psychiatric disorders is the _____ and _____ *Manual of Mental Disorders*, Fifth Edition, Text Revision (DSM-5TR).

4. Anxiety Disorders
    A. Individuals suffering from anxiety disorders are able to tell the difference between fantasy and _____ but frequently experience vague feelings of _____, worry, _____, or dread.
    B. Compulsions, _____ acts performed to _____ anxiety, are frequently accompanied by _____ (persistent thoughts).
    C. Some people have abnormal fears called _____.
5. Cognitive Disorders
    A. Delirium, particularly if related to _____ _____, can be transient and is usually treated by easing the person into _____ from substances or by treating the _____ cause.
    B. Dementia is a progressive disease that robs a person of _____ memory but that sometimes leaves long-term memory intact.
    C. Family members of patients with Alzheimer's disease, a type of _____, also need support.
6. Developmental Disorders
    A. With Down syndrome, a person is born with both _____ and _____ development problems.
    B. Mental retardation is a broad term that includes some individuals who are profoundly unable to _____ in the world and also those who have relatively _____ intelligence but are slow to _____.
    C. Rehabilitation is usually successful at improving the _____ of life for a person with developmental delay but usually does not increase the _____ quotient.
    D. Autism (also known as autism _____ disorder) has a range of symptoms that generally include difficulties with _____ and with forming _____.
7. Dissociative Disorders
    A. Dissociative disorders cause a person to withdraw from _____ and dissociate, or _____ _____, at least temporarily from the life issues that give them anxiety.
    B. Dissociative identity disorder (formerly called _____ _____ disorder) is a(n) _____ dissociative disorder in which the person develops multiple personalities.
    C. These individuals have usually been severely _____ and have developed multiple personalities as a(n) _____ mechanism.

8. Eating Disorders
   A. In anorexia nervosa, individuals develop a(n) _____ self-image.
   B. Individuals may begin to _____ themselves or _____ excessively, continuing to believe that they are _____ even when they have become very thin.
   C. _____ nervosa is another eating disorder, in which bouts of overeating are followed by purging with _____ or _____.
   D. Medications can be used in the treatment of eating disorders, but _____ _____ therapy is usually indicated.

9. Hypochondriasis
   A. Hypochondriasis is a disorder in which the person is preoccupied with fears of _____, or with the idea that one has, a(n) _____ _____, based on a misinterpretation of one of more bodily signs or _____.

10. Impulse Control Disorders
    A. Attention-deficit/hyperactivity disorder (ADHD) is a disorder of _____ control that affects many children and often persists into _____.
    B. ADHD is often treated with _____ that help the patient focus better, in combination with _____ _____ to help the patient learn strategies to improve focus and impulse control.
    C. Other impulse control disorders include those that manifest as excessive _____, _____, or setting _____.

11. Mood Disorders
    A. Bipolar disorder is characterized by mood swings from excessive _____ to profound _____.
    B. Depression is characterized by a lack of _____ in life's usual pleasures, such as food, _____, friends, _____, and hobbies and can be life threatening when accompanied by _____ thoughts.
    C. Mania is characterized by excessive _____, flights of _____ and enthusiasms, weight _____, and cognitive lack of _____.
    D. Depression by itself is a serious mental illness that affects _____ million people in the United States.
    E. Depression can usually be successfully treated with _____ medication.
    F. Treatment for depression also includes talk _____ with a psychologist or counselor to process any issues that may _____ the depression.

12. Personality Disorders

    A. List five behavior traits associated with personality disorders.

       i. _____

      ii. _____

     iii. _____

     iv. _____

      v. _____

13. Psychotic Disorders

    A. Psychotic disorders are severe mental disorders that interfere with individuals' perceptions of _____ and ability to cope with the demands of _____ _____.

    B. List five symptoms of schizophrenia.

       i. _____

      ii. _____

     iii. _____

     iv. _____

      v. _____

14. Somatoform and Factitious Disorders

    A. Somatoform disorders occur when unresolved _____ _____ is displaced into _____ complaints.

    B. In factitious disorders, the person creates _____ to get _____.

    C. If the person injures himself/herself to gain attention, the disorder is _____ disorder.

    D. If the person tries to get attention by injuring _____ _____, it is known as Munchausen's by _____.

III. Substance Abuse Disorders

    1. Addiction is a physiological need for a substance that, in its _____, causes _____ symptoms.

    2. _____ is a psychological addiction to a substance.

    3. Successfully treating substance abuse or dependence is generally _____ as long as the person doesn't recognize the _____ or recognizes it but is _____ to do anything about it.

    4. A medical assistant may need to give information to a substance abuser about local meetings for _____ Anonymous or _____ Anonymous.

5. Supportive groups such as Al-Anon/Alateen are for _____ of substance abusers.

6. Substance abusers may come to a medical office in search of _____ medications.

7. Notify the physician if you suspect drug-_____ _____ in a patient.

8. Symptoms of Substance Abuse (List six symptoms.)

    A. _____

    B. _____

    C. _____

    D. _____

    E. _____

    F. _____

9. Some substance abusers use legal drugs but in a(n) _____ way.

10. The most commonly abused drug in the United States is _____.

11. If a provider in the office is impaired because of substance abuse, report the behavior _____ to the _____ _____ and perhaps notify the state board of _____ or _____.

IV. Treatments for Mental Disorders

1. Psychotherapy includes psychoanalysis, _____ therapies, and family and _____ therapy.

2. Cognitive behavioral therapy helps to change both the way the patient _____ and the way the patient _____.

3. The goal of psychotherapy is to help the patient _____ with _____.

4. Psychoanalysis is a method of obtaining a detailed account of the _____ and _____ emotional and _____ experiences from the patient to determine the source of the problem.

5. Through humanistic therapies, the patient is helped to feel better by building _____ and a feeling that he or she is _____.

6. Family therapy and group therapy are _____ focused.

7. Psychopharmacology

    A. Psychopharmacology is the study of the effects of drugs on the _____ and _____, particularly the use of drugs in treating _____ disorders.

    B. The quality and _____ of the functions of the mind vary with _____ and development.

C. List the main classes of drugs used in the treatment of mental disorders.

    i. _____

    ii. _____

    iii. _____

    iv. _____

8. Electroconvulsive Therapy (ECT)

A. ECT is a procedure occasionally used for cases of prolonged major _____.

B. It is a controversial treatment in which a(n) _____ is placed on one or both sides of the patient's _____, and electric _____ is briefly turned on, causing a convulsive _____.

C. Advocates of this treatment state that it is more effective than the use of drugs to treat _____ _____.

D. ECT carries the risk of some _____ loss.

9. Transcranial Magnetic Stimulation (TMS)

A. TMS is a noninvasive procedure that causes _____ or hyperpolarization in the _____ of the brain.

B. TMS uses electromagnetic induction to induce a weak electric current that rapidly changes the _____ _____ in the brain.

C. List six diseases and disorders treated using TMS.

    i. _____

    ii. _____

    iii. _____

    iv. _____

    v. _____

    vi. _____

10. The Role of the Medical Assistant in Treating Mental Disorders

A. A medical assistant is not usually engaged in psychological _____ of a patient.

B. The assistant may be instrumental in arranging _____ from the medical office to a(n) _____ or psychologist.

V. Erikson's Developmental Stages of Life*

1. Erik Erikson posited that throughout the _____ _____, people go through different developmental stages in which they seek to complete certain _____ _____.

---

*Information related to this section will be covered in activities later in this chapter.

2. List the five main developmental periods identified by Erikson.

A. _____

B. _____

C. _____

D. _____

E. _____

VI. Maslow's Hierarchy of Needs

1. Abraham Maslow developed a hierarchy of needs in which he maintained that people have

special _____ and move through _____ levels in

achieving _____ in life.

2. Describe the five levels of Maslow's hierarchy of needs.

A. Level I— _____

B. Level II—_____

C. Level III—_____

D. Level IV—_____

E. Level V—_____

3. Maslow believed a person cannot move to a(n) _____ level until the basic

needs at each _____ level are met.

VII. Stress

1. Stress is the body's _____ to the world around it.

2. Depending on the level, stress can be energizing, _____, or

_____.

3. A stressor is a real or even a(n) _____ event that _____ stress.

4. List five factors that create a tendency to become stressed.

A. _____

B. _____

C. _____

D. _____

E. _____

5. Post-Traumatic Stress Disorder (PTSD)

A. List five event exposures that might cause someone to suffer from PTSD.

i. _____

ii. _____

iii. _____

iv. _____

v. _____

B. PTSD may affect _____, and the patient may experience

_____ of the event.

6. Coping with Stress

A. The following recommendations help in coping with stress.

   i. Develop a strong _____ _____, including family and friends.

   ii. Find a balance between _____ and fear of _____.

   iii. Eat _____ meals.

   iv. Avoid harmful habits such as _____ and _____.

   v. Get _____ _____ such as walking, jogging, dancing, biking, and swimming.

   vi. Look _____ to develop a social interest by understanding other people's problems and _____.

   vii. Try to see the _____ in situations.

   viii. Limit the number of activities to a(n) _____ few.

B. _____ stress and _____ stress need to be kept separate and should never interfere with one another.

VIII. Assisting a Patient Who Has a Terminal Illness

1. A terminal illness is an illness that is expected to end in _____.

2. Although there is always hope of _____ or finding a cure through research, it is wise to listen to the patient express his or her _____ and concerns rather than to offer _____ _____ for recovery.

3. When there is no hope of recovery and death is expected within _____ _____, the patient may be referred to _____ services.

4. Culture

A. In some cultures, death is considered a(n) _____ end to the life process and is therefore accepted with _____.

B. In other cultures, death may be _____.

C. A terminally ill patient and his family may have already established a very _____ approach or _____ for handling death and dying.

5. Religion

A. Religious beliefs play an important role in how patients handle _____ and _____.

B. It is unacceptable for a medical assistant to attempt to _____ a patient to the medical assistant's _____ faith.

C. Professionalism mandates that medical assistants and other staff members recognize and

_____ the patient's right to embrace his or her own _____

_____.

6. Personal Experience

   A. If a patient has been closely involved with the care of someone who has died a(n)

   _____ death, the patient may _____ the same kind of

   death.

   B. Patients who have had little _____ to death may have a more difficult

   time understanding their feelings or _____ their experience.

7. Age

   A. Elderly people usually have _____ fear of death than younger people.

   B. If a patient wishes to discuss his or her _____ death, a medical assistant

   should be ready to listen.

8. Stages of Grief

   A. Dr. Elisabeth Kübler-Ross devoted much of her life to the study of the

   _____ process and working with _____ ill patients.

   B. Although these stages relate to death, they can also relate to other _____.

   C. People move between these phases but not necessarily in a(n) _____ way.

   D. List the five stages of grief, as identified by Kübler-Ross (see Table 57-3).

      i. _____

      ii. _____

      iii. _____

      iv. _____

      v. _____

KEY TERMINOLOGY REVIEW

Match each of the following vocabulary terms to the correct definition.

   a. adolescence   d. stress
   b. psychiatrist   e. terminal illness
   c. psychologist

1. _____ An illness that is expected to end in death.
2. _____ Occurs between childhood and adulthood.
3. _____ One who is trained in the methods of psychological analysis, therapy, and research.
4. _____ The body's reaction to the world around it.
5. _____ A medical doctor who has chosen to specialize in psychiatry and can prescribe
                   medications.

APPLIED PRACTICE

1. Using information in the textbook, complete the table below as it relates to Erikson's developmental stages of life.

Developmental Stage	Age Range	Developmental Milestones
Prenatal period		
Infancy and toddlerhood		
Childhood		
Adolescence		
Adulthood		

LEARNING ACTIVITY: FILL IN THE BLANK

Using words from the list below, fill in the blanks to complete the following sentences.

antidepressant drugs   addiction

conception   bipolar

delusions   hallucinations

neurotransmitters   hierarchy of needs

psychopharmacology   psychotic

prenatal period   reality

schizophrenia   statistical

tolerance

1. A(n) _____ disorder has two poles: depression and mania.

2. _____ is a physiological need for a substance, which in its absence causes withdrawal symptoms.

3. _____ is a psychotic disorder marked by a variety of symptoms, including _____ (fixed false beliefs), _____ (false sensory perceptions), disorganized and incoherent speech, severe emotional abnormalities, and withdrawal into an inner world.

4. _____ is the study of the effects of drugs on the mind and brain, particularly the use of drugs in treating mental disorders.

5. The Diagnostic and _____ Manual of Mental Disorders, Fifth Edition, Text Revision (DSM-5TR) is the reference manual used by mental health providers to diagnose a wide range of mental disorders.

6. Abraham Maslow developed the _____.

7. The first stage of Erikson's developmental stages is the _____, which covers the process from _____ until birth.

8. _____ alter the patient's mood by affecting the levels of _____ in the brain.

9. _____ disorders are severe mental disorders that interfere with a patient's perception of _____ and his or her ability to cope with the demands of daily living.

10. Patients may develop problems with _____ after taking minor tranquilizers for an extended time.

CRITICAL THINKING

Answer the following questions to the best of your ability. Use the textbook as a reference.

1. Mrs. Leone and her daughter, Tammy, are at the doctor's office to discuss treatment options for Mrs. Leone's recent diagnosis of pancreatic cancer. Mrs. Leone insists that her test results were wrong and wants to have another set of tests performed. When Tammy speaks, she is very short and abrupt. She is visibly angry about her mother's diagnosis. How does this scenario relate to Kübler-Ross's stages of grief?

   _____

   _____

   _____

   _____

   _____

2. Wyatt Sheldon, a 14-year-old boy, is being seen by Dr. Anderson for an increasing fear of germs. He repetitively washes his hands after he touches various items and, as a result, his hands are extremely red and chafed. Based on the information presented, under what major diagnostic category would Wyatt's fear be classified? What is the technical name for his fear of germs? Is his repetitive handwashing a component of his disorder? Explain your answer.

   _____

   _____

   _____

   _____

   _____

RESEARCH ACTIVITY

Use Internet search engines to research the following topic and write a brief description of what you find. It is important to use reputable websites.

1. Visit the Mental Health America website, at www.nmha.org. What information do you find to be most helpful on this website? How could patients with mental health issues benefit from this website? In what ways could you become involved with Mental Health America?

   _____

   _____

   _____

   _____

CHAPTER 58
Professionalism

STUDENT STUDY GUIDE

Use the following guide to assist in your learning of the concepts from the chapter.

I. Professional Skills in the Workplace

1. A physician needs workers to arrive at work on _____, _____ problems, seek _____ with others, think _____, and solve _____ appropriately.

2. Patients expect _____ and _____ help at a physician's office.

3. Good employees show initiative by jumping in to _____ others when they are able and the tasks fall within their scope of _____ and _____.

4. Qualities of a Professional Medical Assistant (List six qualities.)

   A. _____

   B. _____

   C. _____

   D. _____

   E. _____

   F. _____

5. Integrated Systems

   A. An office should have a(n) _____ and _____ manual in place to direct the employees.

   B. It is important for medical assistants to understand how to _____ within the system established in a medical office.

   C. It is important to clarify the _____ in the office where you are employed early in the work relationship.

   D. The patient's _____ and welfare should be the number-one _____ of a health care professional.

   E. Legal problems will be avoided when _____ is foremost.

   F. You must also work well with _____ _____ professionals outside the office and should develop a(n) _____ of peer relationships.

II. Workplace Communication

1. Patients' impressions of the medical office will depend on how they perceive the level of _____ and _____ of the office as a whole.

2. You represent the office with every _____, whether with an individual _____ or with other members of your _____.

3. Active Listening

   A. Active listening requires the full _____ of the person _____ the message.

   B. A medical assistant with good professional skills focuses on the _____ and what the speaker is saying and asks for _____ if needed.

4. Seeking to Understand

   A. A health care professional should enter every _____, whether with patients or colleagues, seeking to _____ the other person.

5. Speaking to Be Understood

   A. When you are presenting difficult concepts, it is a good idea to seek _____ from the _____ to make sure that person understands you.

   B. Always take into account the _____ and _____ of the patient.

   C. Tailor your vocabulary to the age and _____ _____ of the patient.

6. Effective Writing

   A. In the health care environment, communication must be _____, and it must also be well _____ by others.

   B. _____ is more important than brevity.

   C. Communication that is _____ and _____ is essential for patient understanding and to avoid confusion or incorrect assumptions.

III. Critical Thinking

1. Although some decisions or procedures may be _____, many require critical thinking and _____ _____.

2. _____ and _____ issues often require critical thinking.

3. Thinking critically can improve _____ from the insurance company to the medical practice and can greatly relieve a(n) _____ on the patient.

4. Always read laboratory results critically and _____ results that do not seem _____ with the patient's presentation.

5. As a critical thinker, take all _____ into consideration before forming a(n) _____.

6. Distinguishing Fact from Opinion

    A. Critical thinking involves being able to distinguish _____ from opinion or

        _____.

    B. Considering everything that may be affecting a patient's mood can help you deal with the

        patient in a(n) _____ and more _____ way and will also

        allow you to give the physician a more thoughtful _____ about the patient.

7. Making Value Judgments

    A. A medical assistant must make value judgments _____

        _____.

    B. For example, setting the priority for scheduling a patient visit should be based on the

        _____ _____ and not on how much you

        _____ the patient.

    C. Critical thinking should become so _____ that you are comfortable about

        making value judgments.

IV. Teamwork

    1. If one employee gets _____ with responsibilities, the others should be versatile

        enough in their _____ and _____ enough to help until the work

        is caught up.

    2. Medical assistants, within their _____ of practice, should maintain a variety of

        _____ and a(n) _____ attitude toward working with others.

    3. Each team member should demonstrate _____ when needed.

    4. Teams operate best when they make use of the _____ of each team member.

    5. Diversity

        A. In the average medical office, medical assistants and other health care professionals come

            from _____ _____.

        B. It is in everyone's best interest for _____, stereotypes, and

            _____ to be put aside.

        C. Holding grudges or _____ _____ can prevent a team from

            functioning smoothly.

    6. Resolving Conflict

        A. Conflicts may arise with patients or among _____ members.

        B. The first step in resolving conflict is to seek to _____ the situation.

        C. Look at your own _____ or communication to see if perhaps something you

            said or did _____ or _____ contributed to the conflict.

        D. An important soft skill is not to escalate _____.

E. If two workers are in conflict, it may be wise to ask a(n) _____ to resolve the issue.

7. Responding to Criticism

   A. Learning to respond to criticism appropriately is an important skill in _____ and _____ resolution.

   B. If necessary, ask a non-defensive question to _____ feedback.

   C. If you have made a mistake, _____ it, restate the _____ way to do the task, and move on.

   D. If you feel that criticism is not _____, is unreasonably _____, or is not presented in a tactful manner, it is best not to _____ or become _____.

V. Managing Priorities

   1. Patient priorities are usually managed with a combination of efficient _____ and a(n) _____ system.

   2. Because of your _____ as a medical assistant, you may be asked to do multiple tasks in a(n) _____ _____ of time.

   3. Focusing on one task at a time will ensure _____ and _____.

   4. An efficient _____ _____ system or _____ file system helps a medical assistant remember important items that need to be completed by specific dates.

   5. Becoming distracted by your own _____ issues or other personal problems can have a(n) _____ effect on your job performance.

   6. It is best to turn off your _____ _____ during work hours, knowing that if there is a true emergency you can be reached on the _____ phone.

   7. Stress Management

      A. List 13 stress management techniques.

         i. _____

         ii. _____

         iii. _____

         iv. _____

         v. _____

         vi. _____

         vii. _____

         viii. _____

ix. _____

x. _____

xi. _____

xii. _____

xiii. _____

8. Time Management

   A. Time management requires the ability to _____ tasks, _____ them as appropriate, and _____ them on schedule.

   B. A main responsibility is to manage all the peripheral office _____ so the physician is free to concentrate on practicing _____.

   C. Before establishing a time management system, it is important to define the _____ _____ with the physician.

   D. After the goals have been established, tasks necessary to meet those goals can be _____, prioritized, and _____ to the appropriate _____ members.

   E. _____ lists can be created for everyday responsibilities as well as for special new goals.

   F. Each item on the list is assigned a priority designation of _____, _____, or _____, depending on how _____ the item is to completing the task.

9. Persistence

   A. Persistence is being able to stay on task _____ than the usual time when necessary, even after others might have _____ _____.

   B. When you are frustrated, it may seem easier to _____ _____ on a problem than to seek _____ solutions.

   C. A professional medical assistant _____ thinks of an alternative approach to a problem and persists in trying to find a(n) _____.

VI. Changes in Technology

   1. Approach technology updates with a(n) _____ "can do" _____.

   2. Understand that change is rarely _____, and technology changes in hardware and software often present learning curves and _____ challenges.

   3. Take advantage of every _____ opportunity available and offer to _____ the changes to others.

VII. Professional Image

   1. Always wear clean, pressed clothing that does not reveal _____, waist, _____, or underwear.

2. Keep _____ cut short.

3. Avoid _____ nails, which can harbor microbes.

4. Avoid excessive _____ because it harbors _____ and can get in the way when providing patient care.

5. Control hair so that it does not fall on a _____ or onto a(n) _____ field.

6. Practice excellent _____ and avoid perfumes or strong _____.

7. Wear clean shoes with _____ toes.

8. Wear the name tag issued by your _____, which usually includes both your name and your _____.

9. Remember that a(n) _____ is always part of a professional image.

VIII. Lifelong Learning

1. There are constant changes in the field of _____, and one of those is the growing preference for medical assistants who are _____ _____.

2. Once certified, the next step is to maintain that certification through _____ _____.

3. Continuing education credits can be earned through _____, _____, training in the office, or _____ _____.

4. The Internet provides a rich _____ of information.

5. Refer to medical websites that are reliable, meaning that the information has been _____ or _____ by recognized authorities.

KEY TERMINOLOGY REVIEW

Match each of the following terms with the correct definition.

a. affective
b. cognitive
c. tact
d. psychomotor
e. integrity

1. _____ Based on knowledge.

2. _____ Behaviors that come from feelings and emotions and are truly important in the medical office.

3. _____ Coordination of mind and body.

4. _____ Honesty and having strong moral principles.

5. _____ Sensitivity in dealing with others and with difficult issues.

APPLIED PRACTICE

Read the scenario and answer the questions that follow.

> **Scenario**
>
> John Summers is an office manager at Hillcrest Family Medicine. The physicians at the office have voiced concern to John regarding the lack of professionalism among the office staff. They have asked John to conduct a staff meeting to focus on the importance of professionalism. The physicians have asked John to highlight five qualities of a professional in the health care setting. They have also asked John to create a dress code policy so that all employees project a professional image.

1. What five qualities do you think John should choose to discuss during the staff meeting? Explain why.

    _____

    _____

    _____

    _____

    _____

2. How might John go about creating a uniform dress code? What items might he want to include in the new policy?

    _____

    _____

    _____

    _____

    _____

LEARNING ACTIVITY: TRUE/FALSE

Indicate whether the following statements are true or false by placing a T or an F on the line that precedes each statement.

_____ 1. It is important that a medical assistant always engage in active listening.

_____ 2. When communicating in the health care environment, accuracy is more important than brevity.

_____ 3. Stress management involves differentiating fact from fiction opinion.

_____ 4. The first step in resolving conflicts is to seek to understand the situation.

_____ 5. If two workers are in conflict, it may be wise to ask a peer to resolve the conflict.

_____ 6. One of the main responsibilities of a physician is to manage all the peripheral office functions.

_____ 7. A medical assistant must manage time well but is not responsible for prioritizing tasks.

_____ 8. Stress can be caused by pain.

_____ 9. In a busy medical office, many tasks may have to be deferred to a later time.

_____ 10. Insurance and billing issues often require critical thinking.

CRITICAL THINKING

Answer the following questions to the best of your ability. Use the textbook as a reference.

1. A very angry patient asks to talk with the office manager. The patient explains to the office manager that she overheard two staff members discussing the test results of another patient, who happens to be her sister-in-law. How should the office manager handle this situation?

_____

_____

_____

_____

_____

2. Karen, the office manager, has noticed that a medical assistant, Charles, has been answering his cell phone while at work, as well as checking his e-mail between patients. Today, Charles's wife came to the office to talk with Charles during the busy morning hours. How should Karen address Charles's unprofessional behavior?

_____

_____

_____

_____

_____

RESEARCH ACTIVITY

Use Internet search engines to research the following topic and write a brief description of what you find. It is important to use reputable websites.

1. Type the word "professionalism" into an Internet search engine. What are some of the most interesting and helpful results that are returned with your search?

_____

_____

_____

_____

CHAPTER 59
Externship and Career Opportunities

STUDENT STUDY GUIDE

Use the following guide to assist in your learning of the concepts from the chapter.

I. Introduction

    1. U.S. Department of Labor has projected that medical assisting will be one of the _____-growing occupations.

    2. Most medical facilities that employ medical assistants prefer or require that medical assistants have _____ _____.

II. What Is an Externship, or Practicum?

    1. During an externship, which may also be called a(n) _____, the student leaves the confines of the _____ and works, without _____, in a(n) _____ office, hospital, or other _____ care setting.

    2. Schools that are accredited by ABHES or CAAHEP require an externship of a minimum of _____ hours.

    3. The externship experience is carefully monitored by the school's clinical _____ or externship/practicum _____ so that questions or _____ that may arise can be addressed.

    4. The Externship/Practicum Experience

        A. Externship provides the opportunity to see how a(n) _____ office, ambulatory care setting, or _____ operates on a(n) _____-to-_____ basis.

        B. List 13 areas that are evaluated during an externship experience.

          i. _____

          ii. _____

          iii. _____

          iv. _____

          v. _____

          vi. _____

          vii. _____

          viii. _____

ix. _____

x. _____

xi. _____

xii. _____

xiii. _____

5. Student Responsibilities

   A. Preparation for an externship interview includes reviewing _____, updating the _____, and planning how to project a(n) _____ appearance.

   B. Externships may require medical assistants to have their own _____ insurance coverage.

   C. Documentation of a recent physical _____ and immunizations, including _____ and _____ vaccinations, may be required.

   D. The physician or facility providing an externship expects students to be extremely cautious regarding _____ and _____ concerns.

   E. If you find that you are not receiving the _____ you expect and require, bring this to the attention of your school's externship _____.

   F. Keep in mind that your _____ and work performance during your externship or practicum are a direct _____ on the school that prepared you.

6. Finding the Right Site

   A. Most schools have an externship coordinator who screens and selects health care _____ that are appropriate for _____.

   B. The screening process requires the coordinator to conduct a(n) _____ with the physician or _____ _____ at the site to ensure that the student will benefit from appropriate experiences and receive _____ on site.

   C. Generally, students do not _____ externship sites without _____ from the school or its externship/practicum coordinator.

7. The Preceptor Role

   A. A medical assistant at an externship or practicum site always works under the supervision of a(n) _____.

   B. A(n) _____ provides additional instruction and guidance for a student by observing the student performing particular skills.

   C. The preceptor also provides formal written _____ for a student, usually at the midpoint and at the _____ of the extern hours.

8. Externship/Practicum Site Evaluation

   A. You need to provide a(n) _____ of your experience while assigned to the site.

B. List four questions that may be asked on an evaluation form.

    i. _____

    ii. _____

    iii. _____

    iv. _____

III. The Job Search

1. You may ask the externship site supervisor to write a(n) _____ of _____ to assist with your job search.

2. In some cases, facilities do not want to hire medical assistants until they become _____ after taking the required _____.

3. Job Search Mistakes (List six.)

    A. _____

    B. _____

    C. _____

    D. _____

    E. _____

    F. _____

4. Personal Assessment

    A. It is a good idea to perform a personal assessment or evaluation of your own _____ and _____.

    B. Employers often ask about _____.

        i. Briefly state one weakness and _____ what you are doing about it.

        ii. This shows that you are aware of _____ and lets the employer know you are serious about _____ yourself.

    C. Ask your instructors for _____ and observations on your appearance, _____, and _____.

5. Conducting a Job Search

    A. Many websites can help _____ for a job search.

    B. These websites may focus on _____ writing, job _____, interviewing, job _____, and more.

    C. Using the Internet to search for jobs eliminates the need to access the _____ department of an employer you are interested in.

    D. The school's career services office is one of the _____ places to receive _____ with a job search.

E. A job search organizer or _____ is a place to keep a copy of cover letters, résumés, reference list, letters of _____, follow-up _____, and _____.

F. A(n) _____ _____ is a great reference for information about the offices or people you have contacted about a job search.

G. It is important to call prospective employers from a(n) _____ place.

IV. The Résumé

1. A résumé is a summary of _____, including _____ history, experience, training, and _____.

2. The most popular résumé format or style is to present information in _____ order.

3. In this format, education, work experience, and achievements are listed in _____ chronological order.

4. An educational skills résumé might be useful for someone who is just _____ from school and has not had extensive _____ experience.

5. A résumé is most likely to be noticed if it provides _____ and _____ information.

6. A résumé must be neatly _____ and _____ free.

7. It is important to _____ a résumé to make sure it is error free in content and typing.

8. The purpose of a résumé is to make a good _____ _____ and to obtain a(n) _____.

9. What Is Included in a Résumé?

A. List seven standard items included in a résumé.

    i. _____
    ii. _____
    iii. _____
    iv. _____
    v. _____
    vi. _____
    vii. _____

B. Information included in a résumé should never be dishonest, _____, or _____.

C. List eight items *not* to include on a résumé.

    i. _____
    ii. _____
    iii. _____

iv. _____

v. _____

vi. _____

vii. _____

viii. _____

10. Professional References

    A. A professional reference is a statement of someone who has either _____ with you or _____ you for a period of time.

    B. This person can attest to your _____, personal _____, or value system.

    C. Most employers would like a list of at least _____ references, with their _____ addresses, _____ addresses, and _____ numbers.

    D. It is important to obtain _____ to use a person's name as a reference.

11. The Cover Letter

    A. A cover letter is intended to _____ you and your résumé to the recipient—the person to whom you _____ the letter.

    B. The cover letter should clearly state the _____ of the correspondence.

    C. List five common mistakes to avoid when writing a cover letter.

       i. _____

       ii. _____

       iii. _____

       iv. _____

       v. _____

V. The Interview

1. Information from websites can provide a wealth of _____ that can help you be successful during the _____ _____.

2. Services Offered by a Career Services Office (List eight services.)

    A. _____

    B. _____

    C. _____

    D. _____

    E. _____

    F. _____

    G. _____

    H. _____

3. Preparing for Tough Interview Questions

   A. List 10 questions commonly asked during an interview.

      i. _____

      ii. _____

      iii. _____

      iv. _____

      v. _____

      vi. _____

      vii. _____

      viii. _____

      ix. _____

      x. _____

   B. Be prepared to answer difficult questions with great _____ and

      _____.

   C. List seven questions a candidate could ask an interviewer.

      i. _____

      ii. _____

      iii. _____

      iv. _____

      v. _____

      vi. _____

      vii. _____

4. Professionalism in an Interview*

   A. Present a(n) _____, well-_____, professional appearance.

   B. Wear little or no _____ and avoid showy _____, heavy

      _____, bright _____ polish, and bright _____.

   C. Never go to an interview with your _____ wrinkled.

   D. Make sure there is no _____ on your garments.

   E. Make sure your shoes are _____ and _____.

   F. List 10 mistakes commonly made during interviews.

      i. _____

      ii. _____

      iii. _____

      iv. _____

      v. _____

*Carefully review Procedure 59-4 to polish your interviewing skills.

vi. _____

vii. _____

viii. _____

ix. _____

x. _____

5. The Application

   A. An application includes _____ information and previous work

     _____.

   B. Gaps with no apparent _____ or _____ indicated should be

     clarified.

   C. List the documents needed for an application.

     i. _____

     ii. _____

     iii. _____

     iv. _____

     v. _____

   D. Accuracy of _____ and _____ are important on both online

     and paper applications.

   E. Remember that questions related to _____, _____, place of

     birth, and number of _____ are prohibited by law.

6. Follow-up After an Interview*

   A. Immediately following an interview, on the same day if possible, send a(n)

     _____ _____ the interviewer for her time.

   B. You may wish to _____ the office a few days later to ask about the

     _____ made on filling the position.

   C. If you are offered a position and decide _____ to accept it, use the same courtesy

     when turning _____ the offer as you use when _____ one.

VI. What Does the Employer Want?

   1. Employers prefer employees who are _____ and can successfully perform a wide

     variety of _____ and _____.

   2. Skills a Medical Assistant Must Master to Be Successful (List six skills.)

     A. _____

     B. _____

     C. _____

     D. _____

---

* Carefully review Procedure 59-5 for information on preparing a follow-up thank-you letter.

E. _____

F. _____

3. Qualities That Employers Seek in a Candidate (List eight qualities.)

   A. _____

   B. _____

   C. _____

   D. _____

   E. _____

   F. _____

   G. _____

   H. _____

4. The more _____, values, and _____ you have as a medical

   assistant, the more _____ you will be.

KEY TERMINOLOGY REVIEW

Match each of the following terms with the correct definition.

    a. blind ad   d. professional reference

    b. personal assessment   e. proofread

    c. preceptor

1. _____ Does not identify the institution or facility that placed the ad.

2. _____ Statement of someone who has either worked with you or has known you for a period of time.

3. _____ Ensure that your résumé and cover letter are error free in content and typing.

4. _____ Self-evaluation of strengths and weaknesses.

5. _____ Provides additional instruction and guidance for a student during an externship or practicum by observing the performance of particular skills.

APPLIED PRACTICE

As you answer these questions, assume that you are a recent medical assistant graduate preparing to enter the workforce.

1. You have recently received a phone call for an interview for Mountain View Health Care Center. How will you research the medical facility prior to your interview, and why is this important?

_____

_____

_____

_____

_____

2. Considering your current wardrobe, which outfit would you choose to wear to your interview, and why?

_____

_____

_____

_____

LEARNING ACTIVITY: MULTIPLE CHOICE

Circle the correct answer to each of the following questions.

1. When problems or questions arise during an externship, it is best to contact the _____ for assistance.

   a. office manager
   b. mentor
   c. physician
   d. externship coordinator

2. Which of the following is a responsibility of a student medical assistant during an externship?

   a. Be on time.
   b. Dress appropriately.
   c. Act in a professional manner.
   d. All of the above

3. Which of the following should *not* be part of an interview process?

   a. Projecting self-assurance while interviewing
   b. Preparing responses in case the interviewer asks you difficult questions or asks you to describe yourself
   c. Explaining reasons you didn't like working for a previous employer
   d. Preparing a list of references

4. Which résumé component lets the reader know what career goal you would like to achieve?

   a. Objective
   b. Heading
   c. Credentials
   d. Education

5. Which of the following may be a reason that a medical assistant may not be called for an interview?

   a. The résumé contains typographical errors.
   b. The résumé is presented in reverse chronological format.
   c. The résumé is printed on 8½ × 11-inch, off-white paper.
   d. All of the above

6. A résumé should ideally be _____ page(s) in length.

   e. two
   a. one
   b. three
   c. four

7. A thank-you note should be sent to a potential employer after an interview within _____ days.

   a. 1–2
   b. 2–3
   c. 3–5
   d. 6–8

8. Which of the following are places that a medical assistant might look for employment?

   a. The newspaper
   b. The school's career services department
   c. An employment agency
   d. All of the above

9. Which of the following is not an allowed question during an interview?

   a. Why do you want to work for this medical office?
   b. Why should I should hire you?
   c. How many children do you have?
   d. How are you qualified for this position?

10. Which of the following is appropriate dress for an applicant going to a job interview?

   a. Casual attire
   b. Business suit
   c. Scrubs
   d. Any of the above

CRITICAL THINKING

Answer the following questions to the best of your ability. Use the textbook as a reference.

1. Joann Felmer has just completed an externship for her medical assistant course. One of her final assignments is to describe the benefits of the externship experience for incoming medical assisting students. What information might Joann include in her written assignment?

   _____

   _____

   _____

   _____

   _____

2. Corey Rubatino has just completed his medical assistant training and is preparing for his first interview. He is meeting with the director of the career services department at his school for a mock interview. The interviewer says to Corey, "Explain one of your weaknesses." How can Corey best address this type of question, which is common in interviews?

   _____

   _____

   _____

   _____

   _____

RESEARCH ACTIVITY

Use Internet search engines to research the following topic and write a brief description of what you find. It is important to use reputable websites.

1. Using the Internet and other sources, locate prospective job opportunities for medical assistants in your area. Which jobs interest you most? Explain why.

   _____

   _____

   _____

   _____

   _____